Essentials *of* Dermatology *for* Chiropractors

Michael R. Wiles, MEd, DC, FCCS(C)
Provost and Vice President for Academic Affairs
Northwestern Health Sciences University
Bloomington, MN

Jonathan Williams, MEd, DC, DABCI
Associate Professor
College of Chiropractic, Northwestern Health Sciences University
Bloomington, MN

Kashif A. Ahmad, MBBS, MS, PhD
Associate Professor
College of Chiropractic, Northwestern Health Sciences University
Bloomington, MN

JONES AND BARTLETT PUBLISHERS
Sudbury, Massachusetts
BOSTON   TORONTO   LONDON   SINGAPORE

World Headquarters

Jones and Bartlett Publishers
40 Tall Pine Drive
Sudbury, MA 01776
978-443-5000
info@jbpub.com
www.jbpub.com

Jones and Bartlett Publishers Canada
6339 Ormindale Way
Mississauga, Ontario L5V 1J2
Canada

Jones and Bartlett Publishers International
Barb House, Barb Mews
London W6 7PA
United Kingdom

Jones and Bartlett's books and products are available through most bookstores and online booksellers. To contact Jones and Bartlett Publishers directly, call 800-832-0034, fax 978-443-8000, or visit our website, www.jbpub.com.

Substantial discounts on bulk quantities of Jones and Bartlett's publications are available to corporations, professional associations, and other qualified organizations. For details and specific discount information, contact the special sales department at Jones and Bartlett via the above contact information or send an email to specialsales@jbpub.com.

The authors, editor, and publisher have made every effort to provide accurate information. However, they are not responsible for errors, omissions, or for any outcomes related to the use of the contents of this book and take no responsibility for the use of the products and procedures described. Treatments and side effects described in this book may not be applicable to all people; likewise, some people may require a dose or experience a side effect that is not described herein. Drugs and medical devices are discussed that may have limited availability controlled by the Food and Drug Administration (FDA) for use only in a research study or clinical trial. Research, clinical practice, and government regulations often change the accepted standard in this field. When consideration is being given to use of any drug in the clinical setting, the health care provider or reader is responsible for determining FDA status of the drug, reading the package insert, and reviewing prescribing information for the most up-to-date recommendations on dose, precautions, and contraindications, and determining the appropriate usage for the product. This is especially important in the case of drugs that are new or seldom used.

Production Credits
Publisher: David Cella
Associate Editor: Maro Gartside
Production Editor: Daniel Stone
V.P., Manufacturing and Inventory Control: Therese Connell
Marketing Manager: Grace Richards
Composition: D. Johnson, DBS
Interior Design: D. Johnson, DBS
Cover Design: Scott Moden
Photo Research and Permissions Manager: Kimberly Potvin
Cover and Title Page Image: © Marilyn Volan/Shutterstock, Inc.
Printing and Binding: Imago Group
Cover Printing: Imago Group

Library of Congress Cataloging-in-Publication Data
Wiles, Michael R.
　　Essentials of dermatology for chiropractors / Michael Wiles, Jonathan Williams, Kashif Ahmad.
　　　　p. ; cm.
　　Includes bibliographical references and index.
　　ISBN-13: 978-0-7637-6157-8
　　ISBN-10: 0-7637-6157-5
　　1. Skin—Examination. 2. Chiropractic. 3. Melanoma—Diagnosis. 4. Dermatology. I. Williams, Jonathan, 1951 Aug. 15- II. Ahmad, Kashif. III. Title.
　　[DNLM: 1. Skin Diseases. 2. Chiropractic. WR 140 W676e 2010]
　　RL105.W55 2010
　　616.5′075—dc22

2009019554

6048

Printed in Malaysia for Imago

14 13 12 11 10　　10 9 8 7 6 5 4 3 2 1

Contents

Dedication

Dr. Michael R. Wiles

This textbook is published and dedicated with love and deep appreciation to Noreen for her constant and unconditional support and encouragement for this project.

Dr. Jonathan Williams

This textbook is published in memory of Mary, who provided me the strength and encouragement throughout my professional career and especially during the years of her fight against cancer, which she succumbed to on July 15, 2005.

Dr. Kashif A. Ahmad

This textbook is lovingly dedicated to my daughters Aalishba and Alaia, who have inspired me to complete this work and whom I wish to inspire as they begin their life-long journey of learning.

About the Authors

Michael R. Wiles, MEd, DC, FCCS(C)

Dr. Wiles received his Doctor of Chiropractic degree from Canadian Memorial Chiropractic College in Toronto, Canada in 1976. He also received a Bachelor of Science degree from University of Toronto and a Master of Education degree from Brock University. He completed a residency in chiropractic sciences and was awarded one of the first earned Fellowships in the College of Chiropractic Sciences of Canada. He is currently Dean of the College of Chiropractic at Northwestern Health Sciences University.

Jonathan Williams, MEd, DC, DABCI

Dr. Williams received his Doctor of Chiropractic degree from Northwestern College of Chiropractic (currently the College of Chiropractic at Northwestern Health Sciences University) in 1989. He received a Bachelor of Arts from University of Plano and a Master of Education degree from Argosy University. He earned a Diplomate from the American Board of Chiropractic Internists in 1996 and is a Certified Chiropractic Sports Physician. He was awarded the ACA Council on Diagnosis and Internal Disorders 2004 Frank Hoffman Award for Outstanding contributions to the Chiropractic Profession. Dr. Williams is currently Associate Professor of Clinical Sciences at Northwestern Health Sciences University.

Kashif A. Ahmad, MBBS, MS, PhD

Dr. Ahmad received his Bachelor of Medicine and Bachelor of Surgery degrees from University of Karachi. Following this, he earned a Master of Science in Clinical Dermatology from St. John's Institute of Dermatology, King's College, School of Medicine, London, UK. Subsequent to this, he completed his PhD in physiology from National University of Singapore, followed by a postdoctoral fellowship in lab medicine and pathology at the University of Minnesota. Currently, he is an Associate Professor of Basic Sciences at Northwestern Health Sciences University.

Preface

It has been said that chiropractors see more skin than any other health provider. This provides them with a perfect and unique opportunity to regularly evaluate the skin on a patient's face, neck, back, and extremities. Chiropractors also spend a lot of their time observing the skin on their patients' backs, an area notorious for malignant melanomas and an area rarely seen by patients in the course of their daily routines. One of our first considerations for this textbook was the need to have a reliable source of information, written by chiropractors for chiropractors, regarding the early diagnosis of malignant skin lesions, particularly malignant melanoma. Currently available textbooks of dermatology are written for medical students or medical physicians. While these are usually excellent reference books, the fact is that they contain information about diagnostic tests chiropractors cannot perform and chiropractic students must sift through a specialist's level of material for basic screening, diagnostic, and therapeutic information. Furthermore, these texts rarely contain information about conservative or natural approaches to the treatment of skin disease and the maintenance of skin wellness. There has never been a textbook specifically written for chiropractors in the area of dermatology.

There is a worldwide emergence of interest in natural care and hygiene of the skin. Largely born from a rising concern for environmental risk factors such as the increased exposure to ultraviolet light, we are seeing a demand for information concerning not only the prevention of skin cancer, but also regarding natural care of the skin. It wasn't long ago that we used to hear an old joke that dermatologists were the luckiest specialists since their patients never died and they never got better. This reflected the popular notion that most skin conditions were either incurable or required the continual use of either oral or topical corticosteroids. Certainly the science of dermatology has progressed as much as, or more than, other areas of medicine over the last few decades, but the fact remains that many chronic skin problems defy permanent cure and there is a rising interest in natural approaches to these problems as well as natural health for the skin. A recent Google search of *psoriasis* yielded 23,600,000 citations. A search of *psoriasis natural care* resulted in 198,000 hits. While the percentage of internet references relating to natural care is less than 10% of the total references for this condition, one cannot deny that there are almost 200,000 references to natural approaches to care. This is what patients are seeing and reading on a daily basis and they are looking to their natural healthcare providers for information, clarification, and support in their quest for solutions to their skin problems. Here is another interesting reflection of this rising interest in skin health: a Google search of *skin disease* yielded 4,970,000 hits but *skin health* yielded 9,060,000 hits, almost double the number. Lastly, *skin wellness* yielded 272,000 hits and *skin nutrition* yielded 747,000 hits. This is what patients want today—information and treatment that emphasizes natural approaches, nutrition, and skin health. All of these topics are included in our textbook.

Finally, the skin, along with hair and nails, can provide an important reflection of general health. Certainly many systemic conditions include skin manifestations or asymptomatic lesions and in fact, the skin may yield vital information suggesting serious systemic disease. As primary care or primary contact healthcare providers, chiropractors have a responsibility to determine a diagnosis prior to the delivery of care. Chiropractors must often rely on clinical diagnosis skills since they frequently do not have ready access to the expensive array of diagnostic tests that are typically available to physicians, or they do not have the skill or scope of practice to perform invasive testing. In that regard, chiropractors must be either as good or better at their clinical diagnosis skills than other physicians.

Chiropractors also need to be aware of the medical specialty of dermatology and its sub-specialty branches. Dermatology is a branch of medicine that deals with diagnosis and treatment of the pathological conditions of the skin, hair, and nails. Dermatologists are physicians who have undergone advanced training in dermatology at a recognized hospital and have fulfilled established professional requirements such as those prescribed by the American Board of Dermatology here in the United States. Its sub-specialties include:

- Venereology—specialization in the diagnosis and treatment of sexually transmitted diseases.
- Cosmetic dermatology—the branch of dermatology that deals with collagen and Botox injections, dermabrasion, chemical peeling, and nonabrasive laser treatments.
- Dermatologic surgery—scalpel surgery such as Mohs procedure for skin cancer, electro/cryosurgery, cosmetic surgeries such as face lifts, laser surgery, and photodynamic therapy.
- Dermatopathology—microscopic examination of skin biopsies and tissue samples.
- Pediatric dermatology—the branch that deals with diseases of the skin in children.
- Immunodermatology—the branch that views skin as an organ of immunity and is concerned with diseases such as psoriasis and vitiligo.

Dermatologists are busy specialists. It is important that chiropractors know when and when not to refer a patient to a dermatologist. Chiropractors must refer with confidence in order not to waste the valuable time of already busy dermatologists. At the same time, they need to be able to confidently pursue natural approaches to skin health, knowing that they have performed a competent assessment of the skin.

Our textbook provides this information and much more, specifically written for chiropractors and chiropractic students. We have designed this book to truly represent the essentials of dermatology for chiropractors and chiropractic students. Much of the material is presented in point form and there are numerous cross references between conditions and treatments. It is our hope that this textbook will form a common source of relevant dermatological information for our chiropractic college dermatology instructors, chiropractic students, and practicing chiropractors.

Acknowledgments

The authors would like to gratefully acknowledge the case histories and photo-images that were provided by the following individuals:

Drs. James Abeler Sr., Carla Breunig, Renee DeVries, Christopher Edwards, Lynne Hvidsten, Anne Packard-Spicer, Brian Turner, and Jamal Waris

We want to acknowledge our appreciation for, and the contributions of, the chiropractic students enrolled in the dermatology course at Northwestern Health Sciences University, from 2006 to 2008.

The authors would also like to acknowledge Dr. Azeem Khan for kindly providing some of his private dermatological images.

We owe a very special debt of gratitude to Colonel Dr. Nasser Rashid Dar, Assistant Professor and Head of the Dermatology Department at C.M.H. Lahore Medical College in Lahore, Pakistan. He very generously provided us with his personal bank of dermatological images that have enriched this textbook greatly.

The artistic contributions of Amna Ahmad are acknowledged and appreciated. We would also like to acknowledge the assistance and support of Publisher David Cella, Associate Editor Maro Gartside, and Production Editor Daniel Stone at Jones and Bartlett Publishers, and Catherine Ngoju for her editorial assistance.

Reviewers

Daniel DeLapp, DC, DABCO, LAc, ND

Attending Physician
Western States Chiropractic College
Adjunct Faculty
National College of Natural Medicine
Portland, OR

Margaret M. Finn DC, MA, MS-ABD, RN, FACC

Associate Professor
Chiropractic Clinical Sciences
New York Chiropractic College
Seneca Falls, NY

Anne Sorrentino Hoover, DC, CCSP®, ART®

Post-graduate faculty status as Developer
and Lead Instructor
Palmer College of Chiropractic Continuing
Education Department co-sponsorship with
DConline
Davenport, IA

Tobi Jeurink, BS, DC, DABCI

Associate Professor
Cleveland Chiropractic College
Overland Park, KS

Maria Michelin, DC

Associate Professor
Sherman College of Straight Chiropractic
Spartanburg, SC

Seva Philomin MD

Associate Professor
New York Chiropractic College
Seneca Falls, NY

Dr. Beth A. Roraback, BS, DC

Associate Professor
Director of Physical Examination
Sherman College of Straight Chiropractic
Spartanburg, SC

Rickard J. Thomas, DC

Professor
Chief of Staff
Clinical Sciences
Cleveland Chiropractic College
Overland Park, KS

How to Use This Book

This book is designed to be an easy-to-use and practical reference source for both chiropractors and chiropractic students. Once you are able to describe the basic features of a particular skin lesion, you can classify it according to the information provided in Chapter 4, Pathophysiology of Skin Disease. From this classification and the information provided in Chapter 4, you should be able to determine a short list of possible diagnoses.

Each of the 50 most common skin conditions seen in a chiropractic practice are described in easy-to-read sections in Chapter 6. The common format describes the main features of the diseases or disorders and provides the essential information necessary to establish a diagnosis in most cases. The book is supplemented with more than 100 color images of the skin conditions described in the text, enabling visual recognition of the key dermatological elements of each disease.

Next, the various treatments, including natural remedies are described for each condition and cross-referenced to the formulary in Chapter 7. Additionally, in Chapter 7, each treatment modality or remedy is cross-referenced to the 50 conditions in Chapter 6 so that readers can become familiarized with dermatological diagnosis and treatment by either referencing treatments from a given disorder, or disorders from a given treatment.

We believe that it is important for chiropractors to be a resource on wellness to their patients. More and more people are concerned about their skin as a reflection of their overall wellness. Chapter 2 provides a wealth of information about the health and wellness of skin and includes Patient Information Sheets that can be copied and given to patients.

For self-assessment, case studies and discussion questions are presented in Chapter 9 and selected response questions are provided in Chapter 10. These are also referenced to their source in the text.

Finally, for reference purposes, a supplemental list of 50 less common or less important skin conditions are described in Chapter 8. This second tier of skin disorders and diseases includes conditions less likely to be seen in a typical practice than those described in Chapter 6 (such as pseudoexanthoma elasticum) or those less likely to have clinical significance (such as lipoma). We felt that this chapter was important to complete the collection of conditions that might be considered essential for a chiropractor to be aware of, and further, we felt that it is not improbable that some of the more unusual conditions would be seen over the practice lifetime of many chiropractors.

Introduction: The Role of Dermatology in Chiropractic Practice

Why a Textbook of Dermatology for Chiropractors?

Chiropractors, like other primary contact physicians, must make an accurate diagnosis of their patients' presenting complaints before rendering care. While the majority of chiropractic patients present with musculoskeletal complaints, chiropractors still observe many skin conditions either primarily related to the presenting complaint, or as secondary findings (some of which are morbid conditions such as malignant melanoma). It has been said that "the eyes do not see what the mind does not know;" therefore, it is necessary for chiropractic students to study diseases and disorders thoroughly before they can reasonably be expected to identify these conditions clinically. Moreover, chiropractors place a considerable importance on clinical diagnosis and careful observation and examination. More than any other organ, the skin is readily available for examination and its importance in the clinical diagnostic process is often overlooked and underestimated. While the retina is said to be the only place where we can actually see arteries in the body, the skin is the only organ that can be observed directly in its entirety. When a skin lesion is observed (and they frequently are in the course of daily chiropractic practice) the challenge is to determine which of three possibilities exist: a primary and purely dermatologic disorder (which of course must be correctly diagnosed to determine whether it is self-limited, or not self-limited but will respond to simple and conservative care, or whether it requires the attention of a dermatologist, either urgently or non-urgently), an internal disease manifesting itself as a skin condition, a variant of normal (or, perhaps a fourth possibility which is a combination of the first three).

Chiropractors and chiropractic students need a specialized textbook in dermatology for many reasons. First, and most obvious, is the fact that chiropractors probably see more skin than any other health care providers, with the exception of massage therapists. Massage therapists are well aware of what constitutes normal skin and abnormal skin, but they lack training in diagnosis and may not be aware of the significance of a skin lesion, particularly as this may reflect a state of general or systemic illness. Most people do not (and cannot) typically examine the skin on their own posterior surface, especially over the spine. Even spouses or partners do not typically carefully examine this part of the body and, once children reach the teenage years, their parents are very unlikely to see this region of skin or recognize skin lesions on the back. Furthermore, the most common site for melanoma in men is the upper back while in women the most common sites are the lower legs and upper back. Considering the importance of the skin as a reflector of bodily health and disease, the increasing incidence of malignant melanoma, and the ready access and observation of the skin in chiropractic practice, it is actually surprising that this is the first such textbook of its kind.

Next is the fact that the skin, possibly more than any other body part or organ, reflects states of health and disease, particularly generalized and systemic diseases and disorders. Some common examples of these manifestations include conditions such as obstructive bile duct disorders resulting in the yellow tinge of jaundice, or the typical exanthemas of childhood viral afflictions such as measles, or the pallor of anemia, or xanthomas as a reflection of dyslipidemia. Rheumatologic conditions, which frequently present with joint pains bringing patients to chiropractic offices, may include skin lesions. The skin may manifest or reflect metabolic disturbances, nutritional deficiencies, and numerous states of general disease. For example, the excessive dryness or moistness associated with abnormal states of the thyroid gland or the profuse sweating (diaphoresis) associated with psychogenic disorders, some systemic and infectious diseases.

Moreover, one of the chiropractor's primary responsibilities is to rule out conditions which may not respond to chiropractic care or which may require care from another provider, typically a medical physician. Often, the skin may be the first indication that such a condition exists. Chiropractors must be alert to such possibilities and this includes diligence in the examination of their patients' skin.

Chiropractors play an increasingly important role as "watchdogs" for malignant melanoma. This is partly because the incidence of melanoma is steadily rising (it is said that currently, one in 71 persons in the US will develop melanoma in their lifetime). Also, the most likely candidates for melanoma, baby boomers, are the most frequently seen patients in chiropractic practices. The age demographics of chiropractic practice are somewhat reversed from those of medical practice. In medicine, a large proportion of care is provided to infants and children, who, besides receiving well-baby care and immunizations, are often taken to their doctors by concerned mothers for a host of physiological irregularities. Adults, on the other hand, can be in the habit of avoiding medical care for a variety of reasons such as attempting self-care, the cost of care, and avoidance of painful or uncomfortable examinations. Senior citizens, on the other hand, often represent a captive audience for medical care in nursing homes and related institutions.

This pattern is typically reversed for chiropractic practices. Despite a clinical track record of safety and effectiveness, many mothers continue to be hesitant to take their infants and children to chiropractors, except for simple musculoskeletal conditions. Also, elderly patients, especially those in assisted living settings or nursing homes may lack the ability to visit a chiropractic office or the funds to pay for such a visit. On the other hand, adults, particularly baby boomers, can afford chiropractic care, have often grown up with it, enjoy the hands-on care and the fact that they can often avoid costly medications or even surgery. Social studies of chiropractic care suggest that adult patients trust chiropractors and are very satisfied with what they experience in chiropractic offices. For these reasons, they are likely to seek advice from their chiropractors about conditions that may not even be in the chiropractors' scope of practice.

One of the authors (MW) has observed this frequently in practice and has had the opportunity to direct numerous patients to dermatologists with suspected melanomas, many of which proved to be malignant. The following is an account of one particularly interesting such circumstance, at a time prior to the current laws and regulations governing patient privacy, and when he was practicing in a multidisciplinary clinic with many medical specialists. During a visit with a patient suffering from a lower back condition, a large black, irregular mole was noticed in the area just above the pelvic brim about 5 centimeters lateral to the spine. The examining room door was slightly open and the chiropractor observed a colleague, a dermatologist, passing by the room. Without distracting the patient from the therapy she was receiving, the dermatologist was motioned to enter the room, whereupon he observed the lesion, gave a "thumbs down" sign to the chiropractor and left the room. Having had the benefit of this fifteen-second silent consultation, the chiropractor made a strong suggestion to the patient that she should visit with the dermatologist to have the mole examined. After a biopsy, it was determined that the lesion was indeed malignant and luckily, *in situ*. She recovered from surgical excision and was followed for many years showing no signs of recurrence. Of course, not every chiropractor has a dermatologist roaming the halls of his or her clinic as was the case in this unusual situation, but knowledge and awareness of this condition, coupled with the fact that the majority of chiropractic patients (middle aged and older adults) are at risk for melanoma, and the fact that chiropractors will often see the skin where these lesions are found (in areas where patients don't or can't look) make chiropractors ideal observers and indeed, *watchdogs* for melanoma.

To emphasize the importance of early diagnosis of skin cancer, one chiropractor who is a melanoma-survivor has founded a charitable organization whose goal is "to educate chiropractors on how to identify possible skin cancer in patients, so they may refer those patients to the appropriate specialist" (taken from the organization's website, www.chiros-care.com).

In their primary contact role, chiropractors need considerable familiarity with the most common skin diseases, less familiarity with conditions that are less common, and a general or cursory knowledge of virtually any condition that could present in their offices. This often poses a difficulty for practicing chiropractors and especially for chiropractic students since most textbooks of dermatology (written for primary care physicians and dermatologists) are very comprehensive, and usually do not separate the common from the uncommon or rare. Chiropractors must know what is infectious and what is not, what *should* be referred to a dermatologist and what *must* be referred to a dermatologist, and how to distinguish a morbid skin lesion from a simple benign lesion. This textbook contains detailed descriptions of the fifty most common skin conditions (Chapter 6) as well as general descriptions of fifty less common conditions, or common but less significant conditions (Chapter 8). The authors believe that this pre-screening of information will be very beneficial to both busy practicing chiropractors and chiropractic students who need quick access to the most vital and relevant information.

Many skin disorders are either self-limited or respond well to simple, natural remedies or easily available over-the-counter medications. These are described in this text and, in fact, fifty different skin treatments or remedies are mentioned in Chapter 7. For those chiropractors interested in educating and advising their patients about natural approaches to health, this chapter is a goldmine of information.

More than at any other time, patients are seeking information about wellness and health promotion. This is especially related to the skin since to the average person, wellness is often mostly manifested in our outward appearance and in our skin in particular. This phenomenon is clearly evidenced in the retail stores where a never-ending variety of cosmetic and skin health products tries to satisfy the growing consumer market for these products. However, even given this growing consumer need for products and information about skin health and wellness, there still seems to be a lack of reliable information on this subject in textbooks of dermatology.

Health care providers of all types are sought by patients for information about the maintenance and care of their skin (and by extension, their youthful appearance and by further extension, their self-image). The chiropractic paradigm of health care, agreed upon by professional consensus and published by the Association of Chiropractic Colleges in 1996, describes health and disease as a continuum (**Figure 1-1**).

On one extreme end of the continuum is a total lack of health and on the other extreme is total health. An individual's specific state of health, or position on this continuum, is a dynamic phenomenon as we are all constantly moving backward and forward on it. The chiropractic

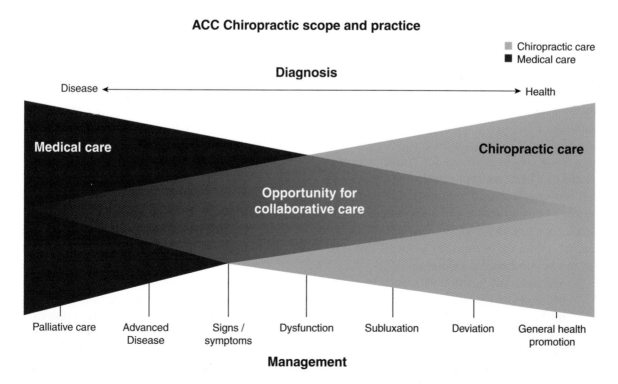

Figure 1-1 Chiropractic Scope and Practice Paradigm, Association of Chiropractic Colleges, 1996.

paradigm model proposes that the primary effort of the medical profession is dedicated to the illness pole of the continuum, metaphorically *pushing patients* away from disease and towards health. Certainly, medicine is equipped to handle all states of disease and illness that may appear at this end of the continuum. Chiropractic, on the other hand, is conceived as functioning mainly at the opposite pole. That is to say, chiropractors want to identify factors associated with health and wellness and *pull patients* to their end of the continuum. It is proposed that this pushing and pulling, when in concert, may function as complementary aspects of the health care system, moving patients away from disease and towards health. While this model was accepted by the profession-at-large in 1996, there has been a paucity of effort to operationalize this in chiropractic education or practice. In fact, most chiropractic research, education and practice still emphasize the role of the profession in dealing with back pain and neck pain rather than in promoting wellness and health. This is unfortunate, because patients, especially wellness-conscious babyboomers, are desperate for information about the promotion of good health (often symbolized by healthy skin). Chapter 2 is dedicated to the subject of skin wellness and provides chiropractors and chiropractic students with professional level, evidence-based information to counsel patients. Also in this chapter are Patient Education and Information sheets on various aspects of skin health and wellness that can be copied and distributed to patients. It is hoped that other chiropractic textbooks will follow suit and promote evidence-based wellness strategies that chiropractors can utilize as they shift their emphasis from disease to health.

A final, and perhaps most compelling reason for a book on dermatology for chiropractors is related to a basic concept of chiropractic science that proposes a clinically important relationship between body structure and body function. The details, mechanisms and evidence for this conceptual model are beyond the scope of this text, but can be summarized as follows:

- The aberrant function of a portion of the musculoskeletal system (especially related to the spine) may result in aberrant, or inappropriate sensory bombardment of one or more segments of the spinal cord. In chiropractic theory, this phenomenon is due to what has been traditionally called a "chiropractic subluxation." In osteopathic theory and practice, this same lesion was formerly known as an "osteopathic lesion" and is currently known as somatic dysfunction.

- Through mechanisms not fully understood, but likely to include segmental facilitation, this sensory bombardment of motoneuron pools result in either spontaneous motor activity or the facilitation of motoneuron pools leading to overt reflex responses following otherwise subliminal sensory stimulation. In fact, it is this motor activity that gives rise to the typical segmental asymmetry and restricted motion that characterizes somatic dysfunction, or the chiropractic subluxation.

- The motor responses associated with this phenomenon are not restricted to only the somatic motor system. At the spinal cord level, segmental facilitation affects both the ventral roots and the lateral horns, thereby affecting sympathetic nerves. A considerable body of evidence exists from early osteopathic research (particularly from the work of Irvin Korr and J.S. Denslow) supporting this idea and demonstrating that the increased segmental sympathetic tone (called segmental sympatheticotonia) is manifested by increased vasomotor tone (resulting in regions of cooler skin, as demonstrated by thermography) and increased sudomotor tone (resulting in regions of hydrated skin, as demonstrated by electrodermography).

- Areas of the body innervated by these sympathetic nerves, and therefore affected by segmental sympatheticotonia are presumed to function abnormally (or inappropriately) since normal autonomic reflex responses are facilitated.

- This very phenomenon was observed by Korr (and previously by Thomas and Korr, and Thomas and Kawahata) by noting the response of sweat gland activity under cool, resting conditions (in other words, no thermoregulatory demand). In these experimental conditions, sweat glands associated segmentally with somatic dysfunction were found to exhibit inappropriate or maladaptive behavior by responding excessively to minor pain stimuli in the absence of thermoregulatory demand. Therefore, the skin was (and remains) the only organ system to be observed to function abnormally in areas segmentally related to the chiropractic subluxation or somatic dysfunction.

As shown in this brief summary of chiropractic theory, the skin has been experimentally observed to function abnormally in the presence of the chiropractic subluxation, or somatic dysfunction. What does this mean for the relationship between chiropractic subluxations and skin disorders? Certainly such relationships have not been demonstrated with evidence greater than anecdotes and suppositions based on case observations; however, the possible and certainly plausible role of sympatheticotonia as a factor in skin pathophysiology is an intriguing one. Both osteopathic physicians (for example, Patriquin who hypothesized a neural basis for the location of warts) and chiropractors (such as Eldred and Tuchin who described a case of atopic eczema that resolved following segmentally related chiropractic manipulative care) have observed the relationship between chiropractic subluxations, or somatic dysfunction, and segmentally related skin disorders. Chronic somatic dysfunction is also thought to be related to increased pigmentation in segmentally related skin (evidently a trophic disturbance). It remains to be seen if clinical observations and, eventually, clinical research will demonstrate this relationship and support the manipulative care of patients with segmentally related skin disorders.

The above model mechanism for manipulative therapy has been called *neuropathogenesis*. When one considers the frequency with which nervous or neurally-related factors are considered in the etiology of dermatological disease (such as acne, "emotional stress may cause exacerbations"; neurodermatitis, "expression of underlying emotional disorder"; seborrheic dermatitis, "tension and diet are often associated with flare-up") we can only speculate and surmise the potential role of chiropractic manipulative care in normalizing the function of the spine to diminish or eliminate segmental sympatheticotonia.

General References

Eldred DC, Tuchin PJ. Treatment of acute atopic eczema by chiropractic care. ACO 1999; 8:96–100.

Korr IM (ed.). The Neurobiologic Mechanisms in Manipulative Therapy. 1977. New York, Plenum Press.

Patriquin DA. Dermal reflections of neural disorders: an hypothesis. Academy of Applied Osteopathy Yearbook. 1967: 83–88.

Thomas PE, Kawahata A. Neural factors underlying variations in electrical skin resistance of apparently non-sweating skin. *J Appl Physiol.* 1962; 17:999–1002.

Thomas PE, Korr IM. Relationship between sweat gland activity and the electrical resistance of the skin. *J Appl Physiol.* 1957; 10:505–510.

Wagner JD, Gordon MS, Chuang TY, Coleman JJ. 3rd. Current therapy of cutaneous melanoma. Plast *Reconstr Surg.* 2001; 105:1774–1799.

Wellness and the Skin

Functions of Skin

The skin, the largest organ of the body, has six major functions. The first and most obvious is protection. It provides a physical barrier to the effects of trauma or penetration from the outside environment, infection from micro-organisms such as bacteria and macro-organisms such as insects. The physical barrier has protective qualities against radiation from the sun, temperature changes and controls movement of moisture across it.

Typically the skin has a regeneration rate of approximately 21 days. This rapid regeneration provides the ability to repair the integument from injury.

Structures within the skin secrete three substances that have protective qualities for the skin and internal structures. Melanin is stored in the melanocytes and secreted into adjacent basal cells as a protection against ultraviolet rays. Sweat is released from eccrine and apocrine glands and helps to maintain body temperature. Sebum from the sebaceous glands flows along the hair follicle providing protection and control of moisture and humidity.

The skin's reticuloendothelial system, along with the inflammatory system and immune system, identify substances that are harmful. Common reactions include hives or urticaria and contact or allergic dermatitis.

Despite the size of the organ, the skin plays a minor but important role in the elimination of toxic and metabolic byproducts. Many times these excretion products are the source of undesirable body odors.

Moderation is essential in all things including exposure to the sun because the irradiation of Vitamin D precursors takes place in the skin. Regular controlled exposure produces sufficient conversion of vitamin D. As a consideration, the darker the skin, the more exposure is required to convert sufficient amounts of Vitamin D.

More information about basic biology of the skin is provided in Chapter 3.

Hygiene

Washing is part of a daily routine. Choosing a soap that meets the skin's need is essential. The normal pH of the skin is *slightly acidic*, in the range of 5 to 7. Most bar-soaps tend to be alkaline with a pH of 7 to 9 that can be irritating and drying, leading to dry itchy skin. Most soft-soaps, especially those that contain oil such as coconut, palm, sesame or other vegetable oils, have a slightly acidic quality, which tends to leave a soft silky feeling to the skin.

Soaps that contain betaine or an extract from beets provide an additional cleansing capability. Betaine acts as a surfactant by providing a lipophilic part and a hydrophilic part. This aspect is beneficial for cleaning very oily skin or very dirty skin. Another commonly found surfactant that is generally nonirritating is polyethylene glycol. (See Patient Guide 1)

The following is a description of proper hand washing techniques using soap and water adapted from the Mayo Clinic for health care practitioners:

- Wet hands with warm running water and apply a liquid soap or use a clear bar of soap, then develop a good amount of lather.
- Rub hands together for 15 to 20 seconds.
- Scrub all areas of hands from the wrists to the tips of the fingers, between the fingers and under the nails.
- Rinse them under warm running water.
- Dry hands with a clean towel, disposable towel or under a hand dryer.

Washing hair is more complicated than skin due to all the cosmetic concerns that need to be dealt with such as dry hair, oily hair, flyaway hair, permed hair, colored hair, and split ends. Choosing a shampoo to meet the cosmetic needs is a very complex question. Rather than addressing all those variables, let's identify the adverse reactions to an improperly chosen shampoo or conditioner. The wrong shampoo or conditioner may lead to any of the following symptoms: increased bacteria or yeast counts leading to dandruff, dry itchy scalp, increased permeability of the scalp leading to dermatitis, increased scalp infections, stinging or itchy scalp, urticaria, and contact or allergic dermatitis. (See Patient Guide 2)

Skin Hydration

Dry skin results from loss of moisture. This results in skin that presents with raised, scaly, itchy patches (as in psoriasis), red itchy papules (as in dermatitis), scaly appearance (ichthyosis), or large areas that are itchy without a red rash (pruritus). The most common causes include cold weather, excessive or hot water bathing, swimming in chlorinated pools, exposure to wind, washing with harsh soaps, inherited factors, changes in metabolism due to pathology of the thyroid or rapid weight loss, medications such as diuretics, chaffing and poor humidity control in air conditioned spaces. (See Patient Guide 3)

The moisturizing lotion should contain some occlusive agent such as lanolin in order to prevent or slow the evaporation of moisture off the skin. A second component could be a substance such as glycerin, urea, a sugar or alpha hydroxy acid which act to bring moisture from the deep layers of the skin to the surface.

Areas of skin that are exposed to the weathering effects of wind and sun should have higher concentrations of occlusive agents such as petrolatum or waxes. For areas of chaffing, heavy oils and petrolatum can help to lubricate the skin to prevent friction induced injury.

Skin that is scaly needs additional care that includes an emollient, which helps to sooth and fill the ridges and cracks. Some of the natural substances are castor oil and almond oil. Some of the milder pharmaceutical emollients include octyl dodecanol, hexyl decanol, isopropyl palmitate and isopropyl myristate. These substances help to sooth the skin as well as retain moisture.

Oily skin results from over active sebaceous glands that produce high amounts of oil, giving the skin a greasy, shiny appearance and increased pore size that makes the skin look rough. The most common causes of oily skin are congenital,

hormonal (including puberty, pregnancy and birth control medications), high humidity and high temperatures, as well as heavy cosmetic use. (See Patient Guide 4)

Weather and Skin Protection

The OSHA Fact Sheet 3166-06R 2003 provides some very good information for people who work outside, but it also pertains to everyone who spends time outside.

Sunlight contains ultraviolet (UV) radiation, which causes premature aging of the skin, wrinkles, cataracts, and skin cancer. The amount of damage from UV exposure depends on the strength of the light, the length of exposure, and whether the skin is protected. *There are no safe UV rays or safe suntans.*

Skin Cancer

Sun exposure at any age can cause skin cancer. Those who tend to burn easily must be especially careful in the sun. An individual who spends a lot of time outdoors, or has any of the following physical features must take extra care to prevent UV injury to the skin:

- Numerous, irregular, or large moles.
- Freckles.
- Fair skin.
- Blond, red, or light brown hair.

Self-Examination

Patients must be informed of the importance of a monthly self-examination because skin cancers detected early can almost always be cured. The most important warning sign is a spot on the skin that is changing in size, shape, or color during a period of 1 month to 1 or 2 years.

Skin cancers often take the following forms:

- Pale, wax-like, pearly nodules.
- Red, scaly, sharply outlined patches.
- Sores that don't heal.
- Small, mole-like growths—melanoma, the most serious type of skin cancer.

Inform patients of the importance of reporting any unusual skin changes (See Patient Guide 5).

The sun delivers three forms of ultraviolet (UV) light rays, UVC which is absorbed by the ozone layer, UVA which causes the stimulation of the melanocytes for tanning but is also associated with aging of the skin, eye problems and reactions from medications, and UVB, which is associated with the burning of the skin, aging and skin cancer. The National Institutes of Health associate both UVA and UVB with increased risk of skin cancer. The best ways to be protected from the sun's UV rays are to limit exposure to the sun, to wear clothing that covers the skin and to use sun screening substances that reduce UV exposure. In the summer, when temperatures are the warmest, 10:00 am to 4:00 pm is peak time for UV exposure. Wearing long sleeve shirts, pants, hats and sunglasses helps protect against UV exposure. However, if the skin can be seen through the clothing, the UV rays are only partially blocked.

Sun screening substances are rated by an SPF (sun protection factor) number. The number is used to calculate the exposure time before the skin starts to burn. For example if skin typically starts to burn in 10 minutes without any protection then following the application of an SPF 15 substance it will be protected for 150 minutes. The time will be reduced or negated if a person is sweating or swimming, so in these cases, frequent reapplication is recommended.

Zinc oxide and titanium dioxide are two substances that block both UVA and UVB. Though these substances are absorbed minutely through the skin, zinc oxide is less toxic and easier to excrete than titanium dioxide. Zinc is a nutritional metal while titanium is a heavy metal that generally is considered toxic.

The cold and wind tend to have very drying effects upon the skin. Moisture is pulled from the outer layers which leads to cracking and itching. There are four basic actions that can reduce the winter drying effect.

- Use a humidifier in the home to maintain the moisture content of the air between 40% to 50%.
- Wash with warm water rather than hot, using a mild pH balanced soap to reduce the loss of the skins natural oils.
- A moisturizing soap can be used to counteract excessive drying.
- Following washing and bathing use a moisturizer that has an occlusive agent to replenish and protect the moisture in the skin.
- Wear protective clothing to prevent chapping of the skin and a lip balm to protect the lips from cracking and drying.

The heat of summer, whether it is humid or dry, will affect your skin. In areas of low humidity, increase the use of high quality moisturizers. In areas of high humidity, increase the frequency of washing to remove the dirt and grime followed by a light oil free moisturizer.

The real danger of summer is the systemic effect of being overheated. The OSHA Quick Card provides an excellent overview of what to look for and how to react.

Heat Exhaustion and Heat Stroke

When the body is unable to cool itself by sweating, a pathophysiologic state known as heat exhaustion and the more severe state known as heat stroke can occur. Severe cases can result in death.

Factors leading to heat exhaustion

- High temperature and humidity.
- Direct sun or heat.
- Limited air movement.
- Physical exertion or poor physical condition.
- Certain medications.
- Inadequate tolerance for hot workplaces.

Symptoms of heat exhaustion

- Headaches, dizziness, lightheadedness or fainting.
- Weakness and moist skin.
- Mood changes such as irritability or confusion.
- Nausea or vomiting.

Symptoms of heat stroke

- Dry, hot skin with no sweating.
- Mental confusion or loss of consciousness.
- Seizures or convulsions.

Preventing heat exhaustion

Patients must be aware of the common signs of heat-related illnesses and can be advised as follows:

- Block out direct sun or other heat sources.
- Use cooling fans/air-conditioning; rest regularly.
- Drink lots of water; about 1 cup every 15 minutes.

- Wear lightweight, light colored, loose-fitting clothes.
- Avoid alcohol, caffeinated drinks, or heavy meals.

Heat exhaustion can become a life threatening situation. Patients exhibiting signs of distress such as weakness, dehydration, confusion or unconsciousness must be immediately treated by emergency personnel. Supportive measures to be taken in the meantime include:

- Moving the person to a cool, shaded area.
- Loosening or removing heavy clothing.
- Providing cool drinking water.
- Fanning and misting the person with water.

For more complete information:
Occupational Safety and HealthAdministration
U.S. Department of Labor
www.osha.gov (800) 321-OSHA

Lip protection is recommended by the American Cancer Society as prevention for squamous and basal cell carcinoma. Summer protection is primarily focused on UV protection while winter protection is compounded by cold dryer climates. Lip compounds should moisturize to prevent cracking, splitting, peeling, chapping, drying and provide sun protection. Most of the lip cosmetics contain moisturizers and sun protection but most contain a staining or coloring compound. The stain or color may act as an irritant causing a contact dermatitis.

Caring for the Skin

Nail care done properly can prevent fungal and bacterial infections, ingrown nails and those ugly nails that cause shame or embarrassment. Patient Guide 6 has tips to keep nails strong and beautiful (See Patient Guide 6).

Soft, weak and brittle nails require special care. When cutting or trimming them, first apply a moisturizer to help prevent splitting or chipping, then cut the nail relatively short. A nail hardener may be applied to protect the nail. Use of a nail glue to repair splits or tears will help. Nail polish remover is very drying and will result in more splits or tears. Rather than removing nail polish, repair any chips by adding an additional layer. This will reduce the exposure and drying effect of the nail polish remover.

Body Art—piercing and tattoos, also includes permanent makeup. The tattoo is a permanent mark produced by the injection of an ink below the skins surface. Regulation of tattooing is under local jurisdiction but the ink is subject to FDA regulation as a cosmetic and color additive. However, the FDA has not investigated the inks or attempted to regulate or test them for toxicity.

Tattoos have been a part of many societies, and are now very popular. Before proceeding, it is highly recommended that a little investigation into tattoos should be done beforehand. (See Patient Guide 7)

Tattoo removal is much more expensive, time consuming and painful than the acquisition process. There are three common methods of tattoo removal.

- Laser surgery is the most effective and leaves the least amount of scarring, however, this process may not remove all the ink.
- Dermabrasion is the process of chilling, then sanding the area to remove the tattoo. This may leave a scar, especially on larger tattoos.
- Surgical removal of the tattooed skin is followed by skin grafting. This process also leaves a scar.

Body piercing other than the earlobe involves the insertion of a hollow needle through the area followed by the piece of jewelry. The risks are very similar to that of tattooing and include:

- Blood borne diseases.
- Localized infections.
- Formation of keloids and granulomas.
- Allergic reactions.
- Dental injury for those who have piercing of tongue and lips.

Good follow up care is essential. Wash the area with warm water followed by the medicated liquid cleanser. Move the jewelry around so that the medicated cleanser may flow through the area. It is best to use the supplied liquid cleansers rather than hydrogen peroxide to avoid drying of the skin.

Hair care following shampooing is drying, then combing or brushing the hair. Hair is a nonliving substance that has an outer layer made up of a tough fibrous protein called keratin. The protein strands can be damaged by heat, chemical, or mechanical action. Brushing and combing are mechanical actions used to control and manage the appearance of the hair. When the hair is wet, it is more susceptible to mechanical damage due to twisting and knotting. Thus, especially for long hair, start combing with a wide toothed comb from the bottom up. Only brush when the hair is almost dry, in long flowing strokes from the top down. (See Patient Guide 8)

Heat damage can occur from sun exposure or from high temperature blow drying. The hair can be protected from the damaging rays of the sun by use of a conditioner that contains a sunblock. Blow drying the hair works well using cooler temperatures. Extra time is required but it leaves more of the natural oils and provides a more natural sheen. (See Patient Guide 9)

Hair coloring is a chemical process to change the color of the hair. This chemical process can dry the hair, causing it to become brittle and break or split. Care needs to be taken to restore the moisture after the coloring process takes place. There are a number of ways to alter the color of the hair. A temporary coloring that will wash out over time typically uses an acrylic dye to coat the hair. Bleaching or lightening the hair uses a bleach or peroxide to damage or destroy the melanin of the hair. A permanent hair coloring splits the hair so the melanin can be destroyed and a new color imbedded into the hair shaft. This type of coloring requires a special follow up conditioner to seal up the hair follicle. Many of the newer permanent coloring systems combine all the steps into a single product (See Patient Guide 10).

Hair removal may be permanent or temporary. The use of lasers and needle electrolysis are considered by the FDA to be permanent hair removal systems because they destroy the hair follicle. The depilatories are creams, lotions or gels that soften and dissolve the hair so that it can be washed off. Waxing and sugaring use substances that dry and harden around the hair allowing it to be pulled out by the root (See Patient Guide 11). Shaving is the most common form of temporary hair removal. It is the least painful, but has the shortest effect (See Patient Guide 12).

Injuries to the Skin

Sunburn is a very common occurrence and should be treated in order to prevent infection, dehydration and shock. The best choice is to prevent it by use of sunscreens and proper dress to block the UV waves that cause the burn.

Mild sunburn presents different from a traumatic burn in that it manifests itself slowly. The skin turns pink to red over a 2 to 6 hour period of time, and reaches peak intensity in 12 to 24 hours. Pealing will generally start in 4 to 6 days after the exposure.

Treatment for mild sunburn consists of cool water baths or cool wet cloths covering the burned area. Other treatments include the use of aloe vera or normal saline followed by oils such as vitamin E, almond, olive, or lanolin to moisturize the skin.

A more severe burn that leads to blistering must be monitored closely in order to prevent sun poisoning, shock, infection, or dehydration. Complications that indicate a severe burn are: fever, chills, dizziness, nausea, vomiting, extremity swelling, flu like symptoms and large blisters. The blisters will peak in 12 to 24 hours, and skin sloughing will begin in 4 to 6 days.

Treatment for severe sunburn may require medical treatment to replenish fluids intravenously and to prevent infections. Home care includes replenishing fluids by increasing water and electrolyte intake, cooling the area with cool baths, and rinsing with sterile saline to prevent infection. Spraying aloe vera diluted with sterile saline solution can cool and reduce the discomfort. Finally, protect the blisters from rupturing too soon by covering them with a dry bandage.

Cuts, lacerations and abrasion, are injuries that involve breaking through the surface of the skin, exposing the dermal layers, muscle, fascia, fat layer, tendon, ligament and even bone. Deep penetrating wounds, avulsions or amputations that require stitching or other medical procedures should be treated by appropriate specialties to prevent serious local and systemic infection.

A cut typically describes a clean slice or incision, while a laceration describes an injury with rough, jagged edges. An abrasion is a wound caused by dragging or sliding on a rough surface.

Treatment for mild cuts, abrasions and lacerations includes:

1. stop the flow of blood;
2. wash the area with an antibacterial soap and warm water;
3. apply an antibacterial agent,
4. cover area with a sterile bandage.

Topical cuts and lacerations that tend to separate due to skin tension may be held together with butterfly tape. Redress and apply antibacterial agent 2 to 3 times per day until wound is healed. At each dressing change, inspect the area for signs of infection, including red inflamed tissue, pus, foul smell, cellulitis and necrosis.

Contusions usually result from a blunt trauma such as a fall or being hit, where the skin is not penetrated but the blood vessels in the area are damaged and ruptured allowing blood to flow into the area. The free blood in the area causes discoloration and can lead to an inflammatory response and local swelling. The subsequent oxidation of heme pigments gives rise to the characteristic color changes seen in bruising.

Treatment for contusions is ice and range of motion exercises. The ice reduces swelling and slows the inflammatory process while slow, pain-free range of motion exercises stimulate fluid motion to allow for the removal of blood, debris and reduce edema in the area.

Severe or deep contusions such as bruising of the bone or bruising that is severe enough to inhibit motion should be treated by an appropriate specialist.

Nutritional Considerations for Skin

Skin is one of the largest organs of the body. It provides a protective barrier against injury, ultraviolet light rays and loss of water. Due to the specialized proteins and oils that are metabolized in the skin, nails and hair, many nutritional deficiencies could be suspected. For example, the hydroxylation process forming the cross links between collagen fibers giving it strength requires vitamin C. Vitamin A is required for proper expression of the keratin formation gene. Also the copper containing enzyme tyrosinase plays a role in the formation of normal melanin.

The formation of the protective proteins of the skin, keratin, melanin and collagen, all require the proper intake of amino acids, along with the vitamins and minerals that act as cofactors or coenzymes.

The lipid film and membrane of the skin requires proper hydration and oils from the diet in order to protect the body from the effects of moisture, dry climates and the variations in temperature. The fatty acids omega 3, 6 and 9 are required to produce healthy cell membranes and sebaceous secretions.

Skin repair and replacement is relatively rapid. In childhood, turnover may be accomplished in as little as two weeks, where an adult may require up to four weeks. During this turnover of skin cells, the metabolism of growth and development moves at a quick pace and requires all the basic building blocks of proteins and fats along with all the coenzymes and cofactors needed for proper formation of the cells. Since this happens relatively quickly, the skin can be an early indicator of nutritional deficiencies or internal disorders (see **Table 2-1**).

General References

Burns DA, Breathnach SM, Cox N, Griffiths CE. *Rook's Textbook of Dermatology,* 7th Ed. Oxford UK. Blackwell Publishing 2004.

Coulston AM, Rock CL, Monsen ER. (ED). *Nutrition in the prevention and treatment of disease.* San Diego, CA. Academic Press 2001.

Fitzpatrick JE, Morelli JG. *Dermatology Secrets.* 3rd Ed. Philadelphia, PA. Mosby. 2006.

Habif TP. *Skin Disease Diagnosis and Treatment.* 2nd Ed. Philadelphia, PA. Elsevier Mosby 2005.

Mackie RM. *Clinical Dermatology* 4th Ed. New York, New York. Oxford Press 2004.

Werback MR. *Foundations of Nutritional Medicine.* Tarzana, CA. Third Line Press 1997.

Further Reading

Hygeine

Bolduc C, Shapiro J. Hair care products: waving, straightening, conditioning and coloring. *Clin Dermotol.*2001 Jul-Aug;19(4):431–436.

Friedman M, Wolf R. Chemistry of soaps and detergents: various types of commercial products and their ingredients. *Clin Dermato.* 1996 Jan-Feb; 14(1):7–13.

Hannuksela A, Hannuksela M. Soaps and detergents in skin disease. *Clin Dermotol.* 1996 Jan-Feb;14(1): 77–80.

Nix DH. Factors to consider when selecting skin cleansing products. *J Wound Ostomy Continence Nurs.* 2000 Sept;27(5):260–268.

Oakley A. Soaps and Cleansers. *DermNet NZ.* December 26, 2006. Available at http://www.dermnetnz .org/treatments/cleansers.html: Accessed February 11, 2009.

Schmid MH, Korting HC. The concept of the acid mantle of the skin: its relevance for the choice of skin cleansers. *Dermatology.* 1995;19(4):276–280.

Strube DD, Nicoll G. The irritancy of soaps and syndels. *Cutis.* 1987 Jun;39(6):544–545.

Trueb RM. Shampoo. *Ther Umsch.* 2002 May;59(5): 256–261.

Trueb RM. Shampoos: ingredients, efficacy and adverse effects. *Dtsch Dermatol Ges.* 2007 May; 5(5):356–365.

Table 2-1 Nutrient and indications of abnormalities

Nutrients	Signs of deficiency	Signs of toxicity
Vitamin A	Corneal scarring / ulcers, dry eyes, xerosis, follicular hyperkeratosis, raised bumps around hair follicles primarily on backs of arms & sides of thighs, night blindness	Peeling skin, headache and arthralgia, alopecia
Carotenoids	Corneal scarring / ulcers, drying of the eyes, follicular hyperkeratosis raised bumps around hair follicles rimarily on backs of arms & sides of thighs	Yellow to orange discoloration of the skin starting with palms of hands
Biotin	Glossitis, angular stomatitis, chelosis, alopecia, dermatitis	Unknown
Vitamin B1 Thiamine	No dermatological findings; Beriberi	Urticaria associated with allergic response as well as headache, weakness and cardiac arrhythmia
Vitamin B2 Riboflavin	Angular stomatitis, swollen tongue, dermatitis	Unknown
Niacin	Rough red scaly dermatitis, glossitis, skin rash due to sun exposure—Casa's collar, Pellagra	Flushing; liver toxicity
Vitamin B6 Pyridoxine	Glossitis, angular stomatitis, chelosis, dermatitis similar to seborrhea	Sensory and motor neuropathy
Vitamin B12 Cobalamin	Glossitis, pallor associated with pernicious anemia, jaundice	Unknown
Folic Acid	Glossitis, pallor associated with macrocytic anemia	May mask B12 deficiency
Vitamin C Ascorbic Acid	Gingivitis, bruising, follicular keratosis, poor wound healing, scurvy	GI disturbances and diarrhea; renal calculi
Vitamin D Cholecalciferol	No dermatological findings	Pruritus, soft tissue calcification
Vitamin E Tocopherol	No dermatological findings	Can interfere with vitamin K therapy
Vitamin K	Bruising	Unknown
Copper	Decreased skin and hair pigmentation, dermatitis, pallor associated with hypochromic anemia	Wilson's disease—Kayser-Fleischer ring
Iron	Pallor associated with hypochromic anemia, glossitis, angular stomatitis, chelosis, spoon-shaped nails	Hemochromatosis
Zinc	Alopecia, dermatitis, poor wound healing	Interferes with copper absorption
Manganese	Dermatitis, hair color changes	Parkinson's-like symptoms
Essential Fatty Acids	Dry skin, pruritis, eczema, psoriasis, acne	Unknown
Protein—Amino Acids	Thinning of skin, decreased pigmentation, thin hair that is dull, easily broken and pulled out	May be toxic in presence of kidney and liver disease

Wolf R, Wolf D, Tuzun B, Tuzun Y. Soaps, shampoos and detergents. *Clin Dermatol.* July-August 2001; 19(4):393–397.

Skin Hydration

Bikowski J. The use of therapeutic moisturizers in various dermatologic disorders. *Cuitis.* 2001 Dec; 68(5 Suppl):3–11.

Draelos ZD. Therapeutic moisturizers. *Dermotol Clin.* 2000 Oct;18(4):597–607.

Katugampola RP, Statham BN. A review of allergens found in current hair-care products. *Contact Dermatitis.* 2005 Oct;53(4):234–235.

Lipozenic J, Pastar Z, Marinovic-Kulisic S. Moisturizers. *Acta Dermatovenerol Croat.* 2006;14(2):104–108.

Loden M. Biophysical properties of dry atopic and normal skin with special references to effects of skin care products. *Acta Derm Venereol Suppl (Stockh)* 1995;192:1–48.

Loden M. Role of topical emollients and moisturizers in the treatment of dry skin barrier disorders. *Am J Clin Dermotol.* 2003;4(7):771–788.

Mayo Clinic Staff. Skin moisturizers, choosing one that works. *Mayo Clin Health Lett.* 2008 Nov; 26(11):6.

Rosado C, Pinto P, Rodrigues LM. Assessment of moisturizers and barrier function restoration using dynamic methods. *Skin Res Technol.* 2009 Feb; 15(1):77–83.

Thune P. The effects of detergents on hydration and the skin surface lipids. *Clin Dermotol.* 1996 Jan-Feb;_14(1):29–33.

Weather and Skin Protection

Broekmans WMR, et al. Determinants of skin sensitivity to solar irritation. *EJCN.* 2003;57:1222–1229.

Skin Cancer

Bikle DD. Vitamin D and Skin Cancer. *J Nutr.* 2004 Dec; 134:3472S–3478S.

Caring for the Skin

FDA Consumer update. Removing Hair Safely. [FDA website] Posted June 27, 2007 Available at http://www.fda.gov/consumer/updates/hair062707.html. Accessed March 10, 2009.

Nutritional Consideration for Skin

Dreizen S. The mouth as an indicator of internal nutritional problems. *Pediatrician.* 1989;16(3-4):139–146.

Goskowicz M, Eichenfield LF. Cutaneous findings of nutritional deficiencies in children. *Curr Opin Pediatr.* 1993 Aug; 5(4):441–445.

Horrobin DF. Essential fatty acid metabolism and its modification in atopic eczema. *Am J Clin Nut.* 2000 Jan; 71(1):367S–372S.

Kuhl J, et al. Skin signs as the presenting manifestation of severe nutritional deficiency. *Arch Dermatol.* 2004 May; 140:521–524.

Office of Dietary Supplements. Dietary supplementation fact sheet: Vitamin A and Carotenoids. [NIH Office of Dietary Supplements Web Site] posted 6/22/2005 updated 4/23/2006 Available at http://ods.od.nih.gov/factsheets/vitamina.asp. Accessed March 10, 2009.

Office of Dietary Supplements. Dietary supplementation fact sheet: Vitamin B6. [NIH Office of Dietary Supplements Web Site] posted 12/9/2002 updated 8/24/2007 Available at. http://ods.od.nih.gov/factsheets/vitaminb6.asp. Accessed March 10, 2009.

Miller SJ. Nutritional deficiency and the skin. *J Am Acad Dermotol.* 1989 Jul;21(1):1–30.

Youmans JB. Vitamin A Nutrition and the Skin. *Am J Clin Nut.* 1960 Nov-Dec; 8:789–792.

Patient Guides

Patient Guide 1 **Pamper and protect the skin when washing:**

- Wash with warm rather than hot water.

- Choose mild soaps that tend to leave the skin soft and silky rather than dry.

- Choose soaps that have the fewest additives which have the possibility of being irritating. Chemicals that tend to be irritating are dyes, fragrances, antiseptics, thickeners, or harsh surfactants such as lauryl sulphate or trimethyl dodecyl ammonium chloride.

- Wash off your makeup first. If wearing waterproof make up, soften it first with an oil based product then follow with a mild soap containing a mild surfactant.

- Rinse with liberal amounts of water to remove all soap and/or makeup residue.

- Pat dry rather than rubbing roughly to reduce the moisture loss. If needed or desired, follow with a moisturizer.

Patient Guide 2 Pamper and protect your hair when washing:

- Use warm water rather than hot to prevent drying. Completely saturate the hair.

- Choose a shampoo that is pH balanced.

- Place a small amount of shampoo in the palm of your hand, sufficient to get a good lather, about the size of a nickel, rub it onto both hands and massage it into the hair starting at the scalp.

- Rinse and repeat only if you have very oily or dirty hair.

- Rinse hair thoroughly with plenty of water.

- Apply conditioner, if desired, starting at midshaft of the hair and work down to ends of hair. Try to prevent conditioner contacting the scalp because it has a very drying effect on the skin.

- Let the conditioner set for about 30 seconds to 3 minutes, depending on the manufacturer's instructions, then rinse thoroughly.

Patient Guide 3 Pamper and protect your dry skin by:

- Washing with warm rather than hot water.

- Reduce the frequency of bathing.

- Shower rather than take a bath.

- Use pH balanced or moisturizing soaps or minimize the use of soaps.

- Wash with bath oils or, after rinsing, apply a bath oil.

- Reduce swimming in chlorinated water.

- Apply a moisturizer after drying.

Patient Guide 4 Pamper your oily skin by:

- Wash with warm water that is warm, but not hot, to help reduce the oil.

- Increase frequency to 2 or 3 times per day but not more. Excessive washing will irritate the skin resulting in more oil production.

- Use a mild oil based soap that has a mild surfactant such as betaine or polyethylene glycol to help remove the oil.

- Use a mild astringent such as witch hazel to remove the oil.

- Avoid the use of moisturizers.

Patient Guide 5 Protection against ultraviolet rays:

- **Cover up.** Wear tightly-woven clothing that blocks out light. Try this test: Place your hand between a single layer of clothing and a light source. If you can see your hand through the fabric, the garment offers little protection.

- **Use sunscreen.** A sun protection factor (SPF) of at least 15 blocks 93 percent of UV rays. You want to block both UVA and UVB rays to guard against skin cancer. Be sure to follow application directions on the bottle.

- **Wear a hat.** A wide brim hat (not a baseball cap) is ideal because it protects the neck, ears, eyes, forehead, nose, and scalp.

- **Wear UV-absorbent shades.** Sunglasses don't have to be expensive, but they should block 99 to 100 percent of UVA and UVB radiation.

- **Limit exposure.** UV rays are most intense between 10 am and 4 pm. If you are unsure about the sun's intensity, take the shadow test: if your shadow is shorter than you, the sun's rays are the day's strongest.

Patient Guide 6 **Nail Care:**

- Keep the nails clean and dry. The toenails are the hardest to protect. Alternate the shoes you wear, and put on clean socks or stockings daily that allow for the removal of sweat. Make sure the shoes and socks are not tight.

- Do not bite your nails or the cuticle area since this habit can damage the bed of the nail and introduce bacteria or funguses which will lead to an infection. Picking or cutting the cuticle can lead to a disfiguring of the nail.

- Trim and moisturize your nails regularly. When trimming, always use sharp manicure scissors or clippers to prevent chipping. Follow up with an emery board to smooth any rough edges. Especially on the toes, square the nail off to prevent an ingrown nail. As you moisturize your hands rub the moisturizer into the nails to help prevent drying and chipping.

- Protect your nails by not using them for tools to pry or pick. When using chemicals or cleaning solutions wear gloves.

Patient Guide 7 Tattoo considerations and care:

- Since a hollow needle with a dye is being driven into the skin there is a chance for blood borne infections to occur including hepatitis B, HIV and tetanus.

- Be alert for redness and other signs of infection.

- In susceptible individuals, granulomas and keloids may develop.

- Allergic reactions may result from the ink producing itching and burning. This may subside, but can be stimulated by sun exposure and heat.

- An MRI (magnetic resonance imaging) may cause burning or swelling in the area due to metallic inclusions.

- Selection of a particular design may date the person in the future.

- The placement of a tattoo in an area that is not easily covered may affect the ability to work in certain areas.

- When it is decided to get a tattoo, ensure that facility and practitioner are reputable and licensed.

Caring for the new tattoo:

- For the first 24 hours, keep it covered as prescribed by the artist.

- Do not pick at any of the scabs over the tattoo.

- Wash the area with antimicrobial soap and pat dry with a soft towel.

- Ice the area if any swelling or redness develops.

- No swimming or long hot showers or bathing until the area over the tattoo is healed.

- Do not expose the tattoo to the sun until the area is completely healed.

- Long term exposure to the sun may fade the tattoo so always use sun block over the area.

Patient Guide 8 Tips for combing and brushing the hair:

- Never brush wet hair.

- Use a comb starting from the bottom and working up, to reduce tangles.

- When hair is almost dry use a brush in long sweeping strokes starting at the scalp.

- Contact a hair stylist to determine the best type of brush needed for the length and style of hair.

Patient Guide 9 Tips for blow drying hair:

- Blow dry hair on a cool setting.

- Leave the hair slightly damp.

- Use a conditioner that has UV protection.

- Start combing the hair to remove tangles when the hair is damp, not dry.

Patient Guide 10 **Tips for coloring hair:**

- Decide how long the color change should last.

- Determine what color is desired and then contact a stylist to determine the base melanin of the hair so that a true color will result.

- Test a small area of hair and scalp to determine for color and sensitivity or allergic responses before proceeding.

Patient Guide 11 Tips for hair removal other than shaving:

- Compare the cost and the effectiveness of each procedure.

- Determine how much pain is tolerable.

- Follow the directions for follow up care to prevent infection.

- Sun exposure following electrolysis or laser treatment may result in an unexpected sunburn.

- Perform the procedure in a small area to determine if an allergy to the procedure is present.

Patient Guide 12 Tips for shaving:

- Soften the beard or area to be shaved with warm water.

- Never shave over a dry area.

- Apply a non-allergenic cream or gel to area to prevent razor burn.

- Shave in the direction of the hair.

- Rinse with warm water after shaving.

- Apply a moisturizer to the shaved area.

Shaving tips to prevent folliculitis and ingrown hairs for those who are prone:

- Use an electric razor, since they do not cut as close.

- Use a single blade razor rather than 2 or 3 blade razors.

- Never pull skin tight when shaving.

- Use moisturizing shave cream.

- Shave every other day when you are experiencing a breakout.

- For more aggressive breakouts stop shaving for a month or longer to allow the area to heal.

- At night, an exfoliation gel may be applied to help prevent build up of dry skin.

Basic Biology of the Skin

The skin is often underestimated for its importance in health and disease. As a consequence, it's frequently understudied by chiropractic students (and perhaps, under-taught by chiropractic school faculty). It is not our intention to present a comprehensive review of anatomy and physiology of the skin, but rather a review of the basic biology of the skin as a prerequisite to the study of pathophysiology of skin disease and the study of diagnosis and treatment of skin disorders and diseases. The following material is presented in an easy-to-read point format, which, though brief in content, is sufficient to provide a refresher course to mid-level or upper-level chiropractic students and chiropractors.

Please refer to **Figure 3-1**, a cross-sectional drawing of the skin. This represents a typical cross-section of human skin and features most of the major components in such a typical section of skin. Most skin disease can be characterized as either epidermal, or dermal, or epidermal and eroding, or spreading, into the dermal layer. As will be seen in Chapter 4, Pathophysiology of the Skin, an understanding of normal anatomy and physiology is essential to understanding pathophysiology and serves as a basis to de-mystify many skin conditions.

Embryology of the Skin

The skin is mainly mesodermal in its embryonic derivation. Specialized skin cells and structures are formed from 3-6 months of gestation.

Types of Skin

- Non-hairy (glabrous)—a skin type on the palms and soles, it has thicker epidermis and lacks hair follicles.
- Hairy—a type of skin having hair follicles and sebaceous glands.

Layers of the Skin

1. Epidermis—the outer most layer of the skin that is divided into the following five layers from top to bottom. These layers can be microscopically identified:

   - Stratum corneum—also known as the horny cell layer, consisting mainly of keratinocytes (flat squamous cells) containing a protein known as keratin. The thick layer prevents water loss and prevents the entry of bacteria. The thickness can vary regionally. For example, the stratum corneum of the hands and feet are thick as they are more prone to injury. This layer is continuously shed but is replaced by new cells from the stratum basale (basal cell layer). The stratum corneum constitutes about 15 to 20 layers.
   - Stratum lucidum—this layer is present in the thick skin of palms and soles and consists of a transparent layer of dead cells. It functions as a barrier and also has water proof properties.
   - Stratum granulosum—also known as the granular layer, consisting mainly of stratified squamous cells arranged in 1 to 3 rows containing lamellar granules and tonofibrils. It is important to note that besides the palms and soles, skin lacks a well defined stratum lucidum and stratum granulosum.
   - Stratum spinosum—also known as the spinous layer consisting mainly of a cuboidal cell arranged in multiple layers and synthesizes keratins that function to support structures. The cells are adherent by specialized cells known as desmosomes.
   - Stratum basale or Stratum germinavatum—also known as the basal cell layer, is the deepest layer of the epidermis. The layer consists of tall columnar cells that are

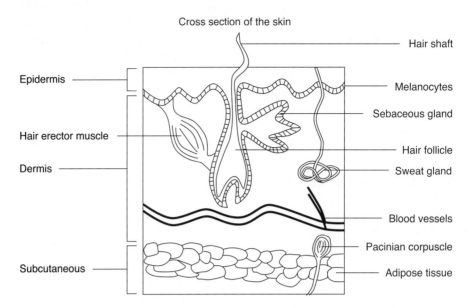

Figure 3-1   Cross-section drawing of the skin showing the epidermis, dermis and subcutaneous layers.

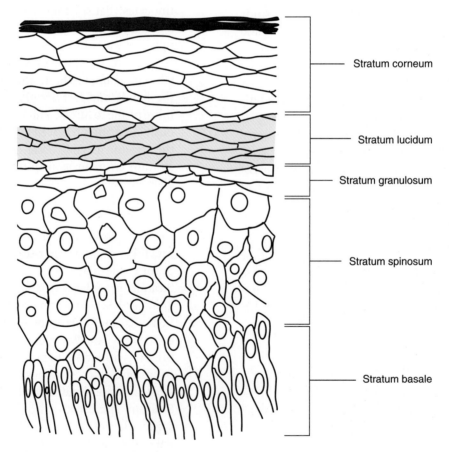

Figure 3-2   Division of the epidermal layers of the skin.

constantly undergoing cell division and help form new keratinocytes (keratinization) that will replace the lost ones from stratum corneum. This process takes about 27 days. Further down the stratum basale, the cell layer is attached to a basement membrane which serves as a demarcation or a boundary between the epidermis and dermis. The layer also contains melanocytes containing melanin, Langerhans cells which recognize antigens and present them to the immune system and Merkel discs which detect pressure on skin.

2. Dermo-epidermal junction—a well demarcated junction that lies between the epidermis and dermis.

3. Dermis—lies between the epidermis and subcutaneous layer. This middle layer of skin contains connective tissue in the form of collagen in bulk and elastin in minimal quantities, with a rich intertwining blood supply. The types of cells located in the dermis are fibroblasts, mast cells and histocytes. Hair follicles, nerves, lymphatic vessels and sweat glands also reside in the dermal layer of the skin.

4. Subcutaneous tissue—also know as the subcutis or hypodermis is the lower most layer comprising mainly of fat (adipose) which provides protection from injury, produces heat and serves as a cushion for the body.

Innervation of the Skin

- Parasympathetic nerves—consisting of cholinergic neurons that release acetylcholine to the sweat glands.
- Sympathetic—consisting of adrenergic neurons that release norepinephrine to the sweat glands, arteriolar smooth muscle and erector pili muscle.

Functions of the Skin

- **Protection and repair** which is provided mainly by keratinocytes while UV protection is offered by melanocytes. The subcutaneous layer protects the deeper body organs. Gentle stroking of the skin with a blunt object can result in white line response caused mainly by capillary constriction. A deeper stroke using a tongue blade will lead to the triple cell response, resulting in a red line, flare and wheal. The wheal is caused by the release of histamine that acts as a vasodilator in local response to injury. The eliciting of the red wheal is known as dermographism that is more pronounced in patients who suffer from hives (urticaria).
- **Skin color** is given by melanocytes that contain melanin.
- **Temperature regulation and excretion of waste products**—sweat glands produce sweat containing urea and water and play a role in temperature regulation. To facilitate heat loss in hot temperatures, the blood vessels in the skin dilate and sweat glands become active. Alternatively, in cold temperatures skin blood vessels constrict to conserve heat and the body burns fat stored in the adipose tissue. The burning of brown fat under sympathetic stimulation is common in infants. In colder temperatures, the sweat glands become inactive and the erector pili muscles become functional to promote trapping of air for insulation of skin. The adrenergic receptors like α_1, innervating the skin blood vessels are responsible for vasoconstriction under sympathetic stimulation.
- **Lubrication** of the skin is provided by sebaceous glands, which produce an oily substance known as sebum. Occlusion and infection of these glands can lead to conditions such as acne.
- **Immunity**—Langerhans cells in the skin are dendritic cells that take up microbial antigens in the skin to transform into antigen presenting cells and provide immunity by interacting with T cells. The name Langerhans comes from the German physician and anatomist that discovered these cells in the skin when he was a medical student.
- **Storage**—the skin is an organ which stores fats to provide insulation. This is mainly in the subcutaneous layer.
- **Sensation**—sensation occurs through specialized structures known as mechanoreceptors:
  - Pacinian corpuscle—vibration.
  - Meissner's corpuscle—tapping and flicker, point discrimination.
  - Ruffini's corpuscle—joint movements and stretch.
  - Hair follicle receptor—speed and direction of movement.
  - Merkel's discs—vertical dimpling of the non hairy skin.
  - Tactile discs—vertical dimpling of the hairy skin.
  - Nociceptors—detection of pain.
- **Vitamin D synthesis**—skin is a rich source of 7-dehydrocholesterol and under the effect of UV light is converted into Vitamin D (cholecalciferol) that is ingested mainly from diet such as milk and dairy products.

Cholecalciferol is converted into 25-hydroxycholecalciferol (25-OH) in the liver and finally to activated 1, 25 hydroxycholecalciferol (1,25 OH) in the kidneys. The activated 1, 25 hydroxycholecalciferol plays a vital role in calcium absorption from the intestine and kidneys.

- **Aesthetic**—skin can be seen as a mode of communication or attraction.
- **Absorption**—the skin has the ability to absorb oxygen and water. Certain drugs such as topical steroids that are applied topically could be absorbed through skin surface.

Skin Types

Skin can be classified based on its reaction to ultraviolet radiation:

Type	Definition	Description
I	Always burns but never tans	Pale skin, red hair, freckles
II	Usually burns, sometimes tans	Fair Skin
III	May burn, usually tans	Darker Skin
IV	Rarely burns, always tans	Mediterranean
V	Moderate constitutional pigmentation	Latin American, Middle Eastern
VI	Marked constitutional pigmentation	Black

Essential Skin Facts

- Largest organ of the body.
- Accounts for 15% body weight.
- The organ of the body that is most exposed to bacteria, UV light, toxins, dust and other environmental stressors.
- Every 24 hours the surface of skin sheds dead layer of cells, and on average 40 kg of skin is shed during lifetime.
- Dead skin cells can become a component of household dust.

Structure of the Nail

- Nail bed—the hard surface of the nail that can be visualized.

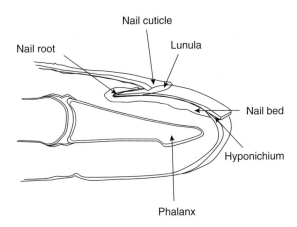

Figure 3-3   Cross section of a typical fingernail.

- Lunula—the half moon shaped structure at the base of the nail.
- Hyponychium—the soft tissue beneath the nail bed.
- Cuticle—the skin that overlaps the nail plate.

General References

Burns DA, Breathnach SM, Cox N, Griffiths CE. *Rook's Textbook of Dermatology,* 7th Ed. Oxford UK. Blackwell Publishing 2004.

Costanzo LS. *Physiology.* 3rd Ed. Philadelphia, PA Elsevier. 2006.

Eady RA, McGrath JA. Recent advances in the molecular basis of inherited skin diseases. *Adv. Genet.* 2001;43:1–32.

Fitzpatrick JE, Morelli JG. *Dermatology Secrets.* 3rd Ed. Philadelphia, PA. Mosby. 2006.

Fitzpatrick TB, Wolff K, Johnson RA, Suurmond R. *Fitzpatrick's Color Atlas & Synopsis of Clinical Dermatology.* 5th Ed. New York, New York. Mc Graw-Hill 2005.

Habif TP. *Skin Disease Diagnosis and Treatment.* 2nd Ed. Philadelphia, PA. Elsevier Mosby 2005.

Mackie RM. *Clinical Dermatology* 4th Ed. New York, New York. Oxford Press 2004.

Richard W, Hunter J, Savin J, Dahl M. *Clinical Dermatology.* 4th Ed Sussex UK. Blackwell Publishers 2008.

Standring S. *Gray's Anatomy.* Elsevier 39th Ed. Philadelphia, PA. Elsevier Mosby 2006.

Pathophysiology of the Skin

In dermatology, it is imperative to identify the type of skin lesions. These terms encompass the language used by dermatologists and are used to described the majority of dermatological conditions. For chiropractors, whether writing a referral letter or having a phone conversation with a dermatologist, observing, learning and understanding these lesions will help formulate a differential diagnosis. Being primary care physicians, chiropractors should learn to avoid simple and confusing terms like rash, bumps, and spots that do not actually aid in skin diagnosis. A more exact description is required using terms from the glossary of the skin lesions.

This chapter summarizes the pathophysiology of skin lesions that comprise a variety of skin diseases.

Classification of Basic Skin Lesions

The presentation of skin diseases can be complex and it is essential for chiropractors to learn and identify the skin lesions. Although identifying skin lesions is a complex process, a systematic approach to diagnose skin diseases can facilitate early treatment of patients. The skin lesions are divided into primary, secondary and special. The most common skin lesions presenting in the majority of the skin diseases are classified as primary skin lesions. The primary lesions can either present with secondary skin lesions or secondary skin lesions could present independently of primary skin lesions. The special skin lesions are categorized separately and can superimpose primary or secondary skin lesions.

The basic skin lesions are summarized in the following table and a pictorial demonstration is shown in the subsequent sections:

Summary of Basic Skin Lesions

Primary	Secondary	Special
Macule	Scales	Lichenification
Patch	Crust	Excoriation
Papule	Ulcer	Comedones
Plaque	Erosion	Cyst
Pustule	Fissure	Milia
Vesicle	Atrophy	Burrow
Nodule	Scar	Telangiectasia
Bulla		Petechiae
Wheal		Purpura

Glossary of Basic Skin Lesions

This section outlines a glossary of basic skin lesions arranged alphabetically:

- Abscess—see pustule.
- Atrophy—shrinking of the skin.
- Bulla—see vesicles.
- Burrows—formation of crevices and tunnels in the skin.
- Comedone—a plug of sebaceous and keratinous material lodged in opening of the hair follicle.
- Crust—a covering over the skin from dried fluid.
- Cyst—closed sac in a tissue that contains fluid or semi-solid material.
- Erosion—superficial loss of epidermis.
- Excoriation—erosions of the skin caused by scratching.
- Fissure—an opening that exists as a groove and is more like a break.
- Lichenification—thickening of the epidermis that appears like tree bark.

- Macule—a change in coloration of the skin, a flat lesion up to 1 cm.
- Milia—a small keratin cyst with no visible opening.
- Nodule—a bigger version of papule, more round and bigger in mass, lesions extra large can be labeled as <u>tumors</u>.
- Papule—a raised lesion <1 cm that could be crusted or scaly and can consists of a variety of shapes on the top.
- Patch—a change in coloration of skin on a wider area than macule (>1 cm).
- Petechiae—a well demarcated deposit of blood <1 cm.
- Plaque—although flat, this lesion is raised and greater than 1cm in diameter.
- Pustule—similar to papule but filled with pus, bigger versions are known as <u>abscesses</u>.
- Purpura—macules or patches that appear as red/purple discoloration of the skin.
- Scale—a flake of epidermis that can be separated from epidermal layer.
- Telangiectasia—superficial blood vessels that are dilated and appear as red strands on the skin.
- Ulcer—an open sore in skin, eyes or mucous membrane.

- Vesicles—similar to papule (<1 cm) but fluid filled and the bigger variety are known as <u>bullae (>1 cm)</u>.
- Wheal—an area of swelling, mostly red in color.

Grouping of Basic Skin Lesions

Skin lesions can be grouped according to their morphological type as:

- Flat lesions—macule, patch.
- Raised lesions—papules, nodules, plaques.
- Fluid filled lesions—vesicles, pustules, bullae, cysts.
- Open lesions—excoriations, erosions, fissure, ulcer.

Skin lesions can present on the human body in a variety of arrangements and shapes. The most common arrangements and shapes are depicted below. Chiropractors should emphasize on the shape, color and arrangement when diagnosing a skin lesion.

Differential Diagnosis in Dermatology

To help chiropractors analyze skin lesions and formulate a differential diagnosis, **Table 4-1**

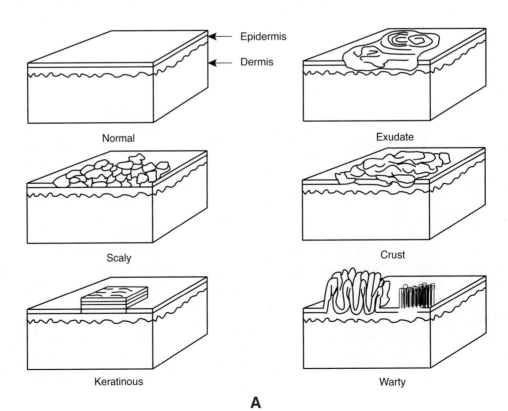

Normal

Exudate

Scaly

Crust

Keratinous

Warty

A

Figure 4-1 (A) Sketches of basic types of skin lesions.

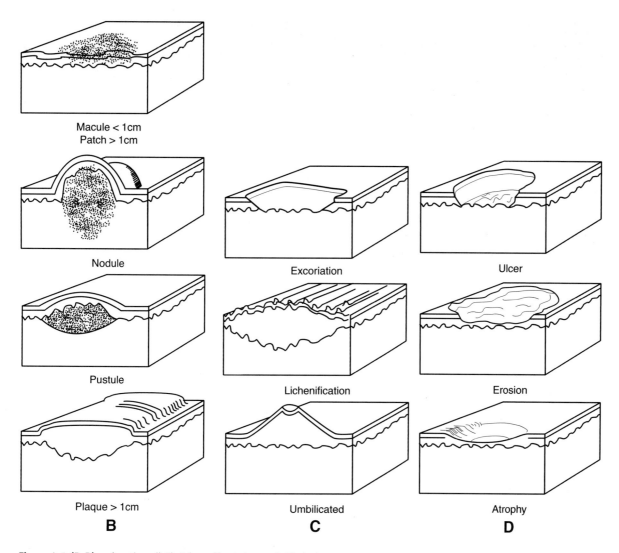

Figure 4-1 (B-D) *(continued)* Sketches of basic types of skin lesions.

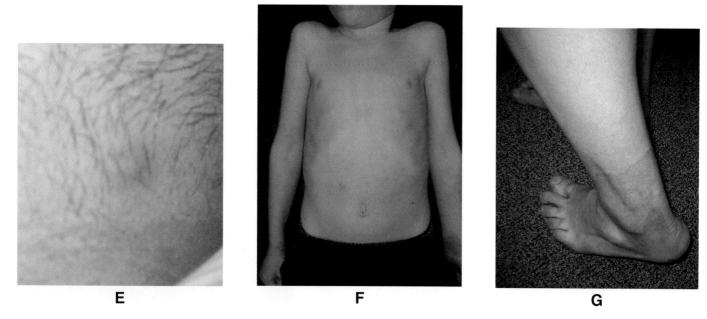

Figure 4-1 (E) Nodular lesion on the posterior surface of the neck.

Figure 4-1 (F) Maculopapular rash on the trunk of a child.

Figure 4-1 (G) Erythematous rash consisting of red patches on the shin and heel.

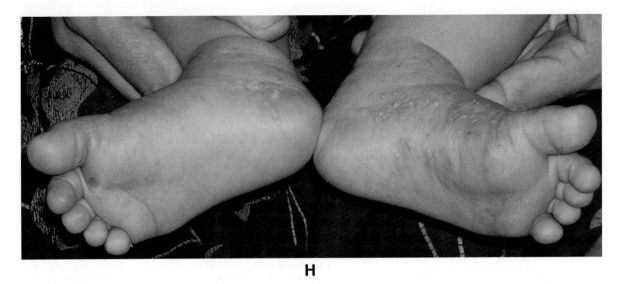

Figure 4-1(H)   Pustules on the soles of the feet of an infant.

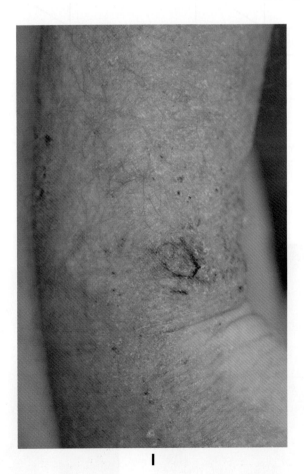

Figure 4-1 (I)   Macular lesion with erosion on the wrist.

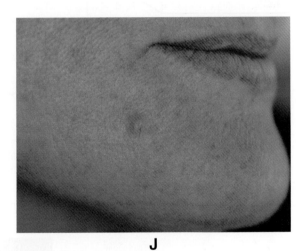

Figure 4-1 (J)   Solitary papule located on the chin.

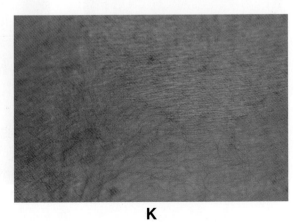

Figure 4-1 (K)   Example of a red patch.

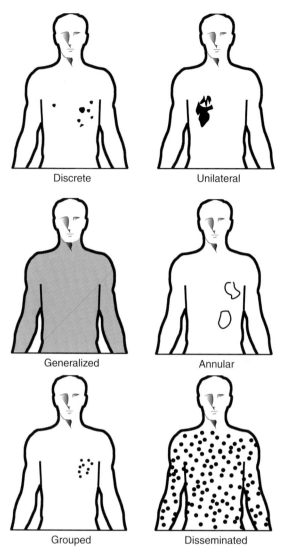

Figure 4-2   Arrangement of skin lesions.

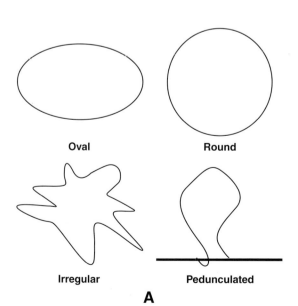

Figure 4-3 (A)   Shapes of skin lesions.

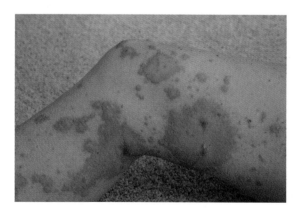

B

Figure 4-3 (B)   Annular shaped lesions.

Figure 4-4   Photograph of a patient suffering from poison ivy dermatitis showing a mixed erythematous rash. The important basic skin lesions can be appreciated.

Table 4-1

Lesions	Major conditions in Chapter 6	Other conditions in Chapter 8
Red Macules/Patches	• Atopic dermatitis • Candidiasis • Contact dermatitis • Fifth disease • Lyme disease • Lymphangitis • Measles • Rubella • Tinea infections	• Bowen's disease • Cutaneous larva • migrans • Dermatomyositis • Erysipelas • Erythema multiforme • Kawasaki's disease • Mastocytosis • Rocky Mountain spotted fever • Stevens-Johnson syndrome • Sweets syndrome • Toxic epidermal necrolysis
Brown Macules/Patches	• Acanthosis nigricans • Melasma • Pityriasis rosea • Post inflammatory hyperpigmentation in acne	• Lentigo • Nevus
Blue Macules/Patches	• Neurofibromatosis (café au lait)	• Mongolian spot (see Nevus)
Hypopigmented/Patches	• Pityriasis alba • Vitiligo • Tinea or pityriasis versicolor	• Idiopathic guttate hypomelanosis • Lichen sclerosus • Morphea • Nevus anemicus (see Nevus) • Scleroderma • Tuberous sclerosis
White or Yellow papules	• Keratosis pilaris • Molluscum contagiosum • Viral warts	• Granuloma annulare • Pseudoxanthoma elasticum • Syringoma
Brown Papules	• Melanoma • Skin tags • Viral warts	• Lentigo
Red papules	• Acne vulgaris • Atopic dermatitis • Contact dermatitis • Eosinophilic folliculitis • Flea bites • Pediculosis • Perioral dermatitis • Polymorphous light eruption • Scabies • Swimmer's itch	• Bee sting • Miliaria • Spider bite
Violet Papules	• Lichen Planus • Melanoma	
Plaque	• Cutaneous lupus erythematosus • Lichen planus • Lichen simplex chronicus • Psoriasis • Pityriasis rosea • Seborrheic Keratosis	• Sweet syndrome
Pustule/Abscesses	• Acne vulgaris • Chicken pox • Impetigo • Rosacea • Skin abscess	• Pseudofolliculitis barbae • Pyoderma gangrenosum

Table 4-1   (continued)

Lesions	Major conditions in Chapter 6	Other conditions in Chapter 8
Vesicle	• Contact dermatitis • Chicken pox • Hand, foot and mouth disease • Herpes simplex • Herpes zoster • Impetigo • Pompholyx • Scabies	• Porphyria cutanea tarda • Dermatitis herpetiformis
Nodule	• Basal cell carcinoma • Carbuncle • Hemangioma • Hidradenitis suppurativa • Keloid • Melanoma • Neurofibromatosis • Pyogenic granuloma • Squamous cell carcinoma • Viral warts • Xanthomas	• Chrondodermatitis nodularis helicis • Erythema nodosum • Kaposi's sarcoma • Keratoacanthoma • Lipoma • Prurigo nodularis
Bulla		• Bullous pemphigoid • Epidermolysis bullosa • Linear IgA disease • Pemphigus
Wheal	• Urticaria	• Mastocytosis
Scales	• Ichthyosis • Psoriasis • Seborrheic dermatitis • Tinea infections	• Actinic keratosis • Cutaneous horn • Grover's disease
Crust	• Atopic dermatitis • Contact dermatitis • Impetigo • Tinea infections	
Ulcer		• Necrobiosis lipoidica diabeticorum • Spider bite • Venous ulcer
Excoriations/Erosion	• Pediculosis	• Bullous pemphigoid • Neurotic excoriation • Pemphigus • Perlèche
Fissure	• Atopic dermatitis • Contact dermatitis • Hyperhidrosis • Psoriasis	
Atrophy		• Lichen sclerosus • Morphea • Scleroderma
Scar	• Acne vulgaris • Chicken pox • Herpes zoster • Hidradenitis suppurativa • Keloid	• Porphyria cutanea tarda
Lichenification	• Atopic dermatitis • Lichen Simplex Chronicus	

(continued)

Table 4-1 (continued)

Lesions	Major conditions in Chapter 6	Other conditions in Chapter 8
Burrow	• Scabies	
Telangiectasia	• Basal cell carcinoma • Rosacea	• Ataxia telangiectasia
Petchiae/Purpura	• Bacterial infections • Henoch Schnolein • Thrombocytopenic • Trauma	• Kawasaki's disease • Rocky Mountain spotted fever
Cyst	• Acne vulgaris • Epidermal • Pilar (wen)	
Milia	• Acne vulgaris	
Comedones (open-blackheads; closed-whiteheads)	• Acne vulgaris • Cutaneous lupus erythematosus • Epidermal cyst	

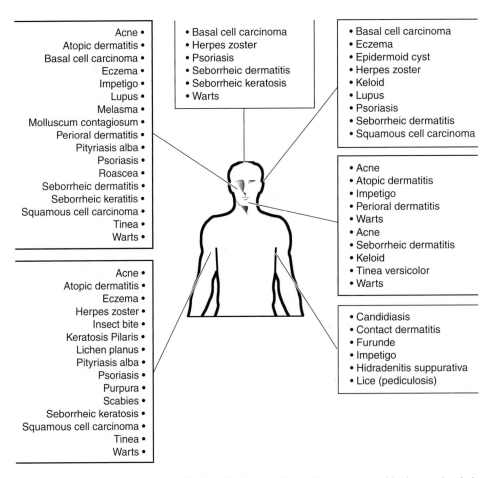

Figure 4-5 Classical regional distribution of diseases that chiropractors could observe in their practice.

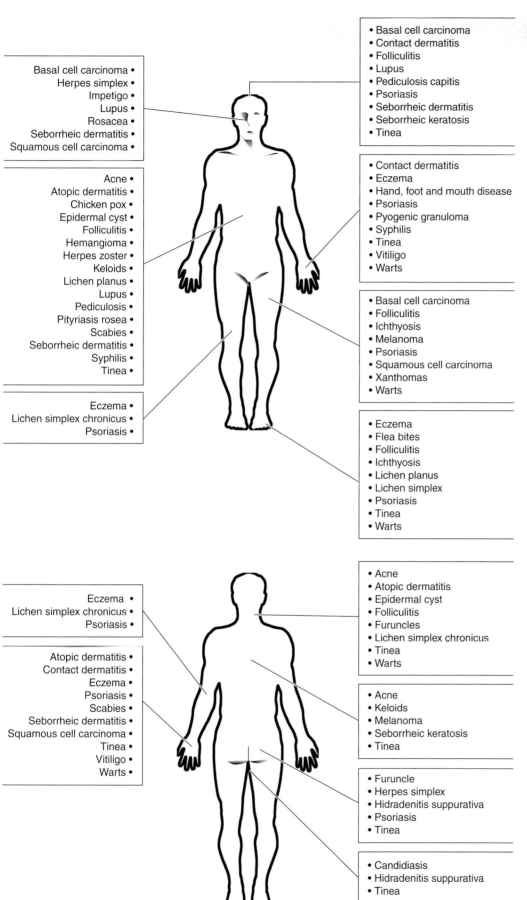

Basal cell carcinoma •
Herpes simplex •
Impetigo •
Lupus •
Rosacea •
Seborrheic dermatitis •
Squamous cell carcinoma •

Acne •
Atopic dermatitis •
Chicken pox •
Epidermal cyst •
Folliculitis •
Hemangioma •
Herpes zoster •
Keloids •
Lichen planus •
Lupus •
Pediculosis •
Pityriasis rosea •
Scabies •
Seborrheic dermatitis •
Syphilis •
Tinea •

Eczema •
Lichen simplex chronicus •
Psoriasis •

• Basal cell carcinoma
• Contact dermatitis
• Folliculitis
• Lupus
• Pediculosis capitis
• Psoriasis
• Seborrheic dermatitis
• Seborrheic keratosis
• Tinea

• Contact dermatitis
• Eczema
• Hand, foot and mouth disease
• Psoriasis
• Pyogenic granuloma
• Syphilis
• Tinea
• Vitiligo
• Warts

• Basal cell carcinoma
• Folliculitis
• Ichthyosis
• Melanoma
• Psoriasis
• Squamous cell carcinoma
• Xanthomas
• Warts

• Eczema
• Flea bites
• Folliculitis
• Ichthyosis
• Lichen planus
• Lichen simplex
• Psoriasis
• Tinea
• Warts

Figure 4-6 Classical regional distribution of diseases that chiropractors could observe in their practice.

Eczema •
Lichen simplex chronicus •
Psoriasis •

Atopic dermatitis •
Contact dermatitis •
Eczema •
Psoriasis •
Scabies •
Seborrheic dermatitis •
Squamous cell carcinoma •
Tinea •
Vitiligo •
Warts •

• Acne
• Atopic dermatitis
• Epidermal cyst
• Folliculitis
• Furuncles
• Lichen simplex chronicus
• Tinea
• Warts

• Acne
• Keloids
• Melanoma
• Seborrheic keratosis
• Tinea

• Furuncle
• Herpes simplex
• Hidradenitis suppurativa
• Psoriasis
• Tinea

• Candidiasis
• Hidradenitis suppurativa
• Tinea

Figure 4-7 Classical regional distribution of diseases that chiropractors could observe in their practice.

Table 4-2

No.	Condition	Classification	Physical Appearance
1	Psoriasis vulgaris	Eczematous	Papulo-squamous
2	Seborrheic dermatitis	Eczematous	Papulo-squamous
3	Atopic dermatis	Eczematous	Papulo-squamous
4	Lichen planus	Eczematous	Papulo-squamous/Erythematous
5	Lichen simplex chronicus	Eczematous	Papulo-squamous/Erythematous
6	Pompholyx	Eczematous	Papulo-vesicular
7	Keratosis pilaris	Eczematous	Papulo-follicular
8	Contact dermatitis–Allergic or Irritant	Eczematous	Papulo-squamous/Papulo-vesicular/Erythematous
9	Pityriasis alba	Eczematous	Macular/Pigmentary
10	Pityriasis rosea	Eczematous	Macular/Pigmentary
11	Ichthyosis	Eczematous	Papulo-squamous
12	Seborrheic keratosis	Tumor	Nodular
13	Xanthomas	Tumor	Nodular
14	Keloids	Tumor	Nodular
15	Hemangioma	Tumor	Nodular
16	Epidermal and Pilar cyst	Tumor	Nodular
17	Skin tags	Tumor	Warty
18	Neurofibromatosis	Tumor	Nodular
19	Squamous cell carcinoma	Tumor	Papulo-squamous
20	Basal cell carcinoma	Tumor	Papulo-nodular
21	Melanoma	Tumor	Nodular
22	Acne vulgaris	Infection	Papulo-nodular/Nodulo-cystic
23	Rosacea	Infection	Papulo-nodular
24	Perioral dermatitis	Infection	Papular
25	Hidradenitis suppurativa	Infection	Nodulo-cystic
26	Eosinophilic folliculitis	Infection	Papulo-follicular
27	Carbuncle	Infection	Nodular
28	Impetigo	Infection	Vesico-bullous /Vesico-pustular
29	Skin abscess	Infection	Nodular
30	Lymphangitis	Infection	Erythematous
31	Pyogenic granuloma	Infection	Nodular
32	Candidiasis	Infection	Maculo-papular
33	Tinea infections	Infection	Maculo-papular
34	Pediculosis	Parasitic	Papulo-nodular
35	Flea Bites	Parasitic	Erythematous skin rash (mix)
36	Scabies	Parasitic	Papulo-nodular/erythematous
37	Lyme disease	Parasitic	Erythematous
38	Swimmer's itch	Parasitic	Erythematous
39	Melasma	Pigmentary	Macular
40	Acanthosis nigricans	Pigmentary	Macular
41	Vitiligo	Pigmentary	Macular
42	Urticaria	Autoimmune	Erythematous

Table 4-2   (continued)

No.	Condition	Classification	Physical Appearance
43	Cutaneous lupus erythematosus	Autoimmune	Erythematous
44	Purpura/Cutaneous vasculitis	Vascular	Erythematous
45	Herpes simplex and Herpes zoster	Viral	Vesicular
46	Viral warts	Viral	Warty
47	Molluscum contagiosum	Viral	Papular
48	Measles, Chicken pox, Viral exanthems	Viral	Papulo-vesicular, erythematous, mix skin rash
49	Polymorphous light eruption	Miscellaneous	Erythematous
50	Hyperhidrosis	Miscellaneous	Sweating

categorizes the diseases that are discussed in this textbook along with other conditions that are not included in this textbook, or considered beyond the scope of this textbook.

Classification of Pathophysiological Conditions

Chapter 6 discusses the fifty most common conditions that chiropractors are likely to encounter in their practices. **Table 4-2** lists those conditions by their dermatological classification and physical appearance.

General References

Ashton R, Leppard B. *Differential Diagnosis in Dermatology*. 3rd Ed. Abingdon UK Radcliff Publishing 2004.

Burns DA, Breathnach SM, Cox N, Griffiths CE. *Rook's Textbook of Dermatology*, 7th Ed. Oxford UK. Blackwell Publishing 2004.

Fitzpatrick JE, Morelli JG. *Dermatology Secrets*. 3rd Ed. Philadelphia, PA. Mosby 2006.

Mackie RM. *Clinical Dermatology* 4th Ed. New York, New York. Oxford Press 2004.

Clinical Dermatology, Part 1: History and Physical Examination

Chiropractors follow the same general principles of diagnosis commonly used by any branch of medicine. The diagnosis of skin disease is a particularly good example of the use of this clinical method, since it is one of the few remaining specialties in which a traditional clinical assessment method is still the most important part of the diagnostic process. In this age of technological wonders, diagnostic investigation is often aided by the use of expensive and specialized testing. However, in the field of dermatology, the clinical art of history taking and physical examination remains the most important factor in arriving at a diagnosis.

The usual components of a medical history are as follows:

- Chief, or presenting complaint.
- History of present illness.
- Past history.
- Family and social history.
- Systems review.

By following this typical pattern, exactly as you would in a non-dermatological case, you can usually identify the general nature of the presenting skin condition. A careful physical examination based on this history should yield the diagnosis in most cases. If the diagnosis is still in doubt at this point, there are specialized tests that can be performed or, more likely in the chiropractic office, the patient will be referred to a specialized medical physician. Unfortunately, it has been suggested in some medical texts that physicians are prone to "guessing" the diagnosis of a skin condition, based on the appearance of the rash or lesion. However, using a formal scheme of history taking and physical examination will enable you to make the correct diagnosis most of the time.

Components of the Patient History

1. Chief Complaint:

It is unlikely that a skin lesion will constitute the chief complaint in a chiropractic practice. In fact, the 2005 Job Analysis of Chiropractic, published by the National Board of Chiropractic Examiners (NBCE) indicated that "acne, dermatitis and psoriasis" and "skin cancer" were "rarely" seen as patient conditions. However, also in this "rarely" seen category were upper respiratory infections, ear infections, pregnancy, menopause, asthma and colic (among 46 different conditions). Many chiropractors report seeing patients with asthma, pregnancy, menopause and colic more frequently than "rarely", defined by the NBCE as "1-10 cases per year", so it is difficult to properly interpret the NBCE data as they apply to a typical practice. Realistically, chiropractors will see few primary chief complaints referring to the skin. However, it is wise to be alert to a number of possibilities such as rheumatic disorders presenting as joint pains along with skin, nail or conjunctival lesions, or, for example, patients presenting with typical musculoskeletal complaints, but with signs of general or constitutional illness as judged by the texture or appearance of their skin. Finally, as has been mentioned previously in this text, chiropractors must always be alert to the possibility of discovering a lesion suggestive of malignant melanoma while examining the skin of the back of a patient for a common musculoskeletal complaint.

2. History of presenting complaint:

The sequence of this section of a medical history typically includes the following subsections:

- Onset and duration.
- Current or prior treatments.
- Prior occurrence.
- Description of presenting symptom (position, character, radiation, frequency).
- Aggravating factors.
- Relieving factors.
- Associated symptoms.

(Another common mnemonic format for this section of the history which will be familiar to many students of chiropractic is "OPQRST": onset, provocative and palliative, quality, region and radiation, severity, timing)

While the nature of a medical history is such that the lines of inquiry are virtually unlimited in scope and direction, there are nonetheless some specific and pathognomonic points relating to dermatological diseases that astute chiropractors should keep in mind.

Onset and duration: In dermatological disease, the most important question has to do with the nature of the onset of the condition, particularly including the duration of the complaint. Clearly, those lesions or conditions that have been present for only a few hours or days are to be distinguished from chronic complaints, which in dermatology can easily refer to decades.

In the diagnosis of musculoskeletal conditions, with which chiropractors are most experienced, the issue of duration is a relatively simple one. A condition is generally acute, sub-acute, or chronic. The definitions and standards for these three terms vary from reference to reference but in general, chronic refers to longer than three months, acute less than three months in duration and more commonly from 0–14 days, and sub-acute is longer in duration than acute, but less than three months. Most chiropractors have an ability to easily gauge a patient's musculoskeletal complaint as acute, sub-acute or chronic and, of course, this aids considerably in the diagnostic process.

In dermatology, however, there are some important distinctions. Skin conditions may be chronic in that they are very long lasting, sometimes decades in duration. However, the same condition may be associated with periodic flare-ups of acute duration. Some conditions are always acute in their presentation but tend to be recurrent and therefore may be confused with chronic conditions. Some true acute conditions exist such as urticaria, in which the lesions may appear and disappear within 24 hours. In other conditions, such as *herpes simplex*, the lesions appear to be acute in nature, that is, lasting 1-2 weeks, but the condition is chronic and recurrent. The nature of the pattern of onset and duration of both the lesions and the condition itself are very important in dermatological diagnosis.

Another consideration related to the onset and duration of a skin lesion is the travel history of the patient. It is important to note a history of travel to areas of the United States known for a high incidence of tick borne diseases such as Rocky Mountain spotted fever (caused by the bacterium *Rickettsia rickettsii*) and Lyme disease (caused by the bacterium *Borrelia burgdorferi*). A travel history can also suggest some common insect infestations such as scabies and pediculosis.

Current or prior treatments: Dermatology is one area in which over-the-counter treatments, home remedies, folk remedies and self medication are very common. Over-medication is also very common and often the cause of chronicity or recurrence of skin conditions. Patients must be carefully questioned as to the nature of previous or current treatment and whether or not they helped or aggravated the condition. Of particular importance to note is the result of self-medication with steroid creams, antibiotic ointments, antifungal agents, and various perfumed moisturizing compounds. Also, skin rashes may be the result of medication for another non-dermatological problem. Medications that are known for causing cutaneous reactions include antimicrobial agents, nonsteroidal anti-inflammatory drugs, cytokines, chemotherapeutic agents, anticonvulsants, and psychotropic agents.

Another reason for concern about patients who have self-medicated is that contact dermatitis may result from the application of an inappropriate over-the-counter product, and steroid creams can be associated with serious fungal infections.

Prior occurrence: As described previously, many skin conditions may appear as an acute condition, but in reality this is an acute flare-up of a chronic condition. A careful history must be made of the prior occurrence of any skin related conditions so that you may discern the possibility of a recurrent or chronic condition.

Description of presenting symptom (position, character, radiation, frequency): One of the main aspects of the description of a skin condition is the presence of itching. Itching can be severe in skin disease and lead to secondary infection caused by scratching. It is characteristic of many skin conditions, particularly those associated with dry flaky skin, but is it variable and not a reliable indicator of any particular condition. Severe itching at night, especially causing sleep disturbance, should lead to a suspicion of scabies, which is caused by an infestation of a mite called *Sarcoptes scabiei*. In fact, the name of this condition comes from the Latin word *scabere*, meaning "to scratch".

It is noteworthy that severe recurrent itching can also be associated with systemic disease, such as obstructive jaundice, as well as pschoneurotic conditions, such as neurodermatitis associated with anxiety.

In addition to a history of itching and scratching, it is important to ask about pain and tenderness, as well as about a history of discharge or weeping from the lesion. Even the odor of a lesion may have a diagnostic significance, with foul purulence suggesting infection and necrosis.

For obvious reasons, pigmented lesions are often identified by patients themselves. In these cases it is important to question the patient about changes in size and color of the lesion or lesions. For example, melanomas may increase in diameter initially, wheras benign nevi may increase in depth or become raised over time.

Aggravating factors: Frequently a skin condition is caused by exposure to a particular physical or chemical agent that is identified by the patient as a specific aggravating factor. An example is solar urticaria (sometimes called sun hives or sun allergy). In this condition, there is a specific and obvious awareness of aggravation (and onset) associated with exposure of the skin to the sun, particularly on the face and other exposed areas such as the arms or backs of the hands. In this condition, the rash will appear within minutes of exposure to sunlight, even through windows. Solar urticaria is usually of short lived duration and disappears within an hour. On the other hand, in porphyria (which is rare), exposure to the sun causes the rash within minutes, like solar urticaria, but the condition usually lasts for days. Again, unlike the more common patterns seen in musculoskeletal complaints, there is often a complex interplay between onset, duration, and aggravating factors in skin disease.

Chemical irritants and allergens are a common cause of contact dermatitis and usually the patient is aware of these aggravating factors. However, this is not always the case and one must carefully question the patient about their habits and activities prior to the onset of the condition to identify the nature of the aggravating factors. Some areas of inquiry to consider are domestic activities, work activities, exposure to cleaning solvents and detergents, hobbies, and cosmetic use. Even hands protected by rubber gloves can develop dermatitis.

Relieving factors: The identification of relieving factors is of considerable importance to chiropractors in the diagnosis of musculoskeletal conditions. However, this is not the case in dermatological diagnosis. For one thing, if a patient identifies a relieving factor (such as an over-the-counter steroid cream) then the lesion may disappear (permanently in the case of a short-lived acute condition, or for a considerable time, in the case of some chronic conditions) so the patient will not seek care at all. Also, the timing of skin symptoms and signs that appear to be relieved by a particular agent or event may be so complex as to confuse both the patient and the doctor. It is unlikely that the patient will report a pattern as noteworthy as we hear in a typical musculoskeletal history, such as aggravated by lifting and bending, and relieved by rest and analgesics.

Associated symptoms: Due to the association of skin lesions with rheumatologic disorders, it is very important that a chiropractor enquire of the possibility of some common associated symptoms. These include ocular symptoms (and signs), skin lesions elsewhere on the body, joint pains, oral or mucous membrane lesions, joint stiffness, swollen joints or fatigue.

3. Past history:

A history of chronic exposure to sunlight may suggest an increased likelihood of skin cancer. The patient should be questioned about living or working in a hot climate or outdoors. Frequent sunburn or particularly blistering sunburn is another clue to the diagnosis of skin cancer. Even a history of blistering sunburn during childhood may herald the onset of skin cancer in an adult or older adult, so the patient must be questioned thoroughly about previous skin health. People with fair skin are more likely to develop skin cancers with chronic exposure to the sun.

Many skin conditions are recurrent, so careful questioning of a patient's past history may reveal similar or related conditions. This information can assist in identifying the nature of the current condition as well as in predicting the outcome of treatment.

4. Family and social history:

In diagnosing musculoskeletal conditions, chiropractors will question patients about family histories of similar complaints, but only rarely are family histories of significant importance in the understanding of back pain. However, many skin problems have a genetic predisposition or a familial tendency. Patients with skin conditions need to be carefully questioned about relatives with eczema, psoriasis and other chronic conditions, including skin cancer. Also, infectious skin conditions, such as fungal infections and scabies may be found in family members.

5. Systems review:
   - General symptoms: fever (infection).
   - General symptoms: wasting, weakness, cachexia (malignancy).
   - General symptoms: obesity (dermatological conditions associated with deep skin folds).
   - Skin, hair and nails: enquire of the skin in other regions than the presenting complaint and note that the health of the hair and nails often reflects both dermatologic conditions as well as the state of general health and the presence of disease in other body systems; the health of the nails in particular may reflect the general state of health and the presence of fungal infections or the habit of biting the nails should be noted when found; symptoms related to the hair include changes in texture (as may be found in hypothyroidism), scalp itching, and changes in the distribution of hair (either increased, as in hirsutism, or decreased, as in alopecia).
   - Eye symptoms: redness (conjunctivitis or iritis, either or both of which may be associated with rheumatologic disease presenting as a skin condition), tearing or excessive lacrimation (allergic conditions such as atopic eczema and generalized urticaria), photophobia.
   - Ear: note that the ear canal is covered by skin and therefore skin lesions such as furuncles may be located in the ear; a history of itching, discharge or foul odor may be significant.
   - Nasal symptoms: rhinitis (allergic conditions), discharge (may suggest infection), bleeding (sometimes associated with rheumatologic diseases).
   - Mouth and throat: mucous membrane lesions may be associated with rheumatologic disease and may suggest a diminished state of general health.
   - Neck: prominent lymph nodes (infection or malignancy), lesions in skin creases which may not otherwise be noticeable to patients, skin conditions in occipital region disguised by hair.
   - Cardiovascular and respiratory systems: indications of general and non-dermatological health concerns; dependent edema (may be associated with ulceration and infection).
   - Gastrointestinal system: association of skin symptoms with dietary habits or food intake (allergies); suggestion of general health concerns; rectal symptoms such as itching may be associated with dermatological disease.
   - Genitourinary system: polydipsia may be present in diabetes mellitus, which in turn may be significantly associated with skin lesions, particularly on the feet; urethritis may occur as part of a rheumatologic condition (in association with ocular or dermatological manifestations); a history of sexually transmitted disease may be significant; many skin lesions occur in and around the perineum and genital region, sometimes associated with infection (hygiene may also play a role in skin conditions of this region).
   - Nervous system: dermatologic disease may be associated with states of anxiety and psychoneurosis (such as nummular eczema); formication as a result of neurologic disease may be confused with a skin condition.
   - Musculoskeletal system: chiropractors should fully investigate this system and seek symptoms suggestive of joint pains, swelling, stiffness or weakness (the enquiry should be thorough: in cases of psoriasis, for example, only the distal interphalangeal joints may be affected, with the patient complaining of morning stiffness).

Finally, there is one more important consideration regarding the taking of a patient history of a skin condition. This factor is the doctor himself or herself. There are several factors that can lead to either misdiagnosis or lack of diagnosis at all. These include fear that even noticing a skin lesion commits you to workup the condition to a final stage of either diagnosis and treatment, or appropriate referral. It is unconscionable to pretend not to have seen a particular lesion on a patient's back but there may be such a temptation during the operation of a busy clinic. The opposite may also occur with overconfidence leading a doctor to underestimate (or overestimate) the nature of a presentation without giving it the proper and due formal examination. Likewise, fatigue, distractions and the pressures of running a busy practice can all contribute to either missing important clues about your patient's health in their skin, or neglecting to follow-up an important observation.

Components of the Patient Examination

The traditional and cardinal elements of a physical examination are inspection, palpation, percussion and auscultation. In principle, one could include all of these components in examining a patient with a skin lesion, however, realistically, other than as part of the differential diagnosis of a potentially vascular lesion, auscultation will very rarely be involved. Likewise, while no rules can ever be made to limit the possibilities in a physical examination, the fact is that percussion will not likely be used in dermatological diagnosis other than in a rare instance of percussing a large dermal mass to determine its constitution as either solid, fluid filled or air filled (if this is still in doubt after inspection and palpation). Therefore the most important aspects of the physical examination of a skin lesion are inspection and palpation. Of course, having said this, it is also worth noting that the skin is the interface through which percussion and auscultation are used to examine deeper tissues and underlying organs.

As a general consideration, gloves should be worn when examining a patient since some fungal infections are highly contagious. Also, before beginning the systematic examination of the patient and the skin lesion, make a note of the general appearance of the patient. Does the general appearance indicate cachexia and generalized illness? Does the appearance suggest nutritional deficiencies and/or poor personal hygiene? Does the appearance suggest depression or anxiety which in turn might be reflected in nutritional deficiency or nummular eczema of psychoneurotic origin?

Thus, the examination of the skin is usually simple: good lighting, careful inspection and confirmatory or exploratory palpation, more superficial than deep. Occasional added information from odors emanating from the patient or the skin lesion.

Inspection: The skin should be observed and inspected systematically and carefully before the patient or the skin lesion is touched and palpated. All that is needed is good lighting, good observational skills, and a thorough knowledge of skin health and disease. As part of a general physical examination the skin is usually examined as the various body parts are examined, however there is merit in initially inspecting the skin as a general measure before commencing a complete physical examination.

The first observation that can be made is the color of the skin. In cases of suspected changes in color, photographs may even be used as a reference to the former color. Color changes may occur so slowly that even patients themselves are not aware of them. Generally, increased or decreased pigmentation in skin that was previously normally pigmented skin is indicative of an abnormal process. Increased pigmentation could indicate postinflammatory hyperpigmentation (also described in Chapter 1 in relation to the chronic neurophysiological effects of the chiropractic subluxation) and decreased pigmentation could suggest vitiligo.

Remember to examine the hair and nails, as part of the same system as the skin. Nail bed infections can be significant and a cause of recurrent itching and/or pain. Note whether the patient has a habit of biting the nails which may be a clue to the presence of anxiety. The texture of the nails is also to be considered as a reflection of general health and wellness. The presence of excessive or unusual distribution of hair (hirsutism) should be noted and may reflect endocrine disease. Patterns of hair loss may be genetic or a reflection of skin disease, as in alopecia areata.

Palpation: Excellent skill in palpation, which is strongly emphasized in chiropractic education, is a tremendous asset in dermatological examination. The ability to pick up very subtle cues such as skin temperature, moistness, texture and the presence of small lesions can considerably enhance the likelihood of arriving at a correct diagnosis.

Examination begins with very light palpation and proceeds through deeper palpation, as with the palpatory examination of other body regions including the musculoskeletal system. Very light palpation is used to determine the temperature of the skin (the back of the hand is most useful for this), the moistness of the skin may be detected by lightly dragging the finger tips (or the back of the hand) over the region being examined and comparing this to other similar regions, and a very slightly deeper palpation may yield information about the texture of the skin, as well as the presence of edema. Chiropractors are particularly adept at this type of palpatory examination in the diagnosis of the chiropractic subluxation or somatic dysfunction (the "T" in the diagnostic mnemonic "PARTS" refers to tissue tone and texture). Careful palpation may also suggest the presence of not only local edema, but also the possibility of a more generalized edema, as may occur in renal disease. One author (MW) had a young patient with Wegener's granulomatosis who was diagnosed with this condition at age 12. The complaints of various recurring joint pains suggested rheumatologic disease but one of the earliest clues was the observation by the patient's mother that he "felt different" when she hugged him. The mother was able to detect a very subtle generalized edema that was not obvious to his examining pediatrician, rheumatologist or chiropractor. This was confirmed with the finding of unexpected weight gain and led to the discovery of nephritis as a consequence of his disease.

Edema, when present may be differentiated as "pitting" (usually indicative of parenchymal and interstitial edema) or "non-pitting" (usually indicative of a more localized phenomenon such as a bite or local infection). As palpation deepens, lesions in the dermis or below the dermis may be palpated. The tissue may be gently manipulated, if it is not fragile or painful, giving the examiner information about elasticity, tissue compliance and underlying muscle tissue.

When skin lesions are discreetly palpable, they should be palpated for several characteristics. Their consistency should be noted, as soft, hard, firm, fluctuant, ropy, or board-like. Next, the temperature of the lesion is to be estimated if possible. Palpation should determine whether a discreet lesion is fixed or mobile. The depth of the lesion should be estimated, particularly the extension of the lesion into the dermis or subcutaneous tissue. Finally, it should be noted if the lesion is painful or tender as it is being palpated and examined. Many skin lesions are painless but the presence of pain may indicate inflammation or an infection.

A special mention must be made of Nikolsky's sign which is virtually pathognomonic of pemphigus vulgaris. The epidermis "sloughs" off when gentle lateral pressure is applied to the lesion. This is a very serious sign requiring urgent referral to a dermatologist.

Special Examinations: There are a number of special tests that are commonly used by dermatolo-

gists, some of which may be used by chiropractors, such as a Wood's lamp examination, depending on experience and training. These include the following:

- Biopsy and dermatopathology examination—this may involve a complex examination of a skin specimen including electron microscopy, immunoflourescence and the use of specialized stains.
- Microscopic and/or microbiologic examination of skin material (such as scales, crusts, exudates or tissue, which may be obtained by scraping)—this may involve direct light microscopic examination using techniques or stains known to facilitate the identification of bacteria (Gram's stain), yeast and fungus (10% potassium hydroxide), spirochetes (dark-field microscopy), or parasites (such as the direct observation of a scabies mite); also, a culture may be used to try to grow and identify an etiologic agent.
- Laboratory examination of blood may be used to perform serologic tests, as well as basic hematology and chemistry.
- Urinalysis and stool examination may be used to determine systemic causes of a patient's skin lesions.
- Wood's lamp examination—this test is based on the unique observations of skin lesions that are noted when skin is exposed to ultraviolet light, in a darkened room. For example, hair shows a green fluorescence under a Wood's lamp in the presence of tinea capitis. Many hyperpigmentation, hypopigmentation and infectious conditions are indicated by unique color under ultraviolet light. These include: bright white (hypopigmentation, vitiligo, leprosy), purple-brown (hyperpigmentation), various shades of green and blue (infections, particularly fungus and yeast), and pink to pink-orange (porphyria).

▨ General References

Bork K. Adverse drug reactions. In: Demis DJ, ed. Clinical Dermatology. *Vol 3. Philadelphia, Pa: Lippincott-Raven; 1998.*

Job Analysis of Chiropractic, 2005. National Board of Chiropractic Examiners, Greeley, Colorado.

Clinical Dermatology, Part 2: Fifty Major Disorders and Their Management

This chapter includes a detailed description of what the authors believe to be the most common and major skin conditions likely to be seen in a chiropractic office. Each section describes the etiology and pathogenesis, symptoms and signs, diagnosis, red flags, and treatment strategies including conventional medical care as well as alternative and complementary approaches. Many of these treatments are cross-referenced to the formulary in Chapter 7.

The 50 conditions in numerical order are (and, as described and categorized in Chapter 4—Pathophysiology):

1   Psoriasis vulgaris
2   Seborrheic dermatitis
3   Atopic dermatitis
4   Lichen planus
5   Lichen simplex chronicus
6   Pompholyx
7   Keratosis pilaris
8   Contact dermatitis—allergic or irritant
9   Pityriasis alba
10 Pityriasis rosea
11 Ichthyosis
12 Seborrheic keratosis
13 Xanthoma
14 Keloid
15 Hemangioma
16 Epidermal cyst and Pilar cyst
17 Skin tags
18 Neurofibromatosis
19 Squamous cell carcinoma
20 Basal cell carcinoma
21 Melanoma
22 Acne vulgaris
23 Rosacea
24 Perioral dermatitis
25 Hidradenitis suppurativa
26 Eosinophilic folliculitis
27 Carbuncle
28 Impetigo
29 Skin abscess
30 Lymphangitis
31 Pyogenic granuloma
32 Candidiasis
33 Tinea infections
34 Pediculosis
35 Flea bites
36 Scabies
37 Lyme disease
38 Swimmer's itch
39 Melasma
40 Acanthosis nigricans
41 Vitiligo
42 Urticaria
43 Cutaneous lupus erythematosus
44 Cutaneous vasculitis (purpura)
45 Herpes simplex and Herpes Zoster
46 Viral warts
47 Molluscum contagiosum
48 Viral exanthemas (incl.measles, chicken pox)
49 Polymorphous light eruption
50 Hyperhidrosis

These 50 conditions in alphabetical order with reference to the condition's number, for convenience, are:

Acanthosis nigricans (40)
Acne vulgaris (22)
Atopic dermatitis (3)
Basal cell carcinoma (20)
Candidiasis (32)
Carbuncle (27)
Contact dermatitis—allergic or irritant (8)

Cutaneous lupus erythematosis (43)
Cutaneous vasculitis (purpura) (44)
Eosinophilic folliculitis (26)
Epidermal cyst (pilar cyst) (16)
Flea bites (35)
Hemangioma (15)
Herpes simplex and zoster (45)
Hidradenitis suppurativa (25)
Hyperhidrosis (50)
Ichthyosis (11)
Impetigo (28)
Keloid (14)
Keratosis pilaris (7)
Lichen planus (4)
Lichen simplex chronicus (5)
Lyme disease (37)
Lymphangitis (30)
Melanoma (21)
Melasma (39)
Molluscum contagiosum (47)
Neurofibromatosis (18)
Pediculosis (34)
Perioral dermatitis (24)
Pityriasis alba (9)
Pityriasis rosea (10)
Polymorphous light eruption (49)
Pompholyx (6)
Psoriasis vulgaris (1)
Pyogenic granuloma (31)

Rosacea (23)
Scabies (36)
Seborrheic dermatitis (2)
Seborrheic keratosis (12)
Skin abscess (29)
Skin tags (17)
Squamous cell carcinoma (19)
Swimmer's itch (38)
Tinea infections (33)
Urticaria (42)
Viral exanthemas (incl.measles, chicken pox) (48)
Viral warts (46)
Vitiligo (41)
Xanthoma (13)

1. Psoriasis Vulgaris

Psoriasis is defined as hyperproliferation of epidermal keratinocytes combined with inflammation of the epidermis and dermis.

Etiology and Pathogenesis

- Alteration of the cell kinetics of keratinocytes with a shortening of the cell cycle from 3 to 36 hours, resulting in 28 times the normal production of epidermal cells.
- Psoriasis is a T cell-driven disease. There are many T cells present in psoriatic lesions surrounding the upper dermal blood vessels.

Signs and Symptoms

- Well-circumscribed, erythematous papules and plaques, covered with thick, silvery, shiny scales.
- Scales are lamellar, loose, and easily removed by scratching. Removal of scale results in the appearance of minute blood droplets.
- Papules grow to sharply marginated plaques, with lamellar scaling that coalesce to form polycyclic or serpiginous patterns. Small papules can appear as drop like lesions on the back in adolescents (guttate psoriasis).
- Psoriatic lesions are most often localized on the scalp, extensor surfaces of the elbows and knees, sacrum, buttocks, penis, soles and feet. Other areas that may be affected are the nails, eyebrows, axillae, umbilicus, and/or perianal region.

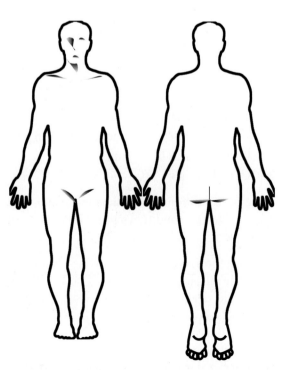

Normal skin.

- The disease can be widespread, involving confluent areas of the skin extending between these regions.
- A psoriatic lesion of the perianal and genital regions usually are not scaly, but is bright red and fissured. This is due to the warm and moist environment.
- Palmoplantar pustulosis is a variant of psoriasis that appears as pustules on the palms and soles.
- Nail pitting is common in psoriasis and distal edge of the nail can separate from the nail bed (onycholysis).
- Psoriatic arthritis. About 10% can suffer asymmetric or symmetric arthritis that could involve the distal interphalangeal joints.

Diagnosis

- Skin biopsy reveals marked, overall thickening of the epidermis, and thinning of epidermis over elongated dermal papillae. There is increased mitosis of keratinocytes, fibroblasts, and endothelial cells.
- On histological examination, parakeratotic hyperkeratosis and inflammatory cells are present in the dermis and in the epidermis, forming microabscesses of Munro in the stratum corneum.
- Serum uric acid is increased in 50% of patients, usually correlated with extent of the disease.

Course and Prognosis

- Some patients develop severe disease with painful arthritis.
- The scaling presented in the disease brings low self esteem.

Treatment

- Topical treatment (emollient creams, ointments, petrolatum, paraffin, and even hydrogenated cooking oils).
- Salicylic acid.
- Coal tar, anthralin, corticosteroids (topically or injected).
- Calcipotriol.
- Tazarotene.
- Methotrexate.
- Retinoids.

- Immunosuppressants.
- UV light therapy.
- PUVA (combination of ultraviolet light therapy and a drug called *psoralen* can also be used in cases that are resistant to ultraviolet light alone).
- Non-inflammatory diet, low in red meats, saturated fats and refined sugars can slow progression of the lesions.
- Zinc oxide can be applied to skin to relieve itchiness in psoriasis.
- Evening primrose oil applied to cracked and sore skin can help promote healing.
- Some clinicians believe that B12 deficiency may contribute to the development of psoriasis, and therefore supplementation is often suggested in treatment.
- Chickweed, Chamomile, Calendula, St. John's Wort, and Goldenseal can be applied topically to promote healing of cracked, painful, or dry skin.
- Herbs may be used as dried extracts (capsules, powders, teas), glycerites (glycerine extracts), or tinctures (alcohol extracts). Teas should be made with one teaspoon herb per cup of hot water. Steep covered 5 to 10 minutes for leaf or flowers, and 10 to 20 minutes for roots.
- Milk thistle (*Silybum marianum*) protects the liver and stops breakdown of substances that contribute to psoriasis.
- Yellowdock (*Rumex crispus*), red clover (*Trifolium pratense*), and burdock (*Arctium lappa*) are other alternatives. Sarsaparilla (*Smilax sarsaparilla*) can be effective in psoriasis. *Coleus forskohlii* (tincture, 1 ml three times a day) has been historically used for psoriasis.

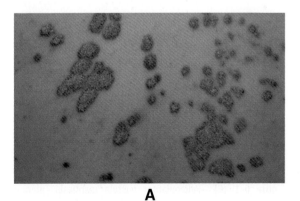

A

Figure 6-1 (A) Psoriatic lesions with an erythematous base.

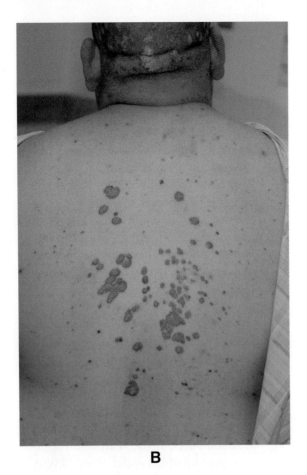

B

Figure 6-1 (B)   Psoriatic lesions on the trunk.

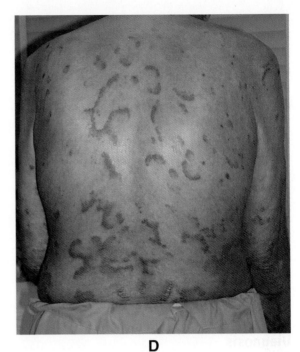

D

Figure 6-1 (D)   Truncal psoriasis.

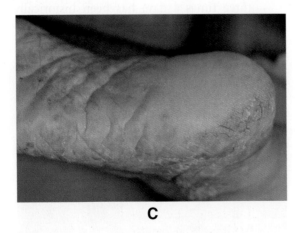

C

Figure 6-1 (C)   Palmoplantar pustular psoriasis (plantar shown).

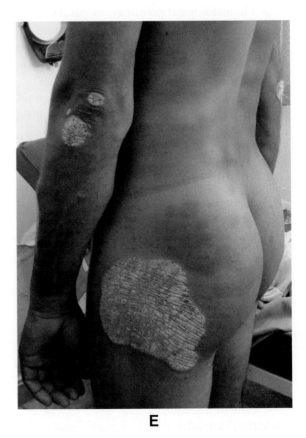

E

Figure 6-1 (E)   Plaque psoriasis.

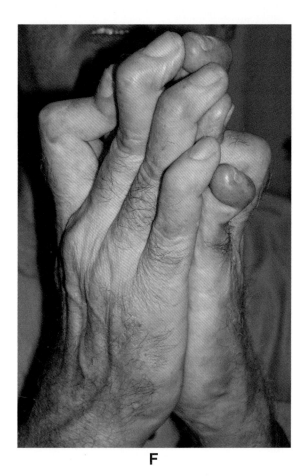

F

Figure 6-1 (F)   Psoriatic arthropathy of the hands.

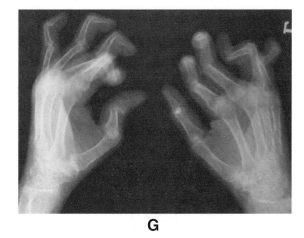

G

Figure 6-1 (G)   Radiographic image of psoriatic arthropathy of the hands.

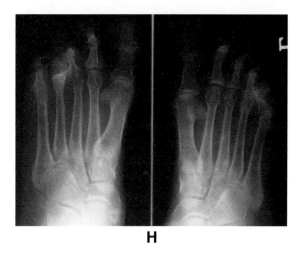

H

Figure 6-1 (H)   Radiographic image of psoriatic arthropathy of the feet.

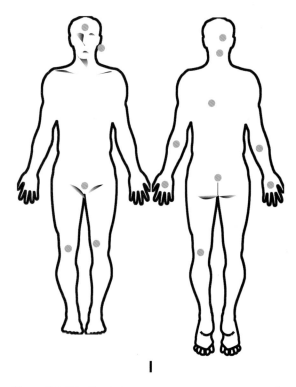

I

Figure 6-1 (I)   Psoriasis.

Red Flags

Psoriasis is rarely life-threatening. Although it is a chronic condition with remission and relapses, it is not contagious.

2. Seborrheic Dermatitis

Seborrheic dermatitis is an inflammatory skin condition that causes flaky, white to yellowish plaques over large areas.

Etiology and Pathogenesis

- The exact cause is unknown, but it can affect infants and adults.
- Slightly more common in males than females, and occurs in persons of all races.

- More common in winter and early spring, with remissions commonly occurring in the summer.
- Could be related to hormones because it often appears in infancy and disappears before puberty.
- Caused by a certain fungus, *Malassezia* and has been linked to conditions like Parkinson's disease and epilepsy.
- It can involve infection and temporary hair loss if the dermatitis is located on the scalp or other skin areas.

Signs and Symptoms

- Seborrheic dermatitis can occur on many different parts of the body, and is presented as dry, flaky skin that is white or yellow in color. Typically, it forms where the skin is oily or greasy.
- Seborrheic dermatitis causes itching due to flaking of the epidermal layer.
- When found on the scalp it is known as "dandruff." In children, it is called "cradle cap".
- Commonly affected areas include the scalp, eyebrows, eyelids, creases of the nose, lips, behind the ears, in the external ear, and along skin folds in the middle of the body.

Diagnosis

- Skin biopsies may be needed in patients with exfoliative erythroderma.
- Fungal culture may be needed to distinguish seborrhea from a superficial fungal infection.

Course and Prognosis

- Seborrheic dermatitis is a chronic, self-limiting condition that can be controlled with treatment.
- If left untreated, seborrheic dermatitis can spread to other areas of the body and secondary bacterial infections can also occur.

Treatment

- Medicated anti-dandruff type shampoos to control the skin proliferation and scaling. These shampoos contain sulfur, selenium sulfide, zinc pyrithione, tar, salicylic acid, or oil of cade.

- Overnight occlusion of tar, bath oil, or Baker's P&S solution may help to soften thick scaly skin, especially helpful when widespread scalp plaques are present. Other options for removing scaly skin involve applying a variety of oils (peanut, olive or mineral) to soften the scales overnight, followed by use of coal tar shampoo.
- Anti-inflammatory topical steroids are used to decrease inflammation. Solutions, lotions or ointments may be used once or twice daily for one to three weeks and discontinued when itching and erythema disappear.

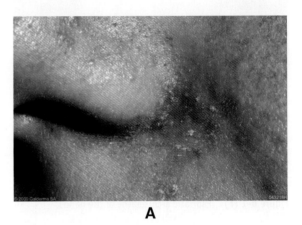

A

Figure 6-2 (A)   A case of seborrheic dermatitis. © *DermQuest. com. Used with permission from Galderma SA.*

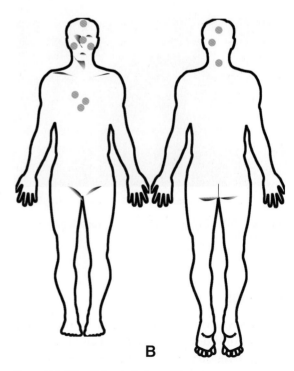

B

Figure 6-2 (B)   Seborrheic dermatitis.

- Ciclopirox is a synthetic agent that has recently been approved as a shampoo to treat seborrheic dermatitis. Ciclopirox was found to inhibit the growth of dermatophyte fungi, *Candida albicans*, and other nonpathogenic fungi. In addition, it has antibacterial and anti-inflammatory properties.
- Patients with a vitamin B2 deficiency have been shown to have a susceptibility to seborrheic dermatitis. Adult patients are recommended to take a multivitamin with 1.2 mg of B2, and infants should receive 300 mcg of B2.

Red Flags

If left untreated, the scales may become thick, yellow and greasy leading to secondary bacterial infection. Scratching and itching can lead to systemic infection. Referrals should be made promptly if diagnosis is in doubt or the patient is non-responsive to treatment.

3. Atopic Dermatitis

Atopic Dermatitis is a chronic skin condition that causes intense itching followed by a red, raised rash. In severe cases, the rash develops clear fluid-filled blisters.

Etiology and Pathogenesis

- Atopic dermatitis may be aggravated by exposure to certain foods, infection, stress, seasonal or climate changes, irritants (such as soaps or chemicals), or allergens such as dust mites or animal dander.
- Normally, the epidermis provides a protective barrier from external irritants, infections, and moisture loss. In a patient with atopic dermatitis, the skin no longer maintains its moisture, and becomes dry and susceptible to infection and irritation.
- Emotional stress.
- Tight clothing.

Signs and Symptoms

- The presentation often varies from person to person. The most common symptoms include red, dry, itchy rashes on the face, elbows, knees, hands and feet.
- Rash on the flexural surfaces like antecubital fossa, popliteal fossa, neck, wrists and ankles is typical.
- Itching is problematic when it occurs at night, resulting in unconscious scratching of inflamed tissue.
- The skin may be red and scaly with small red papules, patches of erythema and scaling. Upon scratching the lesions can leak fluid and become crusty and infected.
- In some patients, atopic dermatitis can affect the skin around the eyes, eyelids, eyebrows and eyelashes. Certain patients will develop an extra layer of skin under their eyelids and can suffer from recurrent staphylococcal, streptococcal, and viral infections.
- Some individuals may develop rashes around the nipples, and adults are prone to developing cataracts.

Diagnosis

- Elevated levels of IgE occurs in majority of patients.
- Patch testing, allergic testing, dietary testing can be considered before deciding on treatment.

Course and Prognosis

- The atopic lesions can get infected with *S.aureus* or could lead to increase in susceptibility of viral infections like herpes.
- Hyperpigmentation can result from previous inflammation.

Treatment

- Atopic dermatitis can be triggered by allergies, irritants, and even emotions. It is important that patients pay close attention to various foods that seem to aggravate their condition, as food sensitivities can stimulate the inflammatory response of the body.
- External irritants can worsen this condition. These irritants include frequent washing of the skin, wool or other coarse fiber, poorly fitting clothing, soaps, detergents, cosmetics, perfumes, dust, sand, and cigarette smoke.

- Stress can trigger an outbreak of atopic dermatitis. Patients suffering should practice stress management techniques and put forth an effort to overcome their emotions.
- Topical corticosteroids are the most common and effective treatment of atopic dermatitis. Creams or ointments of hydrocortisone can be applied directly to the affected area. When treating the face low-strength topical corticosteroids should be recommended.
- Zinc oxide can be applied to relieve itchiness of eczema.
- Evening primrose oil applied to cracked and sore skin can help promote healing.
- Calcium inhibitors such as pimecrolimus and tacrolimus are topical immunosuppressants which are similar to corticosteroids, in that they both inhibit immune function. The FDA recommends caution when prescribing or using Elidel (pimecrolimus) cream and Protopic (tacrolimus) ointment because of a potential cancer risk.
- Antihistamines are used to relieve itching that accompanies atopic dermatitis.
- Oral corticosteroid such as prednisone and prednisolone are used in severe cases when rash covers large areas of the body. Prednisone is a systemic corticosteroid that decreases inflammation and immune response.
- UVA or B can be a very effective treatment for mild to moderate dermatitis in older children (over 12 years old) and adults. A combination of UV therapy and a drug called *psoralen* can also be used in cases that are resistant to ultraviolet light alone. Side effects from long term use of this therapy include skin irritation.
- Cyclosporine is occasionally used in adults if other treatments are unsuccessful.
- Coal tar preparations can be used to control itching. Coal tar is considered safer, though less powerful than topical corticosteroids, and are thus used as a way to wean patients off stronger medications after the condition has been controlled.
- Leukotriene inhibitors, such as zafirlukast (Accolate) and montelukast (Singulair), may have a role in the treatment of atopic dermatitis. These drugs inhibit inflammatory pathways in the body.
- Azathioprine, a known immunosuppressant, has been used in severe atopic dermatitis.
- Interferon therapy.
- Chick weed, Chamomile, Calendula, St. John's wort, and Goldenseal can be applied

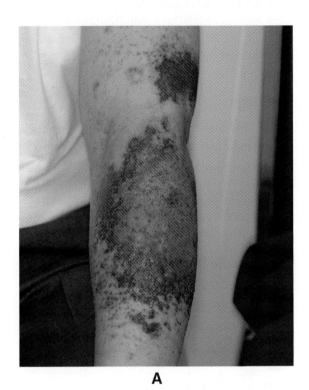

A

Figure 6-3 (A)   A severe case of atopic dermatitis.

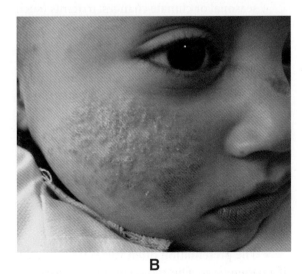

B

Figure 6-3 (B)   Atopic dermatitis on the cheek of an infant.

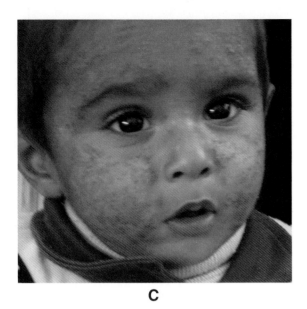

Figure 6-3 (C)   Facial rash of atopic dermatitis.

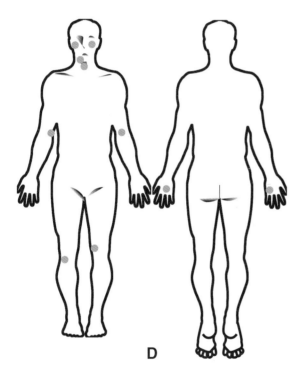

Figure 6-3 (D)   Atopic dermatitis.

topically to the skin to promote healing of cracked, painful, or dry skin.

- Integrate stress management, life style counseling, herbal therapy and vitamin therapy are also recommended.

Red Flags

If a patient experiences a sudden flare up or their condition is no longer responding to treatment,

they should consult their doctor to determine if infection is present and if hospitalization is required.

4. Lichen Planus

Lichen Planus is an inflammatory mucocutaneous condition with characteristic purplish-red colored, shiny, polygonal flat topped papules and plaques. The condition causes severe itching and can be cosmetically destructive in severe cases.

Etiology and Pathogenesis

- The cause of this disease remains a mystery, although some cases appear tied to hepatitis C infection, stress, genetic predisposition, and the use of specific medications for blood pressure and heart disease.
- Cases are seen most commonly in middle age, with a slightly greater predominance in the female population.
- No racial predilections.

Signs and Symptoms

- The patient will present with rash anywhere on the skin, but is most common at the flexor surfaces of the extremities, back, lower legs, and neck.
- Previous traumas often have occurred in close proximity to the outbreak.
- A close examination will allow the clinician to see that these violet flat-topped bumps have very fine scales which cover the surface of the lesions and present them with a shiny appearance.
- There could be intense itching with the rash.
- Lichen planus typically develops on the surface of the skin and may occur in the oral mucosa, nail beds, scalp, and the genital mucosa. The oral form reveals a "white, lacy, reticular pattern" that can be erosive in nature leading to secondary infections and increasing the risk for the development of squamous cell carcinoma.
- Lichen planus of the nail beds is present in approximately 10% of cases and presents with splitting of the nail, longitudinal ridging and grooving, nail thinning, and total nail loss.

- Scalp presentation can damage hair follicles by way of scarring alopecia.
- Genital mucosal infection may show characteristic lesions and become erosive in nature increasing the likelihood of infections and cancer.

Diagnosis

- Skin biopsy.
- Antibodies to hepatitis C virus can be seen in some patients.

Course and Prognosis

- Lichen Planus is not contagious but requires periodic treatment. It appears to be a reaction in response to more than one provoking factor.
- Onset may be gradual or quick, but the cause is unknown.

Treatment

- Lichen planus is a deep-seated and obstinate skin condition which is often resistant to treatment of any form. The total length of treatment varies from case to case, depending on various factors such as the duration of eruptions, the extent of spread of the eruptions, and the general health of the patient.
- The treatment is usually long term. One may expect a change in about three to five months. The total length of treatment may range from six months to two years.
- There is no known cure for this condition unless the source can be located and removed. Medical treatments vary greatly and must be individualized for each case depending upon the severity, area of involvement, and responsiveness to treatments.
- Common treatments begin with corticosteroids, either topical or oral. If the lesions are local, topical applications are more useful, while more generalized cases are better treated with the oral form. Topical applications will be applied for 2–6 weeks depending upon the results.

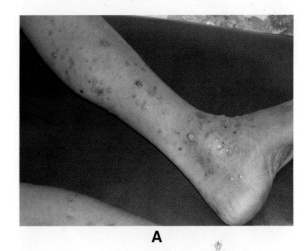

Figure 6-4 (A)   Lichen planus. *I*

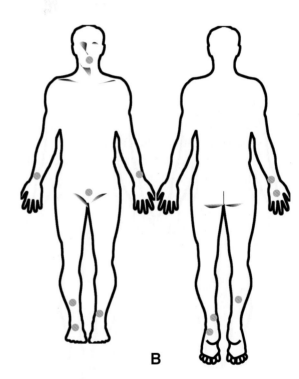

Figure 6-4 (B)   Lichen Planus.

- Other treatments include antihistamines, retinoid drugs and, in unresponsive cases, photo-chemotherapy over the course of weeks to destroy and dry up the lesions.
- Homeopathic medicine has been shown to provide some relief. The homeopathic medicines are prepared from a wide range of substances such as vegetables, herbs, minerals, chemicals, or animal products.

Red Flags

Lichen planus is a relatively common skin disease that comes in episodes lasting months to years but is not contagious.

5. Lichen Simplex Chronicus

This skin disease consists of a chronic plaque, leading to chronic eczema by scratching and rubbing. Another name for the disease is *neurodermatitis*.

Etiology and Pathogenesis

- Common in adults and young children.
- Stress.
- Prurigo nodularis is a nodular form of lichen simplex chronicus from compulsive picking, rubbing and scratching the skin.

Signs and Symptoms

- Well demarcated violet or white plaques with lichenification.
- Due to scratching, the condition can present with pustules and crusting.
- Nodules and lesions can appear behind the scalp, lower legs, wrists, ankles, upper eyelids, ear folds, scrotum or anal skin. The majority of the areas are accessible for pleasurable scratching.
- Itching.

Diagnosis

- Usually on visualization of typical lesions that result from history of scratching.
- The skin is thick and lichenified.

Course and Prognosis

- The condition can become chronic with repeated itching.
- The plaques can become violaceous but do not increase in size.

Treatment

- Reassure the patient and start with the sparing use of moisturizers.
- Areas may be soaked with warm water followed by use of steroid creams.

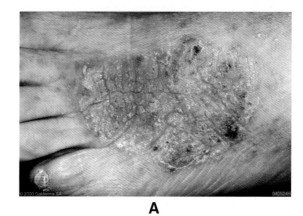

A

Figure 6-5 (A) Lichen simplex chronicus due to excessive scratching. © *DermQuest.com. Used with permission from Galderma SA.*

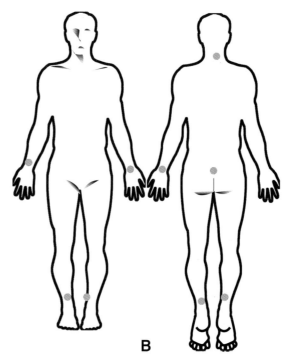

B

Figure 6-5 (B) Lichen Simplex Chronicus.

- Intralesional steroid injections can be used for chronic and nodular plaques.
- Antihistamines may be suggested to break the itch scratch cycle.
- Reduce stress.
- Superficial X-ray therapy has helped in some cases.

Red Flags

Lichen simplex chronicus is a form of eczema and is not a contagious disease. The disease and can be treated effectively.

▮ 6. Pompholyx

Pompholyx is a chronic relapsing vesicular eczema that most commonly present on the palms of the hands and soles of the feet. It is also known as dyshidrotic eczema.

Etiology and Pathogenesis

- Common in young women and middle aged men, especially money handlers, cashiers, and hair dressers.
- Avoid contact allergens.

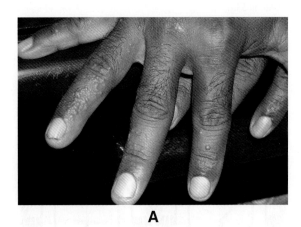

Figure 6-6 (A) Pompholyx.

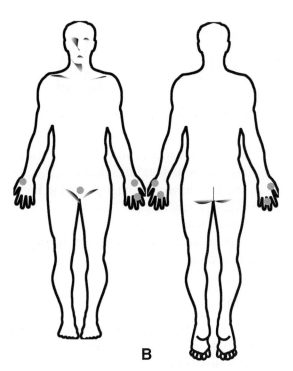

Figure 6-6 (B) Pompholyx.

- Reduce diet containing nickel.
- Pompholyx can be related to fungal infections such as tinea.
- May have a family history of atopic dermatitis.
- Contact allergy from nickel, chromate, rubber, perfumed products.

Signs and Symptoms

- Vesicles that erupt and leave a ring of scales with red cracked base, mainly on both the palms, fingers and soles.
- Moderate to severe itching.
- Brown macules could present suggesting post-inflammatory hyperpigmentation after the vesicles have popped open.
- Hyperhidrosis aggravates or can present simultaneously with these lesions.
- Itching can be intense in cycles.

Diagnosis

- History taking on triggers.
- Usually on visualization of typical lesions that result from history of scratching.

Course and Prognosis

- Mostly, the condition can resolve in three weeks. Relapses happen and can be very frustrating for patients.
- The eczema is rarely superimposed by bacterial infection.

Treatment

- Reassure the patient and start with cold wet dressings of tap water followed by medium potency steroid cream.
- Oral steroids can be considered in severe cases.
- Antihistamines can be prescribed to control itching.
- Reduce stress.
- Tap water iontophoresis or PUVA therapy has helped in some cases.

Red Flags

Pompholyx could become a chronic disease and require a combination of treatments as stated earlier. The disease is not contagious.

7. Keratosis Pilaris

Keratosis pilaris is a common condition with characteristic pin point follicular papules affecting the upper arms, thighs and buttocks.

Etiology and Pathogenesis

- Common in young children and can present in adults.
- Can result from excessive soap washing.

Signs and Symptoms

- Small spiky pin point papules on mainly the upper arms, thighs and buttocks.
- A red halo could appear on the ends of the pin point papule.
- Usually asymptomatic but some itching can occur.

Diagnosis

- Diagnosed by clinical observation and history of scratching.

Course and Prognosis

- A benign condition that when diagnosed properly, can be controlled by avoiding aggravating factors.

Treatment

- Reassure the patient that the condition can be treated and is not contagious.

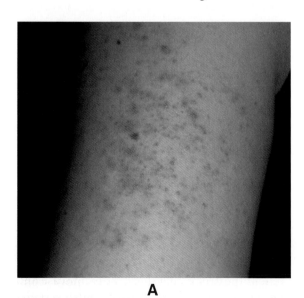

A

Figure 6-7 (A)   Keratosis pilaris.

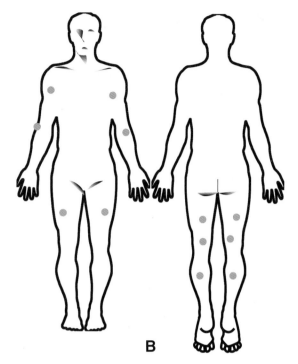

B

Figure 6-7 (B)   Keratosis Pilaris.

- The condition usually resolves by adulthood.
- Retin-A (triretinonin) cream is beneficial.
- Excessive soap washing or hard scrubs should be avoided as this aggravates the condition.
- Moisturizers applied on the affected area may relieve itching.

Red Flags

The condition can be controlled with proper treatment and is not contagious.

8. Contact Dermatitis—Allergic or Irritant

Allergic Contact Dermatitis (ACD) or Irritant Contact dermatitis (ICD) is an inflammation of the skin caused by exposure to an allergen or irritant. The reaction may present as a papular, vesicular or ulcerative lesion. The presentation may involve an acute episode or may be a chronic condition.

Etiology and Pathogenesis

There are many causes of contact dermatitis and the most common are listed below:

- Poison ivy or oak.
- Nickel or chrome plated jewelry.

- Rubber or latex gloves.
- Preservatives or additives.
- Cosmetic, soaps, hair gels, hair dyes, toiletries, fragrances (oil of Bergamot).
- Acids, alkali and wet cement.
- Topical medications.

Signs and Symptoms

- Contact dermatitis begins as a pruritic response to contact with an allergen.
- The eczematous skin changes vary and may range from erythema to blistering to plaques or ulcerations located at the site of exposure. In the acute phase, the erythema and edema will be well-demarcated but may advance to form papules and vesicles.
- In more severe acute cases, erosions and crusts may also be present.
- Chronic plaques may develop, thicken and scale yielding pigmentary changes.

Diagnosis

- Diagnosis is made based upon skin changes and exposure history.
- Patch testing may help rule out an allergen or an irritant but may be inconclusive; a positive test yields erythema, papules and often vesicles.

Course and Prognosis

- Contact dermatitis is not contagious and is self-limiting, beginning acutely and commonly taking about three weeks to completely resolve.
- Chronic cases do occur, lasting weeks to months, however, this is most often due to repetitive allergen triggering.
- Although very uncommon, contact dermatitis may be fatal if the allergen induces an anaphylactic reaction.

Treatment

- The most important recommendation is avoidance of trigger, irritant or allergen.
- Topical treatments are also available including cool compresses and corticosteroids.
- Oral corticosteroids and systemic antihistamines may help to relieve symptoms.

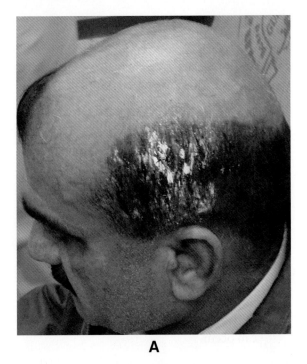

A

Figure 6-8 (A)   Contact dermatitis from hair dye.

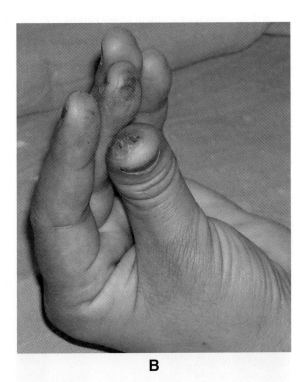

B

Figure 6-8 (B)   Contact dermatitis on finger tips resulting from cutting garlic and ginger.

- Wash with soap and cool water immediately after exposure to remove or inactivate most of the offending substance.
- If blistering develops, cold moist compresses should be applied for 30 minutes three times a day.

- Calamine lotion and cool oatmeal baths relieve itching.
- Ice may be applied either at or in close approximation to the area to reduce pain and inflammation.
- Aggressive physiotherapeutic treatments may actually have a negative affect and can aggravate the reaction.
- Dietary and nutritional advice includes natural antiinflammatory products, such as fish oil, and reducing the amount of red meat, saturated fat and trans fat foods that promote inflammation.

Red flags

Contact dermatitis may be a secondary finding. Any allergy may progress and involve the throat and respiratory system, quickly compromising a patient. The condition must be continually reassessed. If the condition drastically worsens, immediate medical response is indicated.

9. Pityriasis Alba

Pityriasis alba is a common, benign, eczematous disorder usually effecting school aged children. It is characterized by areas of hypopigmented and scaly macules, with borders that fade into the surrounding skin.

Etiology and Pathogenesis

- 90% of incidence are in children during the summer months or in warm climates.
- Can result from excessive soap washing.

Signs and Symptoms

- White hypo-melanocytic patches especially on the cheeks and forehead. In children the patches are about 2–3cm in diameter.
- White patches occur on arms and trunk in adults.
- On close inspection some scaling could be noticed.
- Rarely causes itching and generally is asymptomatic.
- Pityriasis alba is more commonly complained of in summer, as the surrounding skin is darker in pigmentation due to increased sun exposure.
- Pigmenting pityriasis alba is a variant of classic pityriasis alba and appears as a central zone of bluish hyperpigmentation surrounded by a halo of slightly scaly hypopigmentation. The halo may be of varying width, and these lesions usually occur on the face.
- There is apparently a strong association with pigmenting pityriasis alba and a dermatophyte infection, particularly tinea capitis.

Diagnosis

- Diagnosis is made based upon skin changes.

Course and Prognosis

- The condition is not contagious and is self-limiting, with no treatment required for complete condition resolution and re-pigmentation.
- The lesions typically last from several weeks to two years or longer, but usually fade and completely resolve by adulthood.

Treatment

- Reassure the patient that the condition is self limiting and is not contagious.
- 1% hydrocortisone cream can be safely applied twice daily on the affected area for two weeks. This may result in complete restoration of the skin pigment.
- Excessive soap washing should be avoided.

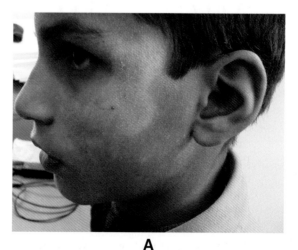

A

Figure 6-9 (A) Pityriasis alba lesions are dry patches on the cheek or other parts of the body mistaken for malnutrition or deficiency of vitamins and minerals.

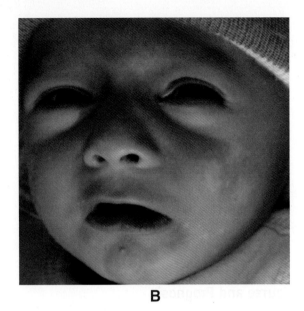

B

Figure 6-9 (B) Pityriasis alba in an infant.

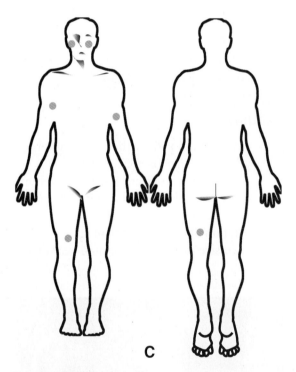

C

Figure 6-9 (C) Pityriasis alba.

- Moisturizers applied on the affected area can enhance healing.
- Pimecrolimus cream, a non-steroid topical cream with apparent immune modulating and anti-inflammatory properties, has been reported to be effective.

Red Flags

No red flag is present in pityriasis alba, as the condition is not life-threatening. The related, but rarer, conditions of extensive pityriasis alba and pigmenting pityriasis alba would warrant a referral to a dermatologist. Extensive pityriasis alba presents as numerous, more persistent lesions on the trunk and extremities that often last into adulthood.

Daycare facilities and schools may voice concern about the possibility of an infectious disease and may request that the child be removed from care and evaluated by a medical professional.

▮ 10. Pityriasis Rosea

Pityriasis rosea (PR) is a self limiting condition that is not fungal in origin and can be identified based on the dermatological findings.

Etiology and Pathogenesis

- No causal agent has been found in PR, though it tends to occur most often during the spring and autumn.
- Some drugs have been found to cause Pityriasis rosea, such as bismuth, barbiturates, penicillamine.
- Limited outbreaks have been reported in military barracks and nursing homes.

Signs and Symptoms

- In 50–90% of the cases, PR begins as a primary plaque called a "herald patch", followed by a generalized rash 1–2 weeks later. The rash lasts approximately 2–6 weeks.
- The classical herald patch measures 1–2 cm and is oval or round with a central wrinkled salmon-colored area surrounded by a darkened zone. There are fine scales along the lesion and the rash will typically follow skin folds. The initial lesion in PR may be mistaken for ring worm, which is contagious and caused by fungus.
- The rash is symmetrical and predominantly on the abdomen, chest, and back. On the back the rash takes on the appearance of a Christmas tree pattern. In PR the face, hands and feet are rarely affected. In more than 75% of cases intense pruritus is present.
- People with PR are more likely to have acne, dandruff, and dermatitis.
- Following the rash, people may experience hypo or hyper pigmentation. In patients

with black skin, hyper pigmentation is more common.

Diagnosis

- A skin biopsy is not necessary but may help to diagnose pityriasis rosea. All blood tests are normal with the exception of a slightly increased ESR.
- Secondary syphilis may present in a similar fashion, should be ruled out by performing a serologic test.

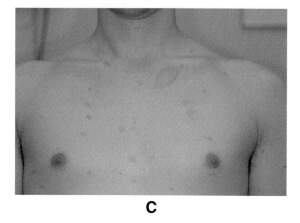

C

Figure 6-10 (C) "Herald patch" at the base of the neck can be noted with brown patches in a patient with pityriasis rosea.

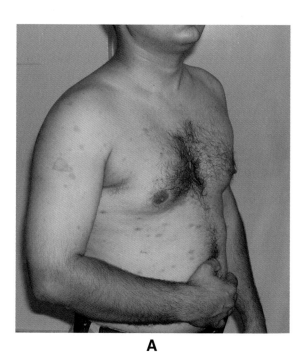

A

Figure 6-10 (A) Pityriasis rosea in a middle-aged man.

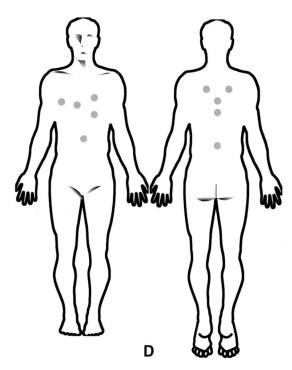

D

Figure 6-10(d) Pityriasis rosea.

Course and Prognosis

- The disease is usually self limiting and lesions can clear in 4–12 weeks.

Treatment

- No treatment is required in the majority of patients because PR will resolve on its own.

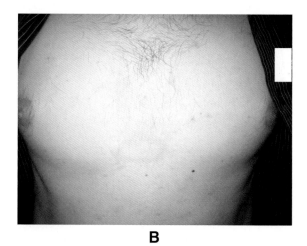

B

Figure 6-10 (B) "Herald patch" in the center of the chest can be noted in a patient with pityriasis rosea.

- Some alternative ways to treat PR are to avoid water, sweat, and soap that can cause irritation early in the disease.
- Zinc oxide and calamine lotion are useful for pruritus.
- If the disease is widespread, topical or oral steroids can be used.
- Ultraviolet light therapy has been demonstrated to be effective for PR, but may leave post inflammatory pigmentation at the site of the lesion.
- Eliminate stress and continue to exercise.

Red Flags

Children do not need to be withheld from school when they have PR, as the disease is not contagious.

11. Ichthyosis

Ichthyosis is a dermatological condition that may be inherited or acquired and is described as dry, scaly skin.

Etiology and Pathogenesis

- The excessive amount of scales is thought to be due to a defect in keratinization or cornification.
- The acquired type of ichthyosis can develop at any point in a person's life and may be a side effect of a medical condition.
- The inherited forms of the disease are rare and symptoms usually appear in early childhood and are present for the duration of a person's life. The inherited forms of ichthyosis are:
  • Ichthyosis vulgaris.
  • X-linked recessive ichthyosis.
  • Congenital ichthyosiform erythroderma.
  • Bullous ichthyosiform erythroderma.
  • Harlequin ichthyosis.
  • Netherton's Syndrome.

Signs and Symptoms

- Ichthyosis is a common skin disorder that presents as dry, scaly skin and is commonly known as fish scale disease.
- The disease may also cause mild itching of the skin and is more noticeable in the winter.

- Overall, a patient will usually present with pruritus, thickening of the skin with cracking and fissuring, decreased range of motion at joints, decreased tactile sensitivity of the fingers and even skin infections. Some patients may also have hypohidrosis with heat intolerance.
- Ichthyosis affects the stratum corneum producing hyperproliferation. It is most common on the legs, but may present on the arms and middle of the body. It may involve the hands, presenting as fine lines on the palm of the hand. The flexural surfaces of the body are usually spared.
- The long term negative side effects of this disease are often associated with the use of the prescription medications. These long term effects include higher risk of chronic skeletal toxicity including calcification of tendons and ligaments, hyperostoses and osteoporosis.

Diagnosis

- Ichthyosis is diagnosed by clinical observation.
- Tests to rule out conditions with similar presentation include routine histopathology, electron microscopy, and even frozen sections of skin biopsy. A genetic analysis may also be done looking for the X-linked recessive form.
- The X-linked recessive form would also be confirmed by blood tests showing elevated

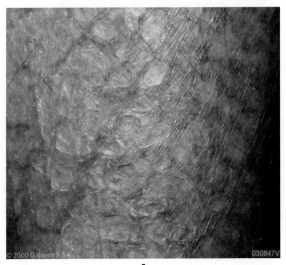

A

Figure 6-11 (A)   Ichthyosis. © *DermQuest.com. Used with permission from Galderma SA.*

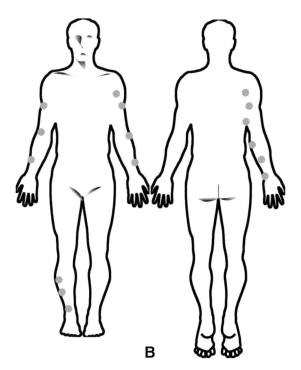

Figure 6-11 (B)   Ichthyosis.

serum cholesterol sulfate levels. The histological findings would include mild hyperkeratosis and a diminished granular layer in the epidermis.

Course and Prognosis

- Ichthyosis rarely affects the overall health of an individual but may come and go over the span of a person's life.
- There is a slight association in men with ichthyosis vulgaris and testicular cancer.
- Patients must be educated that this is a long term chronic disease and treatment is to prevent injury to the permeability barrier of the skin.
- Congenital forms of ichthyosis may be associated with neoplasm or systemic illnesses.

Treatment

- Most treatments for ichthyosis are centered around three mechanisms: hydration, lubrication and keratolysis.
- There is no cure for ichthyosis, but a prescription for alpha hydroxyacid lotion, a keratolytic agent, will increase the moisture content of the skin and dissolve the scales.
- Other keratolytic agents include salicylic acid, urea and propylene glycol.

- Other treatments may include oral retinoids, artificial tears, calcipotriol ointment, topical N-acetylcysteine, and topical cyclosporine. Skin grafts may also be warranted in extreme cases of server abnormalities.
- Products containing camphor, menthol, eucalyptus oil, aloe, and similar substances are very effective as antipruritics.
- Patients need to be educated on lifestyle factors that would help to minimize the symptoms.
- Avoid hot baths or showers.
- It is recommended to avoid harsh exfoliation or forcefully rubbing the area with a towel because this may irritate or damage the skin.
- Soaking in a warm bath is recommended to soften the skin.
- Use pH neutral soap rather than the harsh bar soaps to prevent further drying.
- Living in a warm climate may improve ichthyosis, but if this is not possible, a portable home humidifier or a humidifier attached to the furnace may help.
- It is suggested that food containing chlorophyll should be avoided.

Red Flags

Ichthyosis is mostly an annoyance to a person afflicted with the disease, but a bacterial infection may occur if the individual scratches the infected area enough to cause open sores on the skin. Dermatologists should be contacted if symptoms get worse, symptoms continue despite treatment, skin lesions spread or new symptoms develop.

12. Seborrheic Keratosis

Seborrheic Keratosis is an epidermal tumor that occurs most commonly in middle and older aged people.

Etiology and Pathogenesis

- Unknown, but the reticulated type is often found on sun exposed skin.
- Growth of the lesions may be associated with pregnancy or following hormone replacement therapy.
- The condition is associated with adenocarcinoma of the gastrointestinal tract.

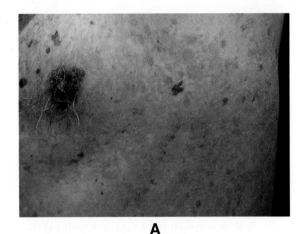

A

Figure 6-12 (A)   Seborrheic keratosis.

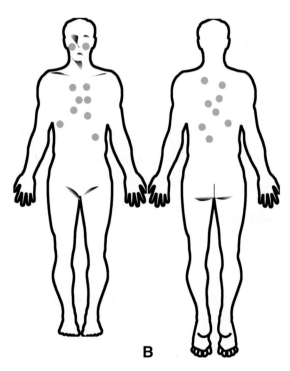

B

Figure 6-12 (B)   Seborrheic keratosis.

Signs and Symptoms

- The raised lesion is evenly dark or tan and is considered a plaque and a benign tumor.
- Lesions are round, flat, coin like, waxy plaques that can be a few millimeters or several centimeters in diameter (35 3 17cm).
- Lesions are uniformly dark, tan, or pink and have a velvety sand-like surface. When the lesions initially present they may feel soft and greasy.
- Close inspection will reveal pores impacted with keratin, which helps to differentiate seborrheic keratoses from melanomas.

- The lesions can number in the hundreds, and cover the trunk, arms and legs. They are itchy and bleed upon scratching.
- The lesions can occur anywhere on the body except the palms, soles and mucus membranes.

Diagnosis

- Shave biopsy will remove the lesion and provide material for histological exam followed by a curette to remove the remainder of the keratotic material.

Course and Prognosis

- Seborrheic keratosis is a chronic but benign condition.
- Other than cosmetic, the lesions present no danger to the patient.

Standard Dermatological Treatment

- Cryotherapy.
- Electrodesiccation.
- Laser surgery.
- Excision with a scalpel.
- Alpha hydroxy acid treatments.
- Trichloroacetic acid.
- Non-inflammatory diet low in red meats, saturated fats and refined sugars can only help slow the progression of the lesions.

Red Flags

The Lesser-Trélat sign is the association of multiple eruptive seborrheic keratoses with internal malignancy. This sign is associated with adenocarcinoma, most commonly of the GI tract.

13. Xanthomas

Xanthomas (also known as xanthelasmas) are a skin disorder in which fat is deposited in an area directly under the skin.

Etiology and Pathogenesis

- Patient has a history of an underlying blood lipid disorder.
- Equal prevalence has been reported amongst males and females. While they may be found at any age, those over the age of fifty are most commonly affected.

- Types:
  - Xanthelasma palpebrarum—the most common type with the lesions being bilateral and asymptomatic. They are soft, flat, yellow, velvety, polygonal papules around the eyelids.
  - Tuberous xanthomas are painless, firm, red and/or yellow nodules. They are often found in extensor regions of the body (knees, elbows, buttocks).
  - Tendinous xanthomas are subcutaneous nodules related to ligaments and/or tendons. The lesions are often related to trauma, and are mostly located on the feet, hands, and Achilles tendons.
  - Eruptive xanthomas are found on the shoulders, buttocks, extensor surfaces of extremities, and oral mucosa. They form crops of small, red/yellow papules.
  - Plane xanthomas are usually macular and rarely form an elevated lesion.
  - Generalized plane xanthoma.

Signs and Symptoms

- Xanthoma can be described as having a flat surface that is soft to the touch. Xanthomas can be found as macules, papules, and nodules. They are yellow in color and have sharp, defined borders.
- Xanthomas are generally painless; however, different subdivisions of cutaneous xanthomas have exhibited pruritus and tenderness. Xanthomas range in size from very small to more than three inches in diameter.

Diagnosis

- Tissue biopsy showing a fatty deposit in the area.

Course and Prognosis

- Xanthomas present as mostly cosmetic disorders, however it is important to note the possibility of disordered lipid metabolism. The xanthoma is generally painless, and is a benign growth of the tissue.
- Those suffering from xanthomas may also have a history of myocardial infarction.
- If there is hereditary hyperlipoproteinemia, a family history of xanthomas may also be encountered.

Treatment

- The main goal for treatment of xanthomas is to control any underlying condition that may be having an impact on the patient's body systems.
- Surgically remove the xanthomas if they become overly bothersome to the patient. However, even with surgical removal, the xanthoma may later reappear.
- There are several natural supplements that are useful in lowering blood lipids:
  - Soluble fiber.
  - B Vitamins.
  - Phytosterols.
  - Niacin.

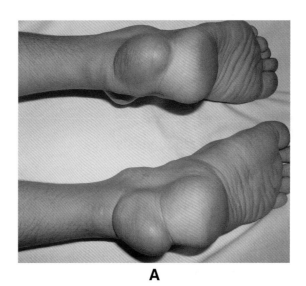

A

Figure 6-13 (A) Tendinous xanthomas.

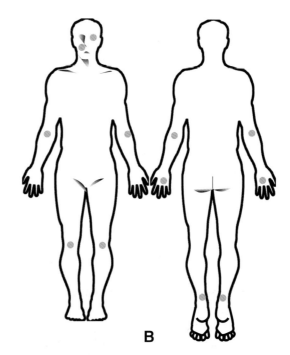

B

Figure 6-13 (B) Xanthomas.

- Dietary intake of fruits/vegetables, grain products, lean meats, fish, and low fat dairy products have shown some benefit.
- Regular, low intensity exercise like walking has also been shown to provide major health benefits.

Red Flags

Xanthomas are not contagious. This condition is generally a cosmetic issue, yet it is advised to seek the help of a health care provider to test for the possibility of an underlying disorder that needs some form of treatment.

■ 14. Keloids

A keloid is a special type of scar which results in an overgrowth of tissue at the site of a healed skin injury.

Etiology and Pathogenesis

- Unknown.
- Following a wound to the skin, both skin cells and fibroblasts begin multiplying to repair the damage. A scar is made up of connective tissue, and fibers deposited in the skin by the fibroblasts hold the wound closed. With keloids, the fibroblasts continue to multiply even after the wound is healed projecting to the surface of the skin.
- Keloids occur as a result of severe scarring, infection at a wound site, repeated trauma to an area, excessive skin tension during wound closure, or a foreign body in a wound. They can also occur where trauma, surgery, blisters, vaccinations, acne or body piercing have injured the skin.
- They generally occur between 10 and 30 years of age, and affect both sexes equally, although the incidence in young female patients has been reported to be higher than in young males, probably reflecting the greater frequency of earlobe piercing among women.
- Studies have consistently demonstrated that persons of African American descent and Asians are more likely to develop keloids.
- Genetic associations for the development of abnormal scars have been found.

Signs and Symptoms

- Keloids are firm, rubbery lesions and vary from pink or flesh-colored to red or dark brown in color. They can be doughy or firm and rubbery to the touch, and they often feel itchy, tender or very uncomfortable. A large keloid in the skin over a joint may interfere with joint function.
- Frequently involved sites are those constantly subjected to high skin tension. Therefore, wounds on the anterior chest, shoulders, flexor surfaces of the extremities anterior neck, and wounds that cross skin tension lines are more susceptible to abnormal scar formation.
- Keloids commonly occur as the result of pimples, insect bites, scratching, or any other skin trauma.
- Keloids are not lethal but when exposed to sunlight can increase the risk of cancer.

Diagnosis

- Diagnosis is by clinical observation of the lesions but skin biopsies can aid in definitive diagnosis.

Course and Prognosis

- Keloids may continue to grow slowly for weeks, months or years. They eventually stop growing but do not disappear on their own.
- Once a keloid develops, it is permanent unless removed or treated successfully.
- It is common for keloids that have been removed or treated to return. People who are prone to keloids should avoid cosmetic surgery.
- When surgery is necessary, precautions to minimize the formation of keloids should be taken.

Treatment

- In a patient with a history of keloid scars, all nonessential surgery should be avoided, especially at sites of predilection. In situations where surgery cannot be avoided, all attempts to minimize skin tension and secondary infection should be made. When possible, preoperative radiation therapy to the wound is a useful form of prevention.

- Corticosteroids has been the most popular treatment of keloids, either as sole treatment or in combination with other therapies. Intralesional steroid injections decrease dermal thickening.
- Silicone gel sheets and silicone occlusive dressings have been used with varied success in the treatment of keloids.
- Mechanical compression dressings have long been known to be effective forms of treatment of keloid scars, especially with ear lobe keloids.
- Simple excisional surgery.
- Radiation can be used as a monotherapy or in combination with surgical excision in order to prevent recurrence.
- Cryotherapy.
- Laser therapy.
- Intralesional injection of INF-alpha, INF-beta, and INF-gamma 5-fluorouracil, bleomycin have been shown to be of help in stubborn keloids that do not respond to other treatments.
- Flurandrenolide tape (Cordran) used on a formed keloid will cause it to soften and flatten over time. This is placed on the keloid for 12–20 hours a day. It is also good at eliminating pruritus. Prolonged use will cause cutaneous atrophy.
- Imiquimod induces local production of interferons at the site of application. It comes as a 5% cream, and is started immediately after surgery and continued daily for 8 weeks.

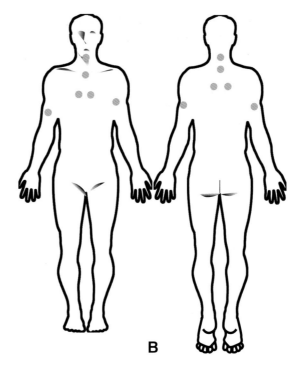

Figure 6-14 (B) Keloids.

- Methotrexate has proven quite successful in preventing recurrences when combined with excision.
- Tacrolimus is a new treatment for keloids.

Red Flags

Keloids are not contagious, or fatal, however they are not self limiting either.

15. Hemangioma

Hemangioma of infancy (HOI) is the most common benign tumor of childhood. The tumor usually takes the appearance of a red macule, although tumors arising from deeper endothelial tissues may appear more bluish in color. The tumor is comprised of plump masses of rapidly dividing endothelial cells.

Etiology and Pathogenesis

- About 83% of hemangiomas appear on the head and neck area, the other 17% appear throughout the rest of the body both internally and externally.
- Hemangiomas can be superficial or deep. Superficial hemangiomas are flat and appear as a reddish color. They are usually a

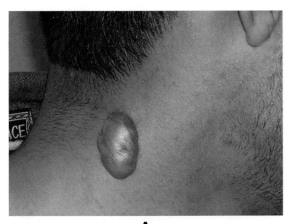

A

Figure 6-14 (A) A single keloid on the back of the neck, note the fleshy nature of the nodule.

well defined, lobulated tumor with minute surface capillaries.

- The deep hemangiomas are deep within the skin and appear bluish in color. These are seen as a poorly defined, slightly raised subcutaneous nodule with normal overlying skin.
- A compound hemangioma is a combination of both superficial and deep hemangiomas.
- An involuted hemangioma is characterized by the development of pale gray regions with ulceration and bleeding.
- Hemangiomas have shown to express GLUT–1 receptors.

Signs and Symptoms

- Hemangioma usually present at birth as a telangiectatic macule surrounded by a pale halo, a pale macule, an erythematous macule, or, less commonly, as a bruise or scratch.
- Most tumors begin during the growth phase in the first couple weeks of life; however, deeper seeded lesions that arise in the reticular dermis or subcutaneous skin may not appear until a few months have passed.
- Lesions are often described as "strawberry hemangiomas" or "strawberry marks." They are also known as cavernous or capillary hemangiomas.
- Hemangioma of infancy (HOI) usually progresses through phases of growth: nascent, proliferating to 9–12 months of age then becoming softer and dull in color leading to involution. The earliest sign of HOI is blanching of the involved skin. However, HOI are widely variable in severity and presentation, ranging from tiny lesions to large lesions that may endanger the child's life.
- The tumor may leave a residual of telangiectasias, which is a permanent dilation of capillaries in the area, atrophic wrinkling, yellowish discoloration, scarring, or alopecia in the area.

Diagnosis

- Diagnosis is made based upon skin changes and skin biopsies are not required.

- Ultrasound can help to determine the extent of the tumor on face or in the midline lumbar regions in infants.

Course and Prognosis

- An infant hemangioma is not contagious. The exact cause is unknown but 10% of infants have a family history. There is nothing that the mother does before or during pregnancy that could play a role in her child developing a hemangioma.
- A hemangioma that occurs in the liver, intestines, airways or brain can be very dangerous and will need immediate intervention.

Treatment

- Most hemangiomas of infancy are self-limiting and will involute.
- Corticosteroids used for 2–3 weeks can have a positive response, including tactile softening, lightening color or slowed growth.
- If the patient is unresponsive to corticosteroids, interferons are used to inhibit angiogenesis and stimulate endothelial cell prostacyclin formulation. This prevents platelet trapping.
- Laser therapy.
- Alternative treatments that have been used are intermittent pneumatic and continuous compression. Both methods have been used to treat symptomatic hemangiomas. The most favorable results are with lesions of the extremities and the mechanism of action is unknown.
- When the hemangioma is present in the diaper area of the child, zinc oxide can be beneficial in protecting the area from moisture to promote healing.
- If the hemangioma is over the eye, clinicians should advise a patch to be worn over the eye to prevent irritation of the hemangioma.
- Topical creams and dressings may be used to decrease the incidence of infection, especially in the case of ulcerative hemangiomas, and decrease pain.
- Psychosocial support for parents and children is important, as parents may undergo accusations of child abuse and express

emotions such as fear and embarrassment that can affect the child.

Red Flags

A hemangioma is severely problematic if it interferes with eating, breathing, seeing, hearing and speaking. When an infant presents with any of these problems, he or she needs immediate aggressive intervention. A hemangioma that grows

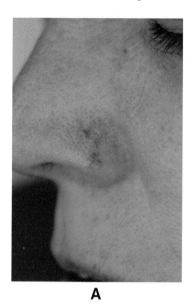

A

Figure 6-15 (A) Cherry angioma on the nose of a female patient.

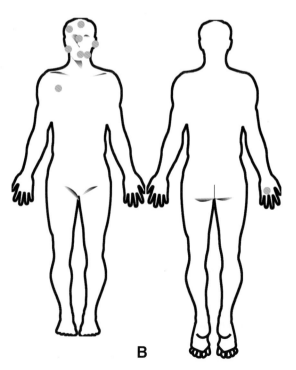

B

Figure 6-15 (B) Hemangioma.

internally is also very dangerous and needs immediate care. When an infant appears to have three or more hemangiomas, an ultrasound should be done of the entire body to rule out internal lesions.

16. Epidermal and Pilar Cyst

An epidermal cyst is a subcutaneous keratin-filled cyst, often originating from a hair follicle, whereas a pilar cyst is a subcutaneous keratin-filled cyst often originating from the sheath of a hair follicle. Another name for pilar cyst is trichilemmal cyst.

Etiology and Pathogenesis

- Arise mainly on the scalp, although can occur on multiple sites like the back, neck and face.
- Arise in puberty in areas of friction.
- Epidermal cysts are single and can be ruptured to extrude keratin like cheesy material, sometimes containing bacteria. A pilar cyst always develops after puberty and rupture less frequently than epidermal cyst. They usually rupture from trauma to the head.
- Epidermal cysts can be mistaken for pilar cysts that are more mobile but difficult to rupture.

Signs and Symptoms

- Nodular subcutaneous cysts ranging from 0.5–5 cm with comedo openings on top.
- Keratinous material is extruded upon rupture and leads to scarring.
- Inflamed cysts are warm, red and tender on palpation.
- Multiple epidermal cysts (Gardener's syndrome) should raise suspicion of colon cancer.
- Pilar cyst are difficult to differentiate from epidermal cysts as they are the same size, subcutaneous in origin, are mobile and do not have a central punctum.

Diagnosis

- Usually on visualization of typical lesions that are present in common skin areas.
- Biopsy is usually not necessary.

Course and Prognosis

- The cysts grow slowly in size and are subjected to repeated trauma.
- If they are not removed, the cysts can exist indefinitely and do not regress.

Treatment

- Asymptomatic cysts should be left alone.
- Surgical excision and debridement under local anesthesia is the best available treatment.

Red Flags

Multiple epidermal cysts occurring on neck, trunk and even the face are suggestive of Garden-

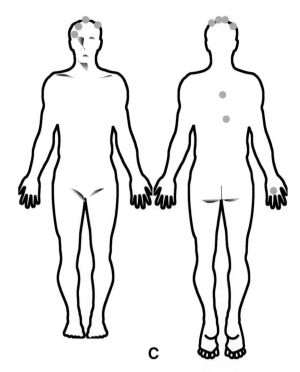

Figure 6-16 (C)   Epidermal and Pilar cyst.

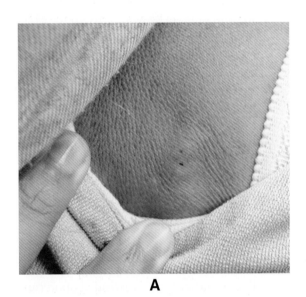

A

Figure 6-16 (A)   Pilar cyst.

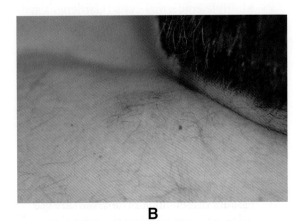

B

Figure 6-16 (B)   Epidermoid cyst.

er's syndrome. This should raise suspicion of colon cancer and chiropractors should promptly refer these cases to a general or plastic surgeon. Pilar cysts do not pose immediate threat and are easily removed by surgery for cosmetic reasons.

17. Skin Tags

Skin tags are fleshy papules that are also known as "acrochordons".

Etiology and Pathogenesis

- Common after 30 years.
- More common in obese.
- Familial.
- Single.

Signs and Symptoms

- 1–5 mm pedunculated papules, fleshy or brown in color.
- Axilla, neck and eyelids are most common sites.
- Asymptomatic but can become irritated upon trauma.
- Depending upon location they may become irritate upon friction with jewelry and clothing.

Course and Prognosis

The tags can become thrombosed or tender upon picking and can remain indefinitely.

Treatment

- Patients seek treatment for cosmetic reasons.
- Asymptomatic skin tags can be excised with scissors.
- Electrocautery.
- Cryosurgery.

Red Flags

Multiple skin tags with fibrous tumor may suggest renal, colon or thyroid cancer

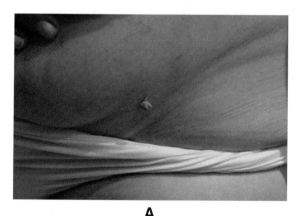

A

Figure 6-17 (A) Skin tags.

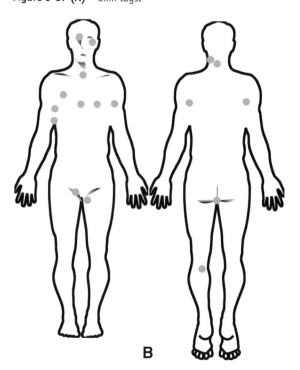

B

Figure 6-17 (B) Skin tags.

18. Neurofibromatosis

Neurofibromatosis (NF) is an inherited condition manifested by changes in the skin, nervous system, bones and endocrine glands. These changes include a wide variety of congenital abnormalities, tumors, skin lesions and hemartomas.

Etiology and Pathogenesis

- The inheritance of NF is autosomal dominant, however approximately 50% of cases of NF arise from new mutations.
- The pathogenesis of NF is believed to be a defect in the neurofibrin gene.
- Two main forms of neurofibromatosis are recognized:
  - classic von Recklinghausen's NF1.
  - central or acoustic NF termed NF2.
- NF1, or von Recklinghausen's disease, is the most common form of NF with the incidence estimated at 1 in 3000 to 4000. In comparison, NF2 has an incidence of approximately 1 in 50,000. Both NF1 and NF2 affect men and women; however, there is a slight male predominance associated with this condition.

Signs and Symptoms

- In 1987, the National Institute of Health developed consensus criteria for the diagnosis of neurofibromatosis. To establish a diagnosis of NF, two or more of the following criteria are required:
- Six or more café-au-lait macules more than 5mm in greatest diameter in prepubertal children and more than 15 mm in greatest diameter in postpubertal people; two or more neurofibromas of any type or one plexiform neurofibroma.
- Freckling in the axillary or groin region; optic glioma; two or more Lisch nodules; a distinctive osseous lesion such as sphenoid dysplasia or thinning of long bone cortex, with or without pseudoarthrosis; and/or a first degree relative with NF1.
- The distribution of the numerous types of skin lesions are often randomly distributed on all regions of the body but can be localized to one region. These are often called regional hemartomas. The axilla and groin region are common locations for tiny and numerous café-au-lait spots.

- Cafe-au-lait macules (CAL) are light or dark brown uniform melanin pigmentation with sharp margination. Lesions vary in size from multiple freckle like macules less than 2mm to very large macules greater than 20cm. CAL macules vary in number from a few to hundreds. Tiny numerous CAL macules located in the axillary or groin region are pathognomic of NF.
- The papules and nodules associated with NF are called neurofibromas. They are the most common cutaneous and subcutaneous skin lesion associated with NF1. They are benign tumors of neural sheath origin that often present during adolescence (only small incidences of malignant change are associated with neurofibromas). They are skin-colored, pink or brown and often present as flat, sessile or pedunculated. They can either present as soft or firm and are occasionally tender.
- In addition to neurofibromas associated with NF, fibroma molluscums are nodules that often present in patients with NF. These are multiple cutaneous nodules that are elevated above the skin surface. They are soft, nipple like, pedunculated or sessile skin tabs that vary in size. They may be widely dispersed or may cover the entire body.
- Plexiform neuromas are soft, drooping, and of a doughy consistency. These may be massive in size and often involve the entire extremity, the head or portion of the trunk. The presence of plexiform neuromas often warrant further investigation into associated bony lesions due to the relationship between these neuromas and bone lesions.
- Although mild to moderate skin manifestations are the predominant manifestation and sign of NF, additional physical findings may present due to the development of tumors of neural origin in other parts of the body.
- Pigmented hemartomas, or Lisch nodules, of the iris present in approximately 20% of children with NF and up to 95% of adolescents with NF present with Lisch nodules. However, Lisch nodules do not correlate with severity of the disease.
- Additional physical findings may include the following: cervicothoracic kyphoscoliosis and segmental hypertrophy; tibial bowing; elevated blood pressure and episodic flushing due to the incidence of an associated adrenal tumor; elephantiasis neuromatosa; optic gliomas; acoustic neuromas; asytocytomas; meningiomas; and neurofibromas.

Skull and Spine

- Blurred vision, scotomas, and transient blindness in a patient with NF suggest a neurofibroma of the optic nerve. A defect in the posterior superior orbital wall may allow drooping of the upper eyelid, dislocation of the eyeball, or pulsating exopthalamos.
- Neurofibromas, similar to skull involvement, can affect spinal nerves and bony structures. Spinal nerve involvement can render localized pain and various motor symptoms and, in advances cases, can lead to paraplegia. In addition to neurofibromas, severe kyphoscoliosis is commonly found in patients with NF and can be asymptomatic but can be complicated by cord compression and paraplegia. In rare circumstances, laxity of the atlantoaxial ligaments occurs and can lead to atlantoaxial subluxation. This can create symptoms of sub-occipital headache and motor weakness to the upper extremities.

Diagnosis

- History and examination.
- Cafe-au-lait spots and neurofibromas are not necessarily diagnostic of NF unless

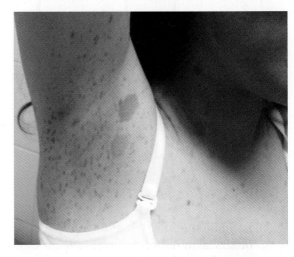

Figure 6-18 Café au lait macules in Neurofibromatosis.

they are associated with other signs and symptoms. Patients should undergo annual examinations including EENT, developmental assessment, scoliosis monitoring, complete neurological examination, and blood pressure screening.

- Often radiographic studies are not a standard procedure in patients and children with NF. However, in children who are experiencing seizures, hypertension, and musculoskeletal conditions further, radiographic workup is required early in the disease.

Course and Prognosis

- In most cases, the symptoms and manifestations of NF are mild, limited to skin lesions, and rarely progressive. Thus, patients are able to live normal and productive lives.
- However, there is variation in the severity of this disorder. In some cases, NF can be severely debilitating. Impaired visual function, cognitive function, and mental retardation have been reported as manifestations of CNS and spinal tumors associated with NF.
- In addition, and predominantly associated with NF2, tumors may affect vital structures such as the cranial nerves and brainstem and lead to life-threatening complications such as seizures, increased intracranial pressure, or vascular complications from hypertension.
- The mortality rate associated with NF is higher than in the normal population, principally because of the development of neurofibrosarcoma during adult life. Research suggests that approximately 3–5% of tumors associated with NF become malignant. This is an important consideration associated with the progression of the disease.

Treatment

- Surgical intervention.
- Neurological consultation if the lesions involve the peripheral and central nervous system.
- For patients with NF, chiropractic care is beneficial in respect to the management of musculoskeletal problems.

- Healthy diet rich in colorful fruits and vegetables and an active, healthy lifestyle is important in maintaining the physical and emotional health in a patient with NF.
- Recommended supplementation for various manifestations includes: white willow bark for pain management; pro-biotic to maintain GI health; bromelain and fish oil for inflammation; glutathione, selenium, Vitamin A, E, and C for antioxidant protection; and calcium and magnesium for associated muscle involvement.

Red Flags

Although NF is often a chronic but self limiting disease, there are specific red flags associated with the condition that require immediate medical attention. A patient with secondary findings associated with NF, such as bony lesions, neuromas, and tumors, and specific symptoms may warrant immediate medical referral. These signs and symptoms include: high blood pressure; visual disturbances; seizures; upper or lower motor weakness; pathological fractures; and severe scoliosis.

19. Squamous Cell Carcinoma

Squamous cell carcinoma (SCC) is the second most common form of skin cancer in the United States with nearly 200,000 new cases presented each year.

Etiology and Pathogenesis

- A thickened keratosis may spread to the deeper layers of the skin causing an invasive, malignant form of the lesion and could be fatal if left undetected.
- SCC forms a crusty, nodular, or scale-like lesion on the skin which may bleed if aggravated.
- It typically manifests in areas exposed to sunlight, such as the nose, ear, top of the head and backs of the legs. The most common SCC is solar keratosis, which is due to unprotected skin in direct sunlight.
- SCC may present on areas of the body that have been severely burned, areas of viral or bacterial infection, or on long standing ulcers. Some people will have SCC on or

around the oral mucosa due to long standing cigarette smoking.

Signs and Symptoms

- SCC may have four different presentations: invasive, in situ, keratoacanthoma, and carcinoma cuniculatum. Invasive refers to cells that have infiltrated the deeper layers of the skin, and perhaps have made their way into the individual's blood stream. This is a very serious form, and once established can be difficult to remove entirely, even with surgical interventions. The clinical form is highly variable, appearing as a red papule, or plaque with a scaly or crusted surface and may become nodular sometimes with a wart-like surface.
- In situ form presents typically on the lower legs in the form of a red scaly patch. "In situ" means that it is limited to the top (epidermal) layer of the skin, with only 5% of cases of this form moving into the invasive category.
- Carcinoma cuniculatum is a very rare form of slow growing SCC that develops on the sole of the foot and probably starts as a plantar wart.

Diagnosis

- Skin biopsy involving the dermis should be preformed to assess the invasion of the tumor.

Course and Prognosis

- SCC varies in size and will sometimes present with just one or two millimeters, or may be several centimeters in diameter. They grow slowly over a period of several months to years.
- Some patients may not notice the lesion until after several months or even years and will present to their doctor with "a sore that won't heal".
- SCC does not spread rapidly and the chance of the lesion metastasizing is small. The most frequent lesions to metastasize are lip and ear lesions which warrant further investigation. In general, lesions that are detected and removed when small have an

excellent prognosis. Some lesions left undetected, however, will eventually metastasize to surrounding skin, lymph nodes, and nearby organ or bone tissue.

- If SCC has metastasized to other tissue, the 5 year survival rate is only 34%.

Treatment

- Surgical removal of the tissue is the standard treatment for detected SCC. After biopsy has confirmed the diagnosis, it is recommended that the lesion be removed as soon as possible.
- There are several methods for removal of the tissue including cryosurgery, radiation therapy, topical chemotherapy, and Mohs surgery, a special procedure in which the cancer is shaved off one layer at a time.
- Metastatic disease responds well to radiation therapy if the lesion is local and maintained; however, SCC does not respond well to chemotherapy regimens.
- Alternative palliative regimens include high quantities of antioxidants such as vitamin E, C, A, selenium and CoQ_{10} but great caution is required in patients receiving chemotherapy.

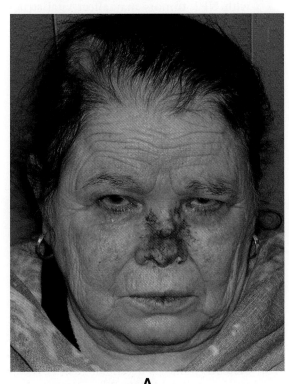

A

Figure 6-19 (A)   Squamous cell carcinoma that developed from radiation dermatitis.

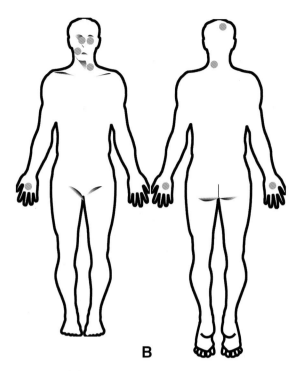

Figure 6-19 (B) Squamous Cell Carcinoma.

- Smoking is the most common cause of the lethal forms of SCC: invasive lingual or perioral mucosa (mucosal). It is best to recommend avoiding smoking.
- SCC typically appears in areas of skin exposed to sun. It is therefore recommended to wear sunscreen with a minimum of SPF 15 at all times when going outside. It is believed that people who consume high quantities of beta carotene have a protective layer in the epidermis that protects the skin from sun damage.

Red Flags

The percentage of SCC on areas of skin exposed to the sun that metastasize is much lower than basal cell carcinoma. However, SCC in areas of lingual or perioral mucosa that metastasizes before being diagnosed is approximately one-third. This is the reason that biopsy of any areas of suspicion are essential to the prognosis. In addition, as noted above in the presentation, the invasive form may manifest in a variety of forms making it difficult to distinguish which is benign and which is malignant. As a general rule, anything that has irregular borders, with a variety of colors, and has grown to larger than 6mm (pencil eraser size) in size should raise red flags.

20. Basal Cell Carcinoma

Basal cell carcinoma (BCC) is the most common form of skin cancer in the world today. It may present in many different forms, but the most common is a small, dome-shaped nodule that is pearly white in color. In dark-haired people, the nodule may be darker in color, and may be mistaken for a mole.

Etiology and Pathogenesis

- Basal cell carcinoma is thought to be caused by overexposure to harmful ultraviolet light from the sun.
- This theory is supported by the fact that there is a higher incidence rate in southern states than in northern states. It is also supported by the higher incidence rate in light skinned individuals.

Signs and Symptoms

There are four presentations that need to be observed:
- The first is an open, non-healing sore that lasts for three or more weeks.
- The second is a reddish patch that may itch or hurt, and sometimes crusts over.
- The third is a pink, elevated growth that has a crusted indentation in the center.
- The fourth is a scar-like area that appears as a shiny white, yellow, or waxy growth.
- Unfortunately, BCC can also mimic such non-cancerous conditions as psoriasis and eczema. BCCs most frequently present either on the face, ears, neck, scalp, shoulders, and back, which are the areas most exposed to direct sunlight.

Diagnosis

- Basal cell carcinoma is usually diagnosed by a tissue biopsy. Once diagnosed, it is recommended that treatment begin immediately.
- Basal cell carcinoma has a very low metastatic rate.
- However, 5–10% of BCCs are resistant to regular treatments or can be aggressive. In these cases, they eat away at the surrounding skin and can reach into cartilage and bone.

Course and Prognosis

- BCC is caused by overexposure to ultraviolet light and is a non-communicable disease.
- BCC is normally a slow growing tumor with a very low mortality rate. All of the medical treatments that are used today have a high cure rate ranging from 85%–95%.

Treatment

There are currently a number of medical treatments available for those who are diagnosed with basal cell carcinoma. The treatment of choice is dependent on where the cancer presents, the type of presentation, and other individual factors. The treatment options include:

- Surgical removal.
- Electrodessication and curettage; cryosurgery.
- Radiation therapy; CO_2 laser therapy.
- Some other treatments that have been used are topical fluorouracil, systemic retinoids, interferona, and photodynamic therapy.
- Controlled Amino Acid Therapy (CAAT) could be helpful where a patient's intake of amino acids is regulated in their diet. There is a specific formula given for each cancer and dietary intake is highly regulated.

- Patient who has BCC is at a 40% increased risk of developing a second BCC and lifestyle modifications are highly recommended. The most effective way to prevent the onset or recurrence of basal cell carcinoma is to avoid direct sunlight, especially

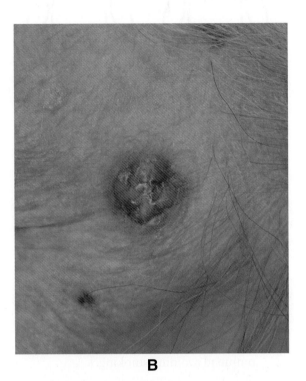

B

Figure 6-20 (B)   Basal cell carcinoma.

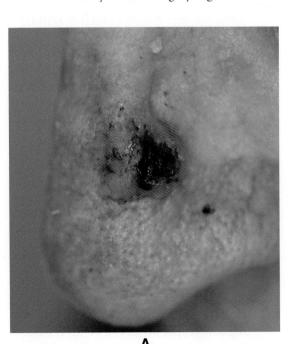

A

Figure 6-20 (A)   Basal cell carcinoma most commonly occurs on the face.

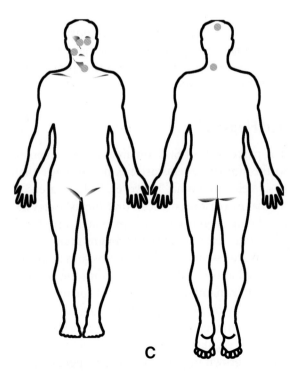

C

Figure 6-20 (C)   Basal Cell Carcinoma.

between the hours of 10:00 a.m. and 4:00 p.m. If a person is out in the sun often, it is recommended that they apply sunscreen of no less than SPF 15 every hour and a half. It is also recommended that a broad-brimmed hat be worn while in direct sunlight.

- Nutritional supplements include parsley, vitamin D, green tea extract, antioxidants, whey protein, grits, niacin, selenium, melatonin, and licorice root extract with pantothenic acid. Before taking any of these nutritional therapies, clinicians should consult a dermatologist since the combinations may increase or decrease the overall effectiveness.

Red Flags

Immediate treatment is nearly always recommended following the diagnosis of BCC. However, the biggest red flag indicating immediate treatment is the presentation of a scar-like area that is white, yellow, or waxy with poorly defined borders. This presentation may mean that the tumor is more aggressive than other presentations.

21. Melanoma

Melanoma is a tumor of the pigment producing cells of the skin known as melanocytes. The cells give skin its color, are located in all parts of the skin, but are much more densely packed in moles. When a melanocyte becomes malignant, it proliferates to form a mole or nevi and undergoes more transformation resulting in a melanoma.

Etiology and Pathogenesis

- Incidence is on the rise and more cases are being reported after lung and breast cancer.
- 1 in every 75 Americans is at a risk of developing melanoma. Occurrence of melanomas is 20 times more frequent in Caucasians as compared to African Americans, and 6 times more frequent than in people of Hispanic descent.
- Melanoma, in its earliest stage, can occur on any part of the body, but it tends to occur in different locations based on the ethnicity of the patient. Fair skin types I and II are more prone to developing melanomas.

- Presence of atypical nevi in the family is a risk factor.
- Ultraviolet light, or sun exposure, in melanoma in the primary stages. Because of this, melanoma tends to occur more frequently on the trunk of males, and the lower legs and back of most females.
- Melanoma, when metastatic, can appear anywhere in the body, not just localized to on particular skin area. When melanoma spreads, it generally appears first as a small tumor in the lymph nodes associated with draining the site of the primary tumor. This is known as lymphatic metastasis. There is also the possibility of hematogenous spread. Should the cells invade the blood vessels, the circulatory system has the potential to carry them around to any and all sites in the body, including remote parts of the skin, the viscera, especially the liver and lungs, the musculoskeletal system, and the brain.
- There are four different types of melanoma: superficial spreading (most common), nodular, lentigo maligna and acral lentiginous melanoma:
  - Superficial spreading melanoma occurs mostly on the trunks and extremities. They are flat and asymmetric and vary in color.
  - Nodular melanoma are more common in males; The tumor grows vertically rather than laterally and can be mistaken for a vascular lesion.
  - Lentigo maligna appears on sun-exposed areas like the face, neck and dorsal arms. They are flat, irregular, can be both flat and nodular and vary in color from red to brown.
  - Acral lentiginous melanoma primarily occurs in the hands, feet and nails and resembles lentigo maligna. Early lesions can be mistaken for insect bites.

Signs and Symptoms

- The most common sites are the plantar surface of the foot as well as sublingual and palmer sites in addition to mucosal membranes such as oral, rectal and vaginal surfaces.
- Melanoma can metastasize to any location, including unusual locations such as the eye, eyelid and genitalia.

- Later signs and symptoms of metastatic melanoma have been known to include a colorless lump or thickening of the skin, unexplained weight loss, melanosis (gray skin), and, most commonly, swollen lymph nodes, especially in the armpit or groin.
- Itching can be present on lesions.
- Metastatic melanoma does not begin as a metastatic disease but as a solitary, primary lesion which then proceeds through four stages of classification:
  - First stage—including primary lesions of 1.0 mm or smaller, which may or may not have ulcerations or primary lesions of size 1.01–2.0 mm without ulceration. However, the common thread is that at this stage there is no lymph node or distant metastases.

- Second stage—there is still no metastases, but the lesions are larger, either 1.01–2 mm with ulceration, or larger than 2.01 mm either with or without ulceration.
- Third stage—first sign of metastasis comes in the third stage, where the tumor will metastasize to lymph nodes or be in the satellite stage, but still lack any metastases to more distant locations.
- Fourth stage—full-blown metastatic melanoma, with tumor spread to distant sites throughout the body.

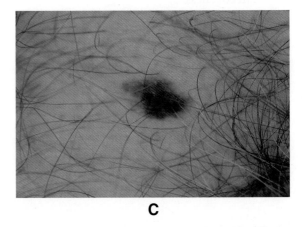

C

Figure 6-21 (C)   Melanoma—note the asymmetry, irregular border, variable color and expanding diameter.

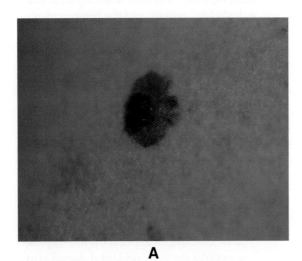

A

Figure 6-21 (A)   Melanoma.

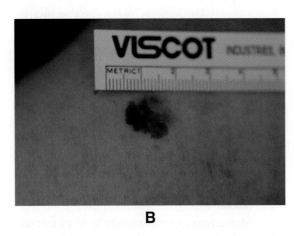

B

Figure 6-21 (B)   ABCD of melanoma (asymmetry, border, color, diameter).

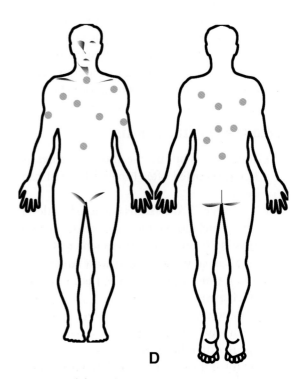

D

Figure 6-21 (D)   Melanoma.

Diagnosis

Diagnosis of Melanoma begins with the ABCDs:

- The first characteristic of this tumor is **A**symmetry, because although normal nevi tend to be round, malignant melanomas tend to lack symmetry.
- "**B**" is for **B**order, because malignant melanomas have irregular borders that are notched, indented, scalloped, indistinct, or blurred.
- **C**olor is the third characteristic, because this tumor tends to present with uneven coloration containing many different shades, as opposed to a more solidly colored mole.
- "**D**" stands for **D**iameter. Standard, normal nevi tend to be smaller than 6 mm in diameter, which is approximately the size of the end of a pencil eraser. Malignant melanomas, however, are nearly always larger than this, especially once they have progressed to the stage where A, B, and C conditions have already been fulfilled.
- Biopsy is essential and is required to determine course of treatment.
- Photographs taken at regular intervals can be a useful tool to assess the extent of progression of melanomas.

Course and Prognosis

- There is potentially a genetic link as it has been noted to occur slightly more frequently in children of patients with melanoma.
- The thinner the melanoma is the better the prognosis. Females and children have a better prognosis.
- Melanomas on the scalp have the worst prognosis.
- Metastatic melanoma is fatal.

Treatment

- In the earlier stages, surgery to excise the tumor and the associated effected tissue is the primary method of treatment. In association with the surgery, either before of after, the patient is often provided with an immunotherapy drug composed of large doses of synthetic interferons.
- Although chemotherapy has been shown to be effective in a variety of cancers, it seems to show no significant survival benefit in metastatic melanoma patients, nor does radiation therapy, retinoid therapy, or vitamin therapy.
- Although the efficacy of such treatments is unsupported in scientific literature, there is significant anecdotal evidence to support the use of acupuncture, herbs, biofeedback, meditation, yoga, and guided imagery, as well as vitamins and nutritional supplements as palliative treatments for metastatic melanoma.
- There are a variety of suggestions for nutritional supplements which can benefit patients, either by minimizing the risks of developing metastatic melanoma, or to improve the chance of survival once the disease has been contracted. Some of these supplements include selenium, which has been shown to have immune-boosting properties, as well as folic acid, vitamins B12 and D.
- Antioxidants such as carotenoids including a-b-carotene, lycopene, and lutein have shown positive effects.
- A standard multivitamin and a combination probiotic cocktail can also serve the patient's health interests.
- Dietary recommendations to help counteract the effects of metastatic melanoma and to allow the body to continue to function well, include limiting intake of red meats, and increasing fiber, in both soluble and insoluble forms. A diet high in fruits and vegetables can contribute antioxidants, but other items which have shown beneficial effects include flaxseed oil, green tea, soy, cauliflower, cabbage, garlic, and onions. As always, caution is to be used in patients receiving chemotherapy.
- Suggested lifestyle modifications include simple things, such as paying attention to the skin, watching for moles that might be appearing or changing.
- Limit the amount of direct sun exposure, and take appropriate preventative actions when in the sun, such as applying and reapplying sun block, even on cloudy days and in winter; wearing a sun hat.
- Chiropractors can play an important role in public health by educating their patients and communities about the "ABCD" of melanoma, and encouraging regular screening for suspicious lesions. Any mole that is

undergoing change should be monitored carefully and suspicious cases should be quickly referred to a dermatologist.

Red Flags

Due to the excessively dangerous nature and the high mortality rate associated with metastatic melanoma, early detection and treatment is key. Chiropractors are in a unique position to help patients screen for this disease so that it can be detected early and treated quickly, ensuring the best of the potential outcomes. Chiropractors are in contact with, and observing, much of the surface of the patient's skin, some of which they are not easily able to see on their own. Through this role, they can serve to inform patients of any suspected melanomas. Melanoma is not a contagious disease and cannot be transmitted from person to person via physical contact or contamination with body products

▊ 22. Acne Vulgaris

Acne vulgaris is a very common skin condition that can ultimately affect 85–100% of the population at some period of life.

Etiology and Pathogenesis

- Acne does not discriminate its prevalence to age and is most common in adolescence and the onset of puberty, but can still affect persons older than 45 and can even affect newborns.
- At young ages (teenage years) it is more common in males but that trend reverses with the progression into adulthood.
- There are four factors commonly attributed to the cause of acne vulgaris:
  - The first is excess sebum and androgen hormones. Because androgens stimulate sebum production and its release into glands, they are grouped together. Acne lesions result from follicular plugging and have been found to contain androgens and are the most numerous when adolescents begin producing amounts of androgens for circulation.
  - Presence of *Propionibacterium acnes* in later lesions. The cell wall and byproducts of this organism are inflammation mediators and can diffuse into the follicle

and destroy the follicle wall creating an environment for inflammatory cells.
  - Epithelial hyperproliferation of the follicle. The cause of this is currently not known but is associated with androgen hormone, lipid composition changes in sebum and general inflammation.
  - Inflammation based on the presence of IL–1α.
- Increased triglyceride, testosterone FSH, LH and dehydroepiandesterone levels and stress are all contributing and aggravating factors.
- Exogenous causes can also be a factor in the severity of acne vulgaris. These include certain cosmetics and hair products, medications such as steroids, lithium, iodides and antiepileptics.

Signs and Symptoms

- The typical manifestations of Acne vulgaris range from small, non-inflamed acne lesions that are not bothersome except for the cosmetic appearance to severe inflammatory nodules that cause pain, physical scarring as well as embarrassment from their appearance.
- The form of the lesions can be papules, pustules, nodules or open or closed comedones (blackheads or whiteheads).
- The condition can present in simple comedonal acne without inflammation and range in severity to inflammatory lesions with painful comedones and large nodules.
- Distribution of acne vulgaris lesions has a tendency to center along areas of sebaceous follicles. They can localize to the face or also be found on the chest, back or upper arm.

Diagnosis

- Hormonal profile for testosterone, FSH, LH and dehydroepiandesterone should be perfomed to rule out excess hormone secretion.
- Bacterial cultures can be performed to rule out other types of folliculitis.

Course and Prognosis

- Acne lesions can subside but late onset acne is difficult to treat.

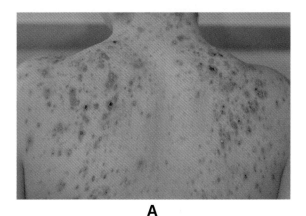

Figure 6-22 (A) Truncal acne.

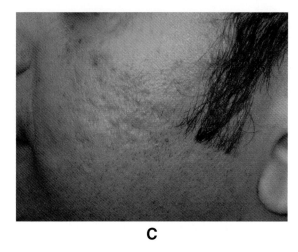

Figure 6-22 (C) Depressed scars resulting from nodulocystic acne.

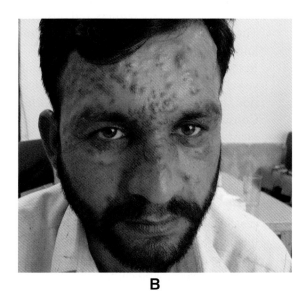

Figure 6-22 (B) Facial acne.

- Scarring depends on skin type. Acne can be long term and can be difficult to control in women after 25 years of age.
- Topical treatment can minimize inflammation but systemic antibiotics and oral drugs best resolve lingering acne.

Treatment

Treatments are often given to reduce symptoms and to reduce appearance of acne. They can be single or combination treatments depending on the desired level of outcome. The most common and usually the first course of action is a topical medication. Following is the list of suggested treatments:

- Retinoids are given to reduce number of lesions and inflammation.

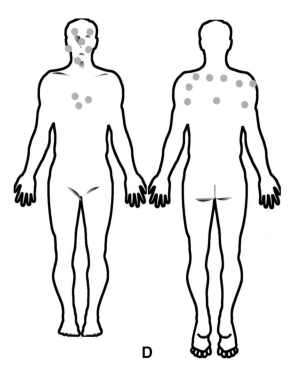

Figure 6-22 (D) Acne.

- Antibiotics are given to combat *P acnes*. Benzoyl peroxide is also given to combat *P acnes* but the microbe has shown resistance to the substance. The advantage of Benzoyl is that it is available over the counter in a lesser dose and in different forms (washes, lotions, creams and gels).
- Systemic antibiotics are given also to combat the presence of *P acnes*. They are more effective than topicals but resistance is becoming more of an issue for these as well.
- Hormone therapies using oral contraceptives can be utilized to decrease circulating

testosterone and androgen receptor competitive inhibitors are also a method.

- Other procedures utilized to treat or reduce acne include manual extraction of comedones, steroids injected into lesions, peels and masks, phototherapy (blue and red light) and laser treatments.
- Psychological counseling to overcome stress.
- Home remedies to reducing the appearance or prevent acne vulgaris include washing the face twice per day with oil-free acne fighting lotions or cleansers and to avoid touching the face with the hands or resting the face on unclean surfaces such as desks, counters or contacting to telephones.
- Herbal spot treatments that are used include tea tree oil, apple cider vinegar, and niacinamide gel.
- Zinc (60–90 mg/day), Copper (to augment Zinc absorption).
- B6 (50 mg/day for premenstrual flare ups).
- Vitamin A (300,000 IU per day) and Vitamin A derivatives like isotretinoin (Accutane).
- Pantothenic Acid, 1–5 g/day.
- Burdock Root tinctures can be taken at 2–4 mL/day.
- Probiotics can be used for general health.
- Acupuncture, chiropractic adjusting and hypnosis can also augment treatment of acne, although very little scientific evidence is available.
- Contrary to several ideas and myths, acne is not worsened by diet (chocolate, fats/oils or greasy foods). One should avoid those foods that are known allergens and a diet high in iodine.
- General patient education and counseling should be done based on severity and the patient's ability to cope with the condition. Advice should be given to avoid complications from too many treatments or herbals and to ensure that they are taken correctly and with or without other products that would cause adverse effects.

Red Flags

There is no life threatening presentation of acne vulgaris that would require immediate medical intervention. The condition, however, can cause permanent scarring, physical discomfort, psy-chological pain and a severely inflamed lesion can lead to fever, redness and systemic symptoms

23. Rosacea

Rosacea is a chronic skin condition characterized by inflammation of the face.

Etiology and Pathogenesis

- Adults between the ages of 30 and 60 often have this condition. Currently, around 14 million Americans have rosacea.
- It is most common in women with fair hair and light skin. These patients will usually have a history of face redness and flushing.
- The cause of rosacea is currently unknown.
- Researchers believe it may be due to a blood vessel disorder, a chronic *H. pylori* infection, or mites living within hair follicles. Consumption of alcohol does not cause rosacea.

Signs and Symptoms

- There is no specific test to diagnose rosacea. Signs that suggest rosacea include visible blood vessels, persistent flushing, pustules, papules, and redness of the nose, forehead, cheeks, and chin.
- Often, people will confuse rosacea with acne, but this is not accurate because people with rosacea do not have whiteheads and blackheads. Rosacea can also be confused with eczema or skin allergies.
- Signs of rosacea are cyclic, with flare-ups and remissions common. Some common rosacea triggers include alcohol, spicy foods, hot beverages, heat, cold, sunlight, stress, anger, embarrassment, strenuous exercise, wind, and some medications.
- The first phase of rosacea is called pre-rosacea. Blood vessels in the face dilate and cause persistent redness, flushing, or blushing.
- Vascular rosacea is the second phase that results dilation of blood vessels on the nose and cheeks. This causes the nose to appear red and bulbous.
- The third stage is inflammatory rosacea. The patient will begin to develop small red bumps or pustules on the nose, cheeks,

forehead, and chin. The skin will begin to have an orange peel texture and roughen over time. Rosacea can affect the eyes by causing a burning or gritty sensation; however, this will not affect eye sight.

- Rosacea has been called adult acne or acne rosacea despite the fact that rosacea is different from acne vulgaris in adolescents. Presentation can vary from one patient to another, but all patients have at least one of the primary signs of rosacea. These primary signs include visible blood vessels, flushing, persistent redness, solid red bumps, and pus-filled pimples.
- Usually several secondary signs occur like eye irritation, burning or stinging, itching, tightness, dryness, raised red plaques, thickening of the nose (rhinophyma), or swelling. These signs are not limited to the face. They may also occur on the neck, chest, scalp, or ears.

Diagnosis

- Usually on clinical signs but bacterial cultures and skin biopsy could be performed to exclude folliculitis and lupus.

Course and Prognosis

- Rosacea is not life threatening, but it does progress if untreated.
- The condition is chronic with many remissions and exacerbations.

Treatment

- Oral antibiotics like tetracycline, erythromycin, and minocycline are usually the first line of medical treatment. The antibiotics reduce inflammation of the blood vessels. They can also help control the papules and pustules. These antibiotics are used first to get the condition under control. After that, the patient is often switched to topical therapy.
- Vitamin A derivatives are often used because they can reduce redness and pimples. The oral retinoid isotretinoin should be used with caution in women of childbearing age because it is known to cause birth defects.
- Patients with rhinophyma may have cosmetic surgery to remove the extra tissue

from their nose. Other techniques used to improve the patient's appearance include mechanical dermabrasion, electrosurgery, and CO2 laser peeling.

- Circular massage to the nose, cheeks, and forehead provides help in some cases.

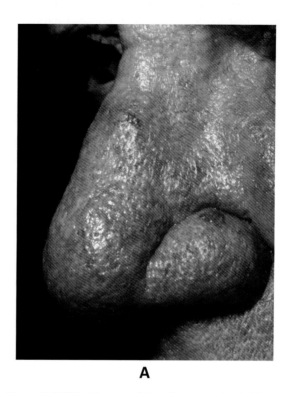

A

Figure 6-23 (A)   Rosacea. © *DermQuest.com. Used with permission from Galderma SA.*

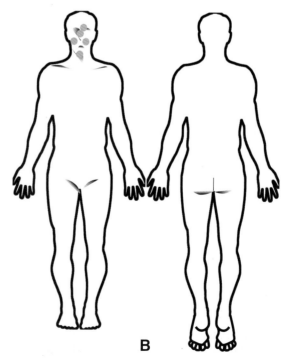

B

Figure 6-23 (B)   Rosacea.

- Riboflavin can be used to help rosacea patients suspected of having B vitamin deficiency.
- The pancreatic enzyme lipase has been shown to decrease indigestion and rosacea symptoms.
- Azelaic acid cream is a natural antimicrobial made from wheat, rye, and barley. It has been used to decrease redness, papules, and pustules.
- Patients should be recommended to avoid foods and beverages that are known to cause flare-ups. Examples include alcohol, caffeine, hot drinks, spicy food, and fatty food.
- Patients should be advised to use sunscreen SPF 15 or higher and avoid environmental factors like excessively hot or cold weather, wind, and direct sunlight.
- During winters, patients should be recommended to use a scarf or mask to protect the face.
- Daily skin care with mild soaps and non-abrasive cleansers should be advised. Non-comedogenic products are useful because they do not clog oil and sweat gland pores. Astringents are contraindicated.

Red Flags

There are no red flags for immediate care as rosacea is not fatal.

24. Perioral Dermatitis

Perioral dermatitis is a red papular eruption occurring mostly in women around the perioral area (around the lips).

Etiology and Pathogenesis

- More common in females and children.
- Fusobacterium points to bacterial etiology.
- Prolonged use of moisturizers and fluorinated products may be a cause.
- Topical steroids can aggravate the condition.

Signs and Symptoms

- Red papules around perioral and perinasal regions with breaks of normal skin known as clear zones around the lips. There could be scaling on the base of papules and pustules.
- Pustules on cheeks and nostrils are common.
- Asymptomatic.

Diagnosis

- Diagnosis is usually made by clinical observation of the typical skin lesions.

Course and Prognosis

- Perioral dermatitis can clear with oral treatment but can relapse and need long-term treatment.

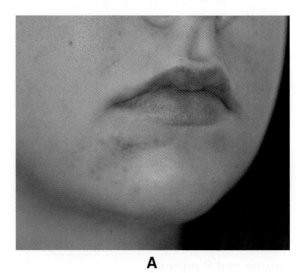

A

Figure 6-24 (A)   Perioral dermatitis.

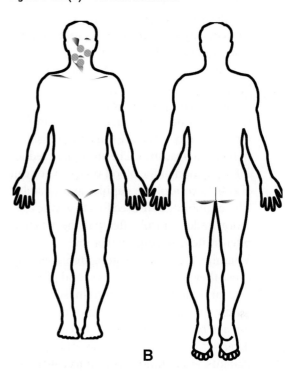

B

Figure 6-24 (B)   Perioral dermatitis.

Treatment

- Metronidazole, Clindamycin, Erythromycin cream twice daily can be used for 4–6 weeks until the lesions resolve.
- Newer creams like tacrolimus (Protopic) and pimecrolimus (Elidel) have emerged as new treatments for perioral dermatitis.
- Oral antibiotics, mainly tetracyclines, are used for a 2–4 week course.
- Azelaic acid cream.
- Glycolic acid peeling can be used in combination with other treatment.

Red Flags

Perioral dermatitis is a benign condition with no systemic symptoms.

■ 25. Hidradenitis Suppurativa

Hidradenitis suppurativa (HS) is a chronic, erythematous skin rash of the apocrine-sweat-gland-bearing skin of the body, most commonly the axillary, inguinal, and anogenital areas. Other names for this condition are Verneuil's disease, acne inversa, and it is occasionally spelled hydradentitis.

Etiology and Pathogenesis

- More common in teenagers and women.
- The hormonal influence in this disease means that it begins soon after puberty and ceases around the fifth decade of life. The condition closely parallels the activity of the apocrine glands and improvement is noted during pregnancy.
- A genetic component most certainly exists, as 38% have a familial history.
- Bacteria contribute to this pathogenesis secondarily, and strains of *staphylococcus aureus, streptococcus milleri,* and *chlamydia trachomatis* may be found.
- Tropical climates are not ideal places for those with HS to live, as heat and humidity can cause outbreaks.
- Smoking and menstruation can trigger HS.

Signs and Symptoms

- Symptoms of this disease include pain in the affected area, serous and purulent discharge, erythema, burning, hyperhidrosis, and malodor. Rarely, fever or sepsis occurs. It presents most commonly as a tender, nodular lesion.
- Recurrent deep seated inflammatory nodules in skin bearing apocrine glands persisting for a minimum period of three months, not always discharging or fluctuating, and with a tendency for cord like coalescence.
- Comedones in skin bearing apocrine glands and the ear lobes.
- Minor criteria include an association with acne vulgaris and, in women, exacerbation with menses.
- Friction from adiposity, sweat, heat, and tight clothes may all contribute to HS.

Diagnosis

- Diagnosis is based on a thorough history and physical exam, and clinical observation.
- For definitive diagnosis, skin biopsy can be performed including the apocrine glands.

Course and Prognosis

- Often HS coexists with acne, pilonidal sinus, and chronic scalp folliculitis, which leads to the term *follicular occlusions tetrad*.
- It is associated with high morbidity and increases the patient's risk for developing nonmelanoma skin cancer.
- Secondary arthritis, infection, dermal contraction, restricted limb mobility from scarring, lymphedema, rectal or urethral fistulas, systemic amyloidosis, and anemia from chronic infection are all potential complications of HS. This skin condition is not contagious, nor is it caused by an individual's poor hygiene.
- The unsightliness, malodorous drainage, and often genital location of the body that this disease occurs add to the tremendous stress and social stigma.

Treatment

Treatment of this condition is often approached medically by two main strategies.

- Antibiotic therapy, which is normally directed at S. aureus. In acute cases, this is only short term care as antibiotics do not treat the underlying primary condition and the infection usually recurs. When a superinfection is suspected, treatment is based on cultures of the drainage from a nodule. High dose oral tetracycline or erythromycin is prescribed to control lesions in acute cases.

- Topical clindamycin.
- Isotretinoin, which functions to inhibit sebaceous gland activity and abnormal keratinization, has also proven effective treatment.
- Azathioprine in severe cases has been proved to be beneficial.
- Patients experiencing substantial symptoms may not benefit from systemic corticosteroids and need a more focused therapy.
- Conservative approaches for medical treatment may include warm baths and hydrotherapy which may be helpful in reducing bacterial growth.
- Nonsteroidal anti-inflammatory drugs are suggested for alleviation of pain and inflammation.
- Oral contraceptive agents containing a high estrogen to progesterone and low androgenicity of progesterone, which may only be clinically appropriate in certain women.
- Radiotherapy has recently been investigated as a treatment option and has shown disease remission and reduction of symptoms in certain individuals.
- CO_2 laser therapy has also been utilized as general surgery for glandular stripping.
- Selective surgical intervention is often necessary for drainage of abscesses, though it is not curative.
- Infliximab, a FDA-approved drug, is a suggested new therapy for severe cases of this disease where antibiotic therapy is ineffective.
- Cryotherapy can assist in decreasing pain and noxious sensory input from skin and give patient some short term relief.
- Ultrasound therapy under water may be useful in decreasing pain and inflammation immune system defense.
- Patients should refrain from scented deodorants, axillary shaving, and depilation should be avoided if they cause irritation.
- Elimination of the use of tight restrictive synthetic clothing may also be important in decreasing pain and discomfort near the affected areas of the body.

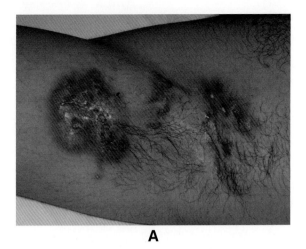

A

Figure 6-25 (A)   Hidradenitis suppurativa.

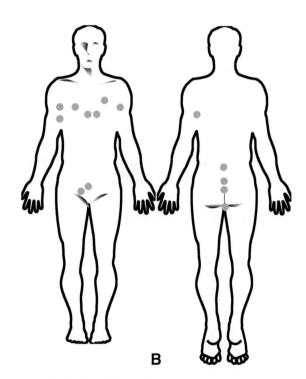

B

Figure 6-25 (B)   Hidradenitis suppurativa.

- The patient should cleanse the skin with antiseptic agents and antibacterial soap on a daily basis.
- Weight reduction and balanced diet could be advised to patients and has shown some positive results.
- Fish oil supplementation may also be beneficial for promotion of healthy skin and maintenance of the impermeable barrier of the skin.
- Smoking has also been identified as a trigger of this disease and often women have increased symptoms during menstruation.

Red Flags

Early detection of a patient with HS, who has developed systemic bacterial sepsis, is considered a medical emergency and important for practitioners to identify. Sepsis left untreated can cause organ failure, septic shock, and possible death from complications.

26. Eosinophilic Folliculitis

For many years, Eosinophilic Folliculitis (EF) was considered a rare skin rash, predominately found on the head and neck of Asian patients. However, with the arrival of AIDS, patients began developing lesions which histologically and clinically resembled this rare disease. Over the past two decades, these cases became known as HIV associated eosinophilic folliculitis.

Etiology and Pathogenesis

- Men are five times more likely to have EF.
- Overgrowth of *Malassezia* or *Demodex* (the hair follicle mite) and *staphylococcus*.
- A deficiency in the immune system.
- Living in a warm, humid climate.
- Exposure to coal tar, pitch or creosote—common among roofers, mechanics and oil workers.
- Infection in the nose, or other recent illness.

Signs and Symptoms

- Eosinophilic folliculitis is an infection that consists of itchy red bumps centered on hair follicles which are predominantly located on the scalp, face, neck, and upper chest.
- The name originates with the predominant eosinophilic cells present, and the involvement of the hair follicle. These pimples often resemble acne, and sometimes contain pus.
- The sores usually spread, may itch, and scratching causes excoriated papules, crusts, bleeding, scarring, and secondary hyperpigmentation in dark skinned patients. Severe cases may cause permanent hair loss and scarring, and even mild folliculitis can be uncomfortable and embarrassing.

- Typically EF is located on the scalp, face, neck, and upper chest and presents as itchy red bumps centered on hair follicles that sometimes contain pus.
- Bumps or papules may progress to a crust and bleeding may occur.
- Skin pigmentation resulting from scarring.

Diagnosis

- Eosinophilic folliculitis is relatively difficult to diagnose but a complete blood cell count reveals leukocytosis and eosinophilia. In many cases, immunoelectrophoresis reveals low levels of immunoglobulin G3 (IgG3), elevated levels of immunoglobulin E (IgE), and low levels of immunoglobulin A (IgA) in pediatric eosinophilic folliculitis.
- HIV associated EF infection appears as levels of CD4 lymphocyte cells drop below 300 cells/mm3.

Course and Prognosis

- Eosinophilic folliculitis is not disabling or life threatening, but it may be extremely itchy.

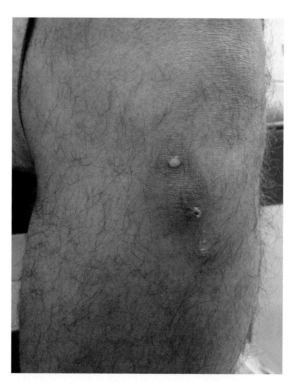

Figure 6-26 Eosinophilic folliculitis.

Treatment

- Topical antifungal creams or the drug Fulvicin may be used.
- Antibiotic treatments include Mupirocin and Dicloxacillin.
- Topical corticosteroids are also used to relieve symptoms, but their mechanism of action is yet to be explained.
- Oral folic acid (vitamin B9) has shown to resolve symptoms associated with folliculitis. The normal dosage is 800 mg twice daily.
- Warm baths and showers may relieve symptoms.
- A diet containing alpha linolenic acid and omega-3 fatty acids should be recommended.

Red Flags

As for immediate care, there are no red flags and the condition is not life threatening or disabling, but rather self-limiting. However, if the patient's condition is affecting his entire body or infection of the sores occurs, referral to a specialist is warranted.

27. Carbuncle

A carbuncle is a local skin infection that is usually caused by the bacteria *Staphylococcus aureus*. It typically begins as a boil or furuncle, a painful infection of a single hair follicle. As the infection spreads deeper into the skin and begins to involve several hair follicles in a location, it is called a carbuncle.

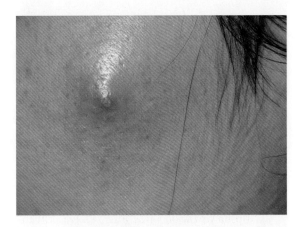

Figure 6-27   Carbuncle.

Etiology and Pathogenesis

- Middle-aged or elderly men and individuals with diabetes.

Signs and Symptoms

- Large cluster of red, inflamed, painful bumps underneath the skin.
- Smaller carbuncles may develop into white or yellow pustules, or they may weep ooze or crust, but usually they are so deep that they do not drain on their own.
- Carbuncle may be accompanied by fever and prostration.
- Anywhere on the body, but are most common on the back and on the nape of the neck.

Diagnosis

- Skin biopsy is usually not recommended and diagnosis is based on clinical observation of the red raised skin lesions.

Course and Prognosis

- A carbuncle caused by the bacteria *Staphylococcus* is contagious. Often it is spread between people living in close and unhygienic quarters.
- It is usually a self-limiting condition; however, it may reoccur. If the infection spreads into the bloodstream it could prove fatal.

Treatment

- Hot compress to allow it to drain spontaneously. A moist heat pack can be applied to the affected area for approximately 30 minutes. If possible, salt water should be applied to the lesion before the compress to help it rupture and drain more quickly.
- Antibacterial soaps are used to help control and stop spread of the infection.
- Topical or systemic antibiotics may be prescribed for larger and more persistent lesions.
- Incision and drainage may be necessary to speed healing.
- Tea tree oil has been found to relieve discomfort and speed healing in some indi-

viduals. The oil should be applied to the carbuncle several times a day for best results.

- Constricting clothing should not be worn to avoid chafing of the skin.

Red Flags

Medical treatment should be sought if a carbuncle does not improve after a week of treatment or if the patient is diabetic, has chills, a spiking fever, a rapid heart rate, or a feeling of being extremely ill. Red lines radiating from the carbuncle suggests underlying cellulitis.

▨ 28. Impetigo

Impetigo is a superficial skin infection seen in children and those involved in contact sports. Impetigo can include impetigo contagiosa, bullous impetigo, impetigo associated with folliculitis or ecthyma.

Etiology and Pathogenesis

- In general, it is an infection caused by group A beta hemolytic *streptococcus* (GABHS) or *staphylococcus aureus.*
- Impetigo is transmitted via direct contact, however, it may spread onto areas where there is no break in the skin.
- Impetigo is very contagious, and in children is commonly spread by contact with contaminated towels, sheets, clothing, toys, or other items.

Signs and Symptoms

- Impetigo contagiosa usually begins with a single 2–4 mm erythematous macule that will become a vesicle or pustule. The vesicle is fragile and may rupture resulting in crusted exudates that looks yellow and honey like. The superficial wound may spread when scratching occurs.
- Impetigo is found usually around the nose and the mouth. The sores begin as small red spots, later changing to blisters. The blisters break open and are not painful but may be itchy. The ooze that comes out of the open blister is crusty and may appear to be later coated with honey or brown sugar. The form of the sore may be as small as a pimple

or as large as a coin. The number of the sores may increase in size and in number.

- Bullous impetigo is a toxin-mediated erythroderma in which the epidermal layer of the skin sloughs off leaving an area of skin loss. Common impetigo is when the infection occurs in an already open wound. Folliculitis, which is the infection of hair follicles, commonly affects a newly shaved area, like the back of the neck or beard.
- Ecthyma, which is a deeper, ulcerated impetigo, is caused by an infection that occurs with lymphadenitis.
- Impetigo may take on alternative forms, depending on the staphylococcal strain that they involve. The presentation also depends on the relative activity of the exotoxin.
- Bullous impetigo presents as a small or large, superficial, fragile bullae. It is usually seen on the trunk and the extremities. Ruptured bullae remnants are seen at the time of the presentation.

Diagnosis

- Clinical observation and cultures of lesions will reveal staphylococcal or streptococcal growth.

Course and Prognosis

- This condition may spontaneously resolve, but usually without treatment, another area will erupt soon after. After treatment, the problem usually resolves within 7–10 days. The condition will rarely resolve in scarring and postinflammatory hyperpigmentation or hypopigmentation.
- Serious complications may include post-streptococcal glomerulonephritis (PGSN), cellulitis, and methicillin-resistant staphylococcus aureus infections. PGSN may cause inflammation of the kidney after a streptococcal infection, and may cause kidney failure. The signs and symptoms of PGSN include; facial swelling—especially around the eyes, decreased urination, blood in the urine and high blood pressure.
- A MRSA infection resists most antibiotics, and may cause severe skin infections, pneumonia or blood infections. These skin infections are very hard to treat.

- Patients with bullous impetigo can develop cellulitis, lymphangitis or bacteremia which will later develop into pneumonitis, septic arthritis, or septicemia. If these conditions occur, hospitalization may be required for IV antibiotic therapy.
- Without treatment, ecthyma may occur and may cause scarring.
- The deep dermal infection may cause scarlet fever, erysipelas, cellulitis, lymphangitis and possibly even bacterial endocarditis.

Treatment

- The best treatment is counseling the patient on prevention.
- Mupirocin ointment has been shown to be as effective as oral antibiotics in limited

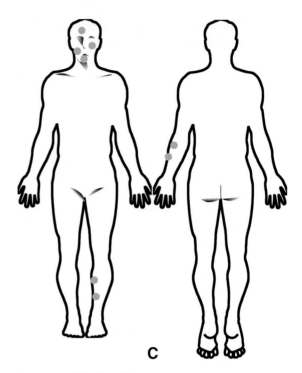

Figure 6-28 (C)   Impetigo.

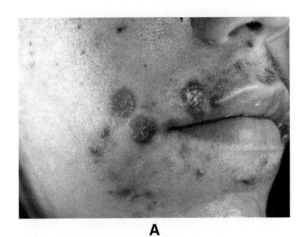

A

Figure 6-28 (A)   Impetigo.

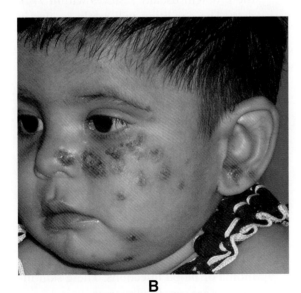

B

Figure 6-28 (B)   Impetigo.

diseases. It may also be used intranasally in patients who are chronic nasal carriers. When used intranasally however, it is applied three times daily for 5 days per month.

- Topical antibiotics are applied to the affected area 2–3 times per day for about a week to a week and a half.
- Oral antibiotics are used on individuals with extensive impetigo and for those diseases refractory to topical treatment. Examples of oral antibiotics include cephalosporin, semisynthetic penicillin or beta-lactam/ beta-lactamase inhibitor.
- One tablespoon of white vinegar to 1 pint of water for 20 minutes. This will make it easier to gently remove the scabs. The treatment choice for impetigo after soakings is an application of topical antibiotic.
- By gently scrubbing the crust with antibacterial soap and a washcloth, this may prevent spreading and recurrences of the disease. Efficacy of this treatment has not yet been proven.
- Echinacea has been shown to decrease the occurrence of cold sores so it may also help with impetigo. Tree oil may also prove to be a good solution for impetigo because it helps with other skin rashes or dryness.

- Recommend that the patient keep their nails short, and their hands clean, which will help prevent the spread of the disease and cross contamination. Washing with antibacterial soap for the recommended time will also provide help in reducing spread of the disease.
- Other recommendations would include avoiding close contact with sheets, towels, or other articles that have been in contact with a person with impetigo. If laundry items are contaminated, wash them in hot water. If toys are contaminated they can be cleaned using a diluted chlorine solution with antibacterial soap, and hot water.

Red Flags

Impetigo typically does not raise any red flags as it is not severe, unless left untreated.

29. Skin Abscess

An abscess is an acute or chronic localized inflammation, associated with a collection of pus and tissue destruction. Abscesses may form in any organ or structure of the body. Abscesses that occur on the skin can arise from the dermis, subcutaneous fat, muscle, or a number of deeper structures.

Etiology and Pathogenesis

- May occur at any age. They are common in children and young adults.
- The cause of abscesses is multi-faceted; however, the most common cause is Methicillin Resistant Straphlococcus Aureus (MRSA) or streptococcal infection.
- Sterile abscess will form in response to a foreign body such as a splinter, ruptured cyst, or injection site.
- Certain conditions increase the likelihood of abscess formation such as diabetes mellitus, HIV, obesity, and chronic bactericidal defects (granuloma formation).

Signs and Symptoms

- Tender, inflamed, and easily compressed nodule which is reddish in color. The center of the nodule may range from a clear center to a pus-filled center.
- Local increase in skin temperature and fever.
- Abscesses can have varying durations and can last from days to months.
- Throbbing pain, tenderness, and increase in temperature in affected area.
- Malaise and fatigue.
- Affected areas of the body include the nostrils, arm pits, the genital areas, the armpits, under the belt line, the front of the thighs, buttocks, and the waistline of an individual.

Diagnosis:

- Clinical diagnosis is best made through physical examination and laboratory examination.
- Positive bacterial cultures and gram staining.

Course and Prognosis

- Skin abscesses include spread of the bacteria through the circulatory and lymphatic systems.
- Rupture of the abscess into surrounding tissues or organs, leading to decrease in organ function, and internal bleeding from vessels worn away by inflammation.
- The abscess either remains deep and is reabsorbed, or points toward the surface and ruptures. A ruptured lesion typically heals with a lowered scar.
- Majority of cases are self-limiting, as they are reabsorbed by the body.

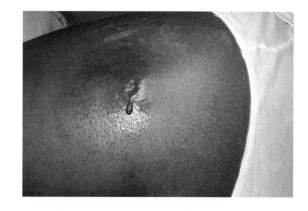

Figure 6-29   Skin abscess.

Treatment

- Keep the area clean and dry, and apply heat.
- Small abscesses may resolve with heat and antibiotics such as Penicillin, Amoxicillin, Cephradine, or Cephalexin.
- Incision and drainage.
- The use of a bar of soap, or body wash containing iodine or benzoyl peroxide in areas of high susceptibility.
- Apply Mupirocin ointment daily to common sites if MRSA has been identified.

Red Flags

If a patient presents with a high fever, the abscess is larger than one half an inch in diameter, if location is near rectum or groin, or if red streaks are radiating out of abscess immediate care is necessary.

30. Lymphangitis

Lymphangitis is an infection involving the lymphatic vessels with ensuing inflammation.

Etiology and Pathogenesis

- Acute and nodular lymphangitis are the two principle forms of the condition. Acute lymphangitis, the more dangerous of the two, is most often caused by the bacterium *Streptococcus pyogenes*, which is the same organism that causes strep throat and infections of the heart.
- To a lesser extent, acute lymphangitis can be caused by staphylococci bacteria, the most abundant normal flora of the skin. In acute lymphangitis, bacteria enter the body through a cut, scratch, insect bite, surgical wound, or other skin injury. Once the bacteria enter the lymphatic system, they multiply rapidly and follow the lymphatic vessels. The infection can reach the bloodstream within hours resulting in septicemia, or blood poisoning, and death. Therefore, acute lymphangitis is a medical emergency and requires immediate antimicrobial intervention.
- Nodular lymphangitis is commonly caused by *Sporothrix schenckii*, a fungus found in various plants, especially roses, and is diagnosed as Sporotrichosis. Infection most often occurs in gardeners who contract the fungus from micro-trauma to their hands and arms. The incubation period is usually 1–2 weeks.

Signs and Symptoms

- Physical examination for acute lymphangitis will demonstrate wide, red, inflammatory streaks which travel from the site of infection along the lymphatic vessel to the armpit or groin.
- A painful abscess may form in the infected area or a generalized infection of the lower skin layers may develop. Blistering of the affected skin is possible. Pyrexia, a general ill feeling, muscle aches, headache, fever, chills, and loss of appetite may be felt.
- Physical examination for nodular lymphangitis involves the presentation of papulonodular lesions spreading along the path of a lymphatic vessel. The lesions are most often painless, although mild tenderness and ulceration may occur.
- Fever is usually absent, as are other systematic complaints.
- Nodular lymphangitis usually occurs on the arms, due to the mode of infection. The lesions are inflamed, elevated, and vary in size and diameter.
- Acute lymphangitis will present with an infected injury site at some part of the body, with red streaks that are visible below the skin surface traveling along the path of a lymphatic vessel. If the injury is on the extremities, the red streaks will travel towards the armpit or groin.

Diagnosis

- Clinical observation of painful, red streaks just below the skin surface with a fever of 100–104°F are diagnostic for the acute condition.
- Culturing for fungus and bacteria from the lesions can help determine the course of treatment for lymphangitis.

Course and Prognosis

- Both conditions are not contagious, although immunocompromised patients should avoid direct contact with the infected individual.

Treatment

- The only treatment for acute lymphangitis is very large doses of intravenous antibiotic, usually penicillin.
- For sporotrichosis nodular lymphangitis, a saturated solution of potassium iodide (SSKI) or itraconazole, an antifungal, are effective treatments. The treatment lasts until all lesions are healed, taking 1–3 months.
- Oral proteolytic enzymes, proteases, cleave kinins and pro-inflammatory prostaglandins.
- Bromelain is a proteolytic enzyme used to reduce inflammation.
- Proline, lysine, and vitamin C supplementation will aid in soft tissue repair that may have occurred from the infections.
- Regarding lifestyle, immunocompromised patients must be diligent to avoid tissue damage and ulceration.
- Diabetics are advised to immediately treat any skin lesion.
- Gardeners are advised to wear gloves when working in their gardens to avoid tissue puncture and possible infection.

Red Flags

Diagnosis of acute lymphangitis is a medical emergency and warrants immediate antibiotic therapy. A patient with nodular lymphangitis and bone, joint, lung, or eye complaints and central nervous system involvement may indicate extra-

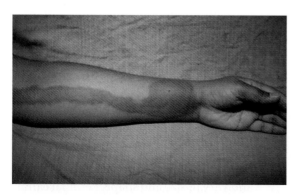

Figure 6-30   Lymphangitis.

cutaneous sporotrichosis and warrants more aggressive therapy.

31. Pyogenic Granuloma

Pyogenic Granuloma is a common benign growth of the skin. It is classified as a vascular lesion and usually results from an injury to the skin that causes a proliferation of the vascular bed under the skin.

Etiology and Pathogenesis

- The cause is unknown but some predisposing factors are trauma, hormonal influences, growth factors, infections and microscopic arteriovenous anastomoses.

Signs and Symptoms

- Pyogenic Granuloma is observed as a red, fleshy nodule averaging half an inch in diameter and grows rapidly in the first few weeks following injury.
- The nodule feels soft and mushy with bleeding that often presents due to the vascular growth in the nodule. There is a thin layer of dermis surrounding the vascular and fibrous growth. The nodule is usually moist, is fleshy and bleeds with pressure or picking.
- They most commonly occur on the gingival, lips, mucosae of the nose, trunk, fingers and toes. Presentation of this condition in many patients occurs after an injury to the area, even if not remembered by the patient.
- The nodule is not contagious, does not spread, does not itch, and does not create a rash. Some concerns that occur with the patient are the nodule's rapid growth and red hamburger-like appearance. It can also bleed spontaneously or after minor trauma to the area.
- "Pregnancy tumors" are pyogenic granulomas that may be slightly larger and can occur on the gums of the mouth.

Diagnosis

- Skin biopsies.
- Histological examination of the lesion aids the diagnosis of the disease.

Course and Prognosis

- The size of the nodule is most often self limiting to 1 inch in diameter and is usually removed by choice of the patient for cosmetic reasons.

Treatment

- Nodules are often tested to evaluate for cancer and more than half of the lesions reoccur at the original site. The majority will disappear on their own without intervention but most are removed surgically.

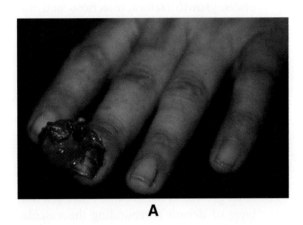

Figure 6-31 (A) Pyogenic granuloma on the index finger.

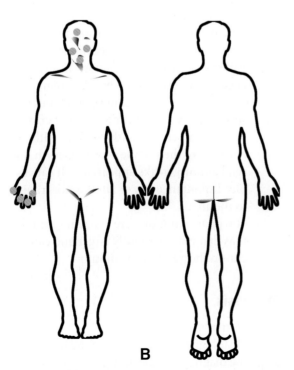

Figure 6-31 (B) Pyogenic granuloma.

- The best chance to eliminate recurrence is to have a full excision of the nodule down through the skin, cauterized and sewed up with stitches. Laser treatments of granulomas have been effective but no evidence shows that it is better than excision.
- There are no documented alternative treatments for pyogenic granuloma. Studies suggest that supplements supporting vascular health may be preventive. Proper nutrition for collagen repair and remodeling may help prevent a removed lesion from recurring.

Red Flags

Pyogenic granulomas are benign and have no clinical consequences. However, they must be differentiated from cancerous lesions by biopsy. The condition is not contagious.

▓ 32. Candidiasis

Cutaneous candidiasis is a skin infection most commonly from the *Candida albicans* fungus.

Etiology and Pathogenesis

- Most infections are of the skin and mucous membranes. Candida is a group of about 150 yeast species and *Candida albicans* is responsible for about 75% of all infections.
- Yeast infections may affect nearly any skin surface on the body, but are most likely to occur in warm, moist, creased areas including the armpits and the groin. The classic form is a red, scaling, itchy rash on the skin or white and patchy in the mouth.
- Candida infection is common among people who are obese, have diabetes or who take antibiotics. Patients will usually have a rash or pimples that ooze clear fluid and causes itching and burning.

Signs and Symptoms

- The signs of the infection are defined as areas of intense itching, well-demarcated patches that are usually reddened in color and vary in size and shape. Perianal candidiasis produces white maceration and itching. Vulvovaginal candidiasis causes itching and white cottage cheese like discharge.

- Signs of yeast infection are also seen in nail beds. This causes pain, swelling, and pus formation. Then a white or yellow nail will separate from the nail bed. If the infection is in the mouth the classic presentation is white patches on the tongue and inside the cheeks and will be painful.

Diagnosis

- Diagnosis is by clinical observation and by findings of yeast and pseudo-hyphae in potassium hydroxide wet mount lab slides that have been taken from an infected area on the skin.

Course and Prognosis

- Yeast infections are self-limiting and do not cause mortality, but those infections in the blood or systemic can be fatal if not treated early.
- The progression of the fungus infection starts off as a harmless yeast area on the skin. As the skin becomes damp and heated, the environment turns into a fertile growth zone. The infection thrives in areas where warmth and dampness are present like the inner thigh and genital regions.
- Candida folliculitis can be found in the hair follicles.
- The fingernail bed when infected with *Candida* becomes inflamed and may demonstrate secondary nail thickening, ridging, and discoloration.

Treatment

A wide array of treatment options is available to treat candidiasis. Options include anti-fungal creams, lotions, tablets or capsules, and lozenges.

- Azole antifungals inhibit the synthesis of ergosterol, a crucial material of the yeast cell wall. Without ergosterol, the yeast cell wall becomes leaky and the yeast dies. Fortunately, ergosterol is not a component of human membranes, and azoles do not harm human cells.
- Nystatin (named for the New York State Public Health Laboratories) is used for thrush and superficial candidal infections.

- Prescriptions for amphotericin B are reserved for more serious systemic fungal infections. These antifungals work by attaching to the yeast cell wall building material, ergosterol, resulting in cell wall defects and cellular death.
- There are some alternative methods that may decrease growth and severity of Candida. *Lactobacillus acidophilus*, a gastrointestinal probiotic, discourages candidal growth, and garlic is considered to have antifungal effects.
- Symptoms of itching and intense burning can be alleviated by cryotherapy.
- Diet restriction with simple carbohydrates. Foods that should be avoided entirely include fruit, sugar, yeast, and mushrooms because they increase growth of the Candida infection.
- Consuming 1 teaspoon–1 tablespoon of soluble fiber twice a day can be beneficial for people suffering from candidiasis.
- Lifestyle changes may include discussions about alternatives to oral contraceptives for birth control.
- Avoidance of alcohol and smoking is recommended.

Red Flags

A red flag would be a patient with an advanced immunodeficiency due to HIV infection. In these

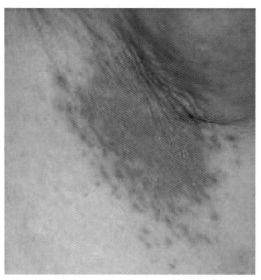

A

Figure 6-32 (A) Candidiasis in the axillary region (note the satellite lesions).

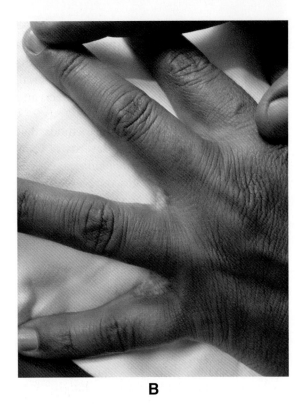

B

Figure 6-32 (B)   Interdigital candidiasis.

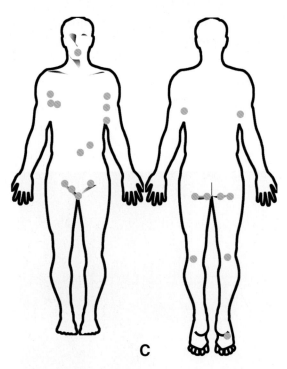

C

Figure 6-32 (C)   Candidiasis.

cases, the infection becomes immune to antifungal therapy and may lead to severe oropharyngeal and esophageal candidiasis that initiates a terrible cycle of poor oral intake, malnutrition, and early death.

▌ 33. Tinea and Cutaneous Fungal Infections

Tinea are fungal infections known as dermatophytosis that affects many body parts such as the head, hair follicles, trunk, crural folds and nails.

The following are types of tinea infections:

- Tinea capitis—affecting the head or scalp.
- Tinea barbae—affecting the hair follicles mainly of the chin.
- Tinea manuum—affecting the hand.
- Tinea corporis—affecting the whole body.
- Tinea cruris—affecting the inner thighs.
- Tinea pedis (Athlete's foot)—affecting the feet.
- Tinea versicolor—upper arms, neck and abdomen. Mainly caused by *Malassezia furfur*.

Etiology and Pathogenesis

- Causative organisms are zoophilic and anthropophilic dermatophytes such as *microsporum*, *trichophyton* and *epidermophyton*.
- Fungal infections are very contagious, and can be passed through direct contact or through contact with body, combs, shoes, stockings.
- Heat and humidity predispose to the infection.
- Locker room floors or communal baths are areas from where the fungi can be contracted.
- Malnutrition, stress, immunosuppression are all predisposing factors.
- Tinea capitis is most common in children.

Signs and Symptoms

Tinea capitis

- Inflamed areas of alopecia.
- Appearance of patchy scaling in the scalp.
- Could accompany with fever and lymphadenopathy.
- The fungi weaken the hair and cause a "black dot" appearance due to break of hair from scalp.

Tinea barbae

- Affect hair follicles mainly of the chin and neck although it can occur all over the face and neck.
- Superficial lesions can form annular plaque that are classical to diagnose the disease.

- In severely affected patients, tinea barbae may occur all over the face and neck.
- Occasionally the infection results in indurated nodules and plaques.
- The presentation most commonly appears as an inflammatory, deep, kerion like plaque and non-inflammatory superficial patch or bacterial folliculitis.
- Hair becomes brittle and loose with pruritus unilaterally, along with scaly patches. The inflammatory tinea barbae is associated with symptoms such as malaise, fever and lymphadenopathy.
- Tinea barbae seems to be controllable and practically eliminated now that single use razors have been developed.
- Tinea barbae has been known to be most commonly found with men who work close to animals.

Tinea manuum
- Affects both dorsal and palmar surfaces of the hands.
- Classical ringworm pattern.
- Hyperkeratotic tinea presents with scaly, dry thick hands and feet.
- Can be accompanied by onychomycosis.

Tinea corporis
- Affecting the body with classical ringworm annular lesions.
- Central area becomes brown and hypopigmented.
- Advancing border of the lesion is scaly or could be inflamed and red due to the severity of the disease.
- Lesions may be itchy or asymptomatic.

Tinea cruris
- Appears mainly in the groin area, in the crural fold, but can migrate to thighs and buttocks.
- Rash is symmetrical and consists of red patch that can alternate with reddish brown color.
- Compared to other tineal infections the rash is less scaly.

Tinea pedis
- Typically, it initially involves the third and fourth interdigital spaces, and later the plantar surface of the foot.

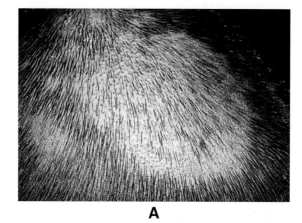

A

Figure 6-33 (A)   Loss of hair (alopecia) from tinea capitis.

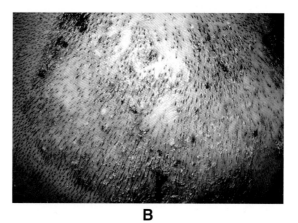

B

Figure 6-33 (B)   Tinea capitis with infection.

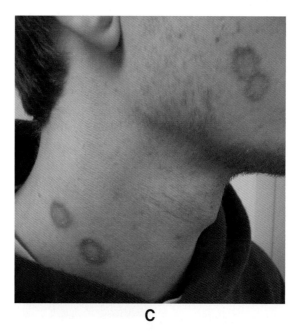

C

Figure 6-33 (C)   Tinea facei (note the annular shaped lesions).

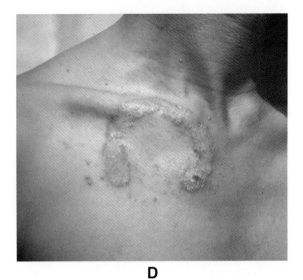

D

Figure 6-33 (D)   Tinea corporis near the neck and chest.

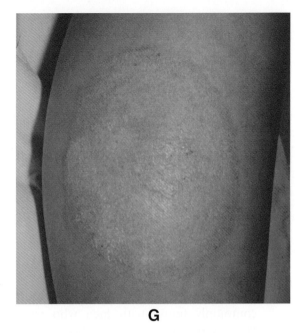

G

Figure 6-33 (G)   Tinea pedis.

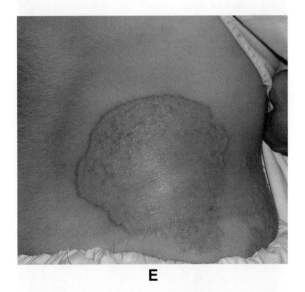

E

Figure 6-33 (E)   An actively progressing annular ringworm lesion.

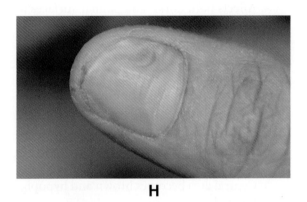

H

Figure 6-33 (H)   Tinea unguium.

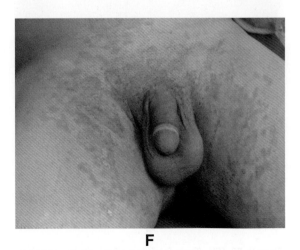

F

Figure 6-33 (F)   Tinea cruris.

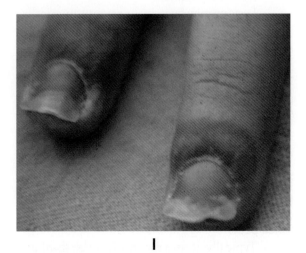

I

Figure 6-33 (I)   Onychomycosis progressing to infection of phalanges.

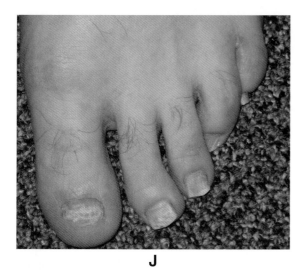

Figure 6-33 (J) Loss of nail tissue from onychomycosis.

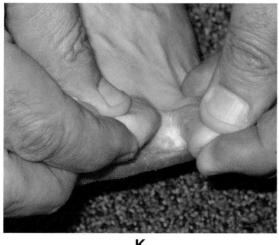

Figure 6-33 (K) Interdigital tinea resulting from tight shoes and excessive sweating.

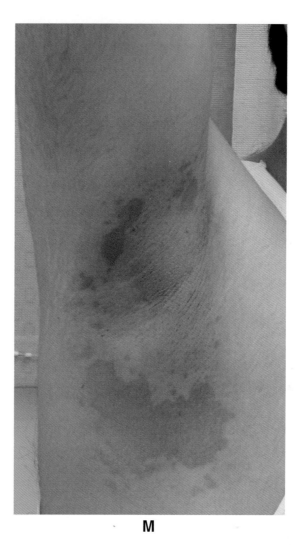

Figure 6-33 (M) Tinea or pityriasis versicolor in the axilla (compare to Fig 33, L).

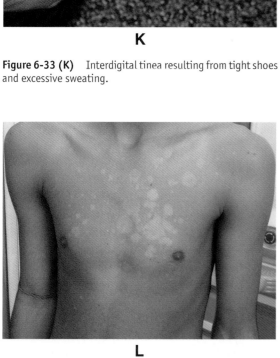

Figure 6-33 (L) Tinea or pityriasis versicolor (lesions are commonly mistaken for vitiligo).

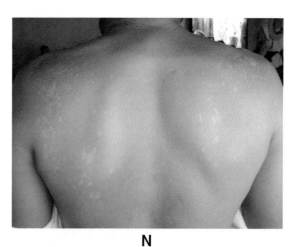

Figure 6-33 (N) Loss of pigmentation in tinea or pityriasis versicolor.

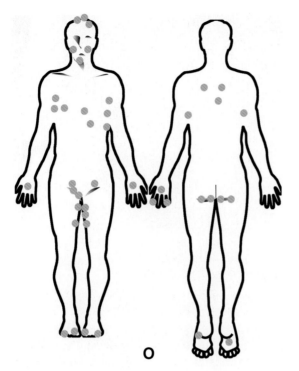

Figure 6-33 (O)   Tinea.

- The toe web lesions may be vesicular, which are macerated, and have scaly borders. During warm weather, flare ups can result in vesicles and bullae. This infection has a pinkish to reddish color.
- If the infection persists it may spread to the toenails, which become thickened and distorted.

Tinea unguium (onychomycosis)
- affecting the thumb and finger nails resulting in greenish yellowish discoloration.
- fungi invade the distal area of the nail, nail plate or the cuticle.

Tinea versicolor
- Appear as white scaling papules on the body that may not necessarily itch mainly on the upper trunk but can involve the upper arms, neck and abdomen.
- Cause by the lipophillic yeast *Malassezia furfur*.
- Lesions are hypopigmented in tanned skin and pink in untanned skin.
- Mild to moderate pruritus is characteristic of tinea but many times it can be asymptomatic.
- Inflammatory lesions undergo spontaneous remission within a few months,

whereas, non-inflammatory lesion are more likely to be chronic and may tend not to resolve spontaneously.

Diagnosis
- Diagnosis is aided by mycological examination that includes direct microscopy and culture.
- A wood's lamp examination has been found to be very beneficial in diagnosing tinea infections, in which there is a dull green fluorescence appearance of the infected hairs upon examination.
- Tinea versicolor caused by *pityrosporum* yeast produces a pale white to yellow fluorescence on Wood light examination.
- Potassium hydroxide staining aids in revealing the hyphae of the fungi.
- Fungal culture is necessary for hair and nail infections. Various culture media can be used to differentiate yeast from tinea infections.

Course and Prognosis
- This condition must be treated before it will resolve. Scarring and permanent alopecia frequently follows spontaneous resolutions of nodules and plaques.
- Athlete's foot may become fatal if complications such as lymphangitis, cellulitis, or pyoderma arise.

Treatment
Oral treatments are preferred over topical treatment because hair follicles respond better to oral treatment.
- Elimination of the source of infection is crucial, especially for those who are in close contact with animals.
- Sole use of corticosteroids should be avoided because fungal infections do not respond well to corticosteroids. However, they can be used in combination with antifungal treatment.
- Topical antifungal like ketoconazole 2%, clotrimazole, miconazole, itraconazole (shampoos and cream) should be used for 10–14 days and can be easily applied to the hair, hands, feet and trunk.

- Zinc pyrithone soap, selenium sulfide (lotion and shampoos) can be sparingly used for two weeks to eliminate the fungus depending upon site of infection.
- Terbinafine (Lamisil) has been very beneficial in treating tinea barbae and all cures have been recorded within 4 weeks of initiating therapy. Terbinafine is used in a dosage of 400 mg/d divided into 2 doses a week and/or, 250 mg/day is also considered a beneficial treatment (Baran, 2004).
- Griseofulvin is a widely used medication. Griseofulvin is given in 20 mg/kg/day dosages until 2 weeks after clinical lesions have resolved and no less than 8 weeks. Pediatric dose is suggested as 5 mg/lb/day.
- Burrow's wet dressings applied 30 minutes several times each day.
- For Tinea Barbae, it is recommended to shave with an electric razor to limit irritation of the skin and help prevent a folliculitis. Warm compressions seem to be beneficial at times to remove crusts and debris.
- Powders absorb moisture and can be applied to the feet before wearing shoes.
- Tinea pedis may be treated with some herbs that include garlic, tea tree oil, chinese worm wood, and black walnut.
- Patients should avoid sharing combs, towels and bedding.
- Recommend that patients change socks daily.
- Recommend that patients choose shoes that allow feet to breathe and stay dry. If using public pools or showers, sandals should be used to prevent feet from touching floors contaminated with fungi.
- Household members should be treated to prevent re-infection.

Red Flags

Immediate treatment should be provided to slow the progression and reduce the duration of symptoms in patients. Tinea barbae is more of a personal appearance and comfort level than it is a need of immediate emergency care.

The use of topical corticosteroids sparingly over fungal skin lesions can alter the classical ringworm shape of the lesions to more diffused, red, inflamed and uniform lesions. This condition is known as *tinea incognito.*

34. Pediculosis

Pediculosis, also known as lice or crabs, are very tiny insects that mainly infest the scalp, body and pubic hair. They survive by feeding on human blood.

Etiology and Pathogenesis

- Lice are pinhead sized, oval, wingless insects with three pairs of legs and depending upon site they are classified as:
  - pediculus capitis (head lice).
  - pediculus corposis (body lice).
  - phthirus pubis (pubic lice).
- The disease is frequently seen in children and girls are affected more than boys.
- Lice most often spread by close or sexual contact.
- Contact with infested bedding or clothing, toilet seats, sharing combs, hats and ear phones.
- Lice feed on human blood every 3–6 hours.
- Females lay eggs, known as nits, that hatch every 10 days.
- Lice require human blood to survive, so it buries its head inside the skin and excretes a substance into the skin that causes itching.

Signs and Symptoms

- Moderate to severe itching in the area affected. The itch is frequently worse at night.
- Crusted excoriations are commonly seen in the scalp, body and pubic but can migrate to the armpits and eyebrows.
- If itching persists and excoriations are torn open, secondary bacterial infection is possible and should be treated immediately.
- Adenopathy can occur in severe cases.

Diagnosis

- Carefully observe the lice and nits using a magnifying glass. Repeated examinations are recommended.
- Patient will complain of itching in the affected area.
- The lice can be seen with the naked eye, and are grayish in color, but appear brown-red when filled with blood from the host.

- The tiny white eggs pubic lice lay are called nits, and are most often seen at the base of pubic hair.
- Wood's light is used to screen children to observe the nits.

Course and Prognosis

- Pediculosis is a treatable condition and can be prevented.
- Intense itching can lead to secondary bacterial infection.

Treatment

- Getting rid of the lice and eggs is critical in the treatment of pubic lice. Everyone in the family or group, whether showing symptoms or not, should be treated at the same time to stop the spread of lice. This also includes sexual partners, close friends, and classmates.
- Nits could be removed by combing or using egg remover gels.
- Hair could be saturated with 50:50 ratio of water and vinegar to help dislodge the lice from hair shafts.
- 1% permethrin lotion or rinse is applied to the scalp, body or pubic area usually overnight. For pediculosis corporis, or body lice,

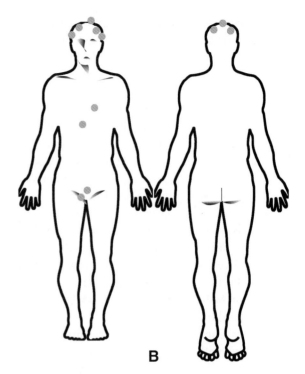

Figure 6-34 (B) Pediculosis.

dermatologists recommend that the cream be applied to cool, dry skin over the entire body (including the palms of the hands, under finger nails, soles of the feet, and the groin) and left on for 8 to 14 hours.
- Lindane shampoo is left for 5 minutes and washed out.
- A second treatment one week later is highly recommended to ensure all nits are hatched and removed.
- Antipruritics can be used concurrently to control itching.
- Oral antibiotics can be given if secondary infection persists.
- Ivermectin (Stromectol) taken orally as a single dose for 10 days selectively paralyzes the nerve and muscle cells of the parasites without affecting humans.
- Good personal hygiene should always be recommended.
- Change and wash all clothing, bedding, towels and underwear daily.
- Avoid sexual or intimate contact with infected people.
- Vaseline, or pomades can be applied to scalp overnight and washed next day with a shampoo. Multiple treatments are required.
- Shaving the scalp or combing the hair to remove nits is helpful in the week during or after treatment.

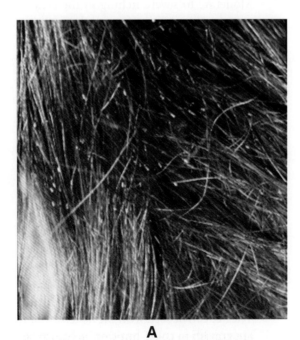

Figure 6-34 (A) Pediculosis capitis, note the fine nits attached to the hair shafts.

■ Neem oil and tea tree oil applications are beneficial.

Red Flags

School teacher or nurse can diagnose pediculosis and children can be sent home until the condition is treated effectively, as the disease is transmissable.

■ 35. Flea Bites

Fleas (Bartonella) are parasites which most frequently live on cats, dogs, rats, and rabbits and are increasingly associated with a range of human and animal diseases. These pests can easily infect the human home, and use any vertebrate as their host.

Etiology and Pathogenesis

■ Adult fleas are about 1/16 inch long, reddish brown, wingless, hard bodied, with three pairs of legs. Fleas are excellent jumpers, leaping vertically up to seven inches and horizontally thirteen inches.

■ A female flea can lay up to 600 eggs in a lifecycle, which is completed between 2 weeks and 8 months. The flea eggs are laid in the fur or hair of almost any vertebrate and hatch between 2 days and 2 weeks after they are implanted.

■ The adult flea can survive for several months without a blood meal. This resilience and fast multiplication is the reason

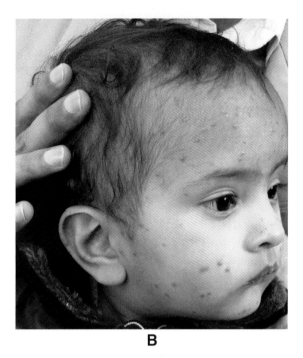

B

Figure 6-35 (B)   Insect bites on a child's face.

the household flea is very difficult to exterminate.

■ Flea eggs can lie dormant for one year and can reactivate with vibrations from foot steps.

Signs and Symptoms

■ The rash starts as a small, hard, red, slightly-raised, swollen itchy papule.

■ Single puncture point in the center of each papule. This differs from a nodule left by a spider or ant in which there are two puncture points in their bites.

■ The lesions produced by bites vary from small papules to large ulcers, with swelling and acute pain.

■ Flea bites may be numerous, found in groups, and mostly located on the feet and legs.

■ Serious consequences result from hypersensitivity reactions or infection; in sensitized people they can be fatal.

Course and Prognosis

■ The condition is self-limiting but can progress to a severe allergic reaction from flea bite allergens.

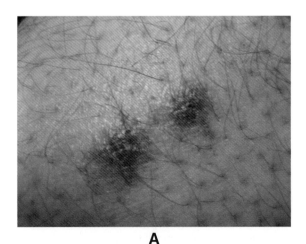

A

Figure 6-35 (A)   Fleas can survive in the seams of clothing resulting in bites which appear as papules containing a punctum.

Treatment

- Relief from itching can be obtained by applying carbolated vaseline, menthol, camphor, calamine lotion or ice.
- Topical steroids, antibiotics and antipruritics can help.
- Advise patients to remove fleas from the home. Be sure to wash pets and their bedding. Additional chemicals to kill the fleas and larva may be necessary.
- Eucalyptus oil, pennyroyal oil balsam, lavender oil, calendula, comfrey, rosemary, tea tree oil and yucca have shown some benefit.

Red Flags

Infested bedding and rugs must be treated to avoid potential spread of fleas. The lesions resolve completely with treatment.

▨ 36. Scabies

Scabies is a skin disease caused by the parasite *Sarcoptes scabiei*. Scabies is transmitted through close physical contact with a person who is infected or prolonged contact with infested linens, furniture, or clothing.

Etiology and Pathogenesis

- Spreading of the mite comes from prolonged, skin-to-skin contact with a person already infested with scabies.
- Contact must be prolonged (a quick handshake or hug will usually not spread infestation). Infestation is easily spread to sexual partners and household members.
- Infestation also occurs by sharing clothing, towels, and bedding.
- Pets become infested with a different kind of scabies mite. If the household pet is infested with scabies and has close contact with the family, this can result in itching and skin irritation. However, the mite dies in a couple of days and does not reproduce. The mites may cause itching for several days, but no treatment is required to kill the mites.
- Attracted to warmth and odor, the female mite burrows into the skin, lays eggs, and produces toxins that cause allergic reactions.

Larvae, or newly hatched mites, travel to the skin surface, lying in shallow impressions where they will develop into adult mites. If the mite is scratched off the skin, it can live in bedding for 24 hours or more. It may take up to a month before a person will notice the itching, especially in people with good hygiene and who bathe regularly.

- For a person who has never been infested with scabies, symptoms may take 4–6 weeks to begin. For a person who has had scabies, symptoms appear within several days.

Signs and Symptoms

- In adults, classic scabies presents as a pruritic, papular rash with excoriations. The itching in scabies is caused by a delayed hypersensitivity reaction to mites, eggs, and fecal pellets.
- Papules and burrows generally follow a characteristic distribution, with the head and neck typically spared. In infants and small children, the scabies rash may include vesicles, pustules, or nodules, and the head and neck may not be spared.
- The lesions are generally distributed but are concentrated especially on hands and feet, buttocks, in body folds and genital organs.
- Scabies should be suspected when an elderly patient has an intensely pruritic condition. In the elderly, scabies lesions may be bullous. The rash often is misdiagnosed

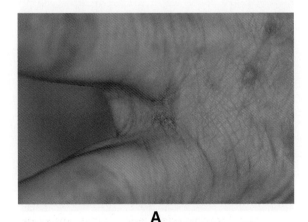

A

Figure 6-36 (A) Scabetic burrows in the interdigital spaces.

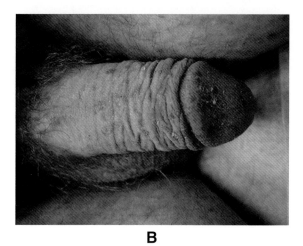

B

Figure 6-36 (B) Penile scabies.

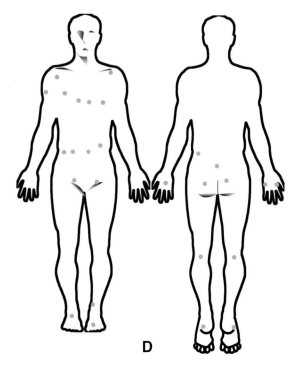

D

Figure 6-36 (D) Scabies.

Diagnosis

- Diagnosis is by clinical observation of the burrows or rash.
- A skin scraping may be taken to look for mites, eggs, or mite fecal matter to confirm the diagnosis.
- If a skin scraping or biopsy is taken and returns negative, it is still possible that the patient could be infested. Typically, there are fewer than 10 mites on the entire body; this makes it easy for an infestation to be missed.

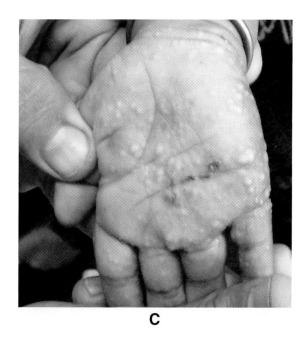

C

Figure 6-36 (C) An infected hand in an infant with scabies.

Course and Prognosis

- If left untreated, scabies can cause life-threatening illnesses like rheumatic heart disease.

Treatment

- Getting rid of the mites is critical in the treatment of scabies. Everyone in the family or group, whether itching or not, should be treated simultaneously to stop the spread of scabies. This includes close friends, day care or school classmates, or nursing homes. Change and wash all clothing, bedding, towels, underwear, etc. daily. Children

and treated with a topically administered steroid, which leads to crusting and diffuse erythema. Papules are often scant. Excoriations are frequently prominent on the buttocks and back.

- Immunocompromised patients with scabies may have crusting of lesions, and itching may be absent. The crusting may be localized or generalized. Patients with human immunodeficiency virus infection sometimes have papular or even nodular eruptions.

should not share clothing or other personal articles such as hair brushes, combs or towels with one another. When an outbreak of scabies or mites is reported be alert for symptoms in members of your family. Keep contact with family members and friends at a minimum until the outbreak is cured.

- 1% permethrin cream is applied to the skin from the neck down at bedtime and washed off the next morning. Dermatologists recommend that the cream be applied to cool, dry skin over the entire body (including the palms of the hands, under finger nails, soles of the feet, and the groin) and left on for 8 to 14 hours.
- Previously, 1% lindane lotion was the standard treatment for classical scabies. Although lindane is generally effective, treatment resistance has occurred. The best advantage of lindane is its low cost. The primary disadvantage is the potential for neurotoxicity, if misused, which may be increased in patients with major breaks in their skin. Lindane should not be used on infants, small children, pregnant or nursing women, or people with seizures or other neurological diseases, and has been banned in the state of California. Lindane lotion is applied like permethrin cream, but it is washed off after six hours and re-applied for one week of treatment.
- A second treatment one week later may be recommended. Side effects of permethrin cream include mild transient burning and stinging. Lesions can heal within four weeks after the treatment. If a patient continues to have trouble, re-infestation may be a problem requiring further evaluation by the dermatologist. 10% sulfur ointment and crotamiton cream, be used for infants.
- Ivermectin is an oral medicine which may be prescribed for the difficult to treat crusted form, but should be avoided in infants, pregnant women or the elderly.
- Antihistamines may be prescribed to relieve itching, which can last for weeks, even after the mite is gone. Pregnant women and children are often treated with milder scabies medications.
- Topical steroids can be used to treat itching and inflammation.
- Unlike other scabies medications, Dexoprin™ attacks the lesion from every direc-

tion. It not only knocks out the scabies mites that are already living under the skin, but it also kills the eggs, putting an end to the infestation and protecting the body from future infestations.

- Bedding and clothing must be washed or dry cleaned.
- Outside of topical treatment for mites, hygiene is the single most important part of the treatment regimen. Since mites can live off of the body for 4–7 days, it is very important to treat your environment for mites.

Red Flags

People with weakened immune systems and the elderly are at risk for a more severe form of scabies, called Norwegian or crusted scabies. This allows the mites to proliferate into the millions.

37. Lyme Disease

Lyme disease is a tick-borne bacterial infection caused by the spirochete *Borrelia burgdorferi*.

Etiology and Pathogenesis

- This disease can be transmitted through the saliva of the tick while it is ingesting blood from a host. The bacteria enter the

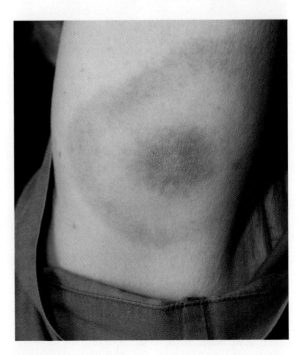

Figure 6-37   Lyme disease.

skin through the bite and eventually make their way into the hosts lymphatic system or bloodstream.

- Lyme disease is spread when an individual is bitten by a deer dick. Not all ticks carry this spirochete, and all bites from infected ticks do not lead to Lyme disease. Re-infection is possible.
- The disease is common in the New England, Mid-Atlantic, and Great Lakes regions of the United States, especially during the summer and early fall. Lyme disease has also been reported in Europe, Asia, and Australia.
- The general population of all ages and both sexes are at risk for Lyme disease, especially those who live in highly wooded areas that lie in infested geographic locations.

Signs and Symptoms

This systemic disease progresses into three different stages. Each stage has its own unique symptoms.

- The first stage begins with infection of the lymph or bloodstream within 3–32 days of the tick bite. The individual may develop cold and flu-like symptoms, pain and stiffness in muscles and joints, and may also develop a bull's eye rash (erythema migrans). A small, red macule or papule may appear within a few days to a month at the site of the tick bite—often in the groin, belt area or behind the knee. It may be warm to the touch and mildly tender. Over the next few days, the redness expands, forming a rash that may be as small as a dime or as large as 12 inches across. This rash affects about 80 percent of infected people. If a patient is allergic to tick saliva, redness may develop at the site of a tick bite. The redness usually fades within a week. This is not the same as erythema migrans, which tends to expand and get redder over time.
- The second stage occurs between the 2nd and 12th weeks after the tick bite. The individual experiences carditis with dysrhythmias, dyspnea, dizziness, or palpitations, as well as central nervous system disorders. This includes meningitis, facial paralysis, and peripheral neuritis.
- The third stage is considered the chronic and persistent stage that occurs at 6 weeks to 2 years after the initial tick bite. During this stage, arthritis, enlarged lymph nodes and neurologic problems, can result. Most, if not all, arthritic and neurologic symptoms that develop from Lyme disease will return to normal once the disease is properly treated.

Diagnosis

- Laboratory tests can be performed to identify antibodies. Enzyme-linked immunosorbent assay (ELISA). This test is the best diagnostic test; it measures the levels of specific IgM antibodies. The ELISA test is usually confirmed by performing a Western blot.
- Immunofluorescent lyme antibody titer is another test that identifies antibodies to a spirochete, Borrelia burgdorferi. If Lyme's disease is not treated with an antibiotic early during the infection, it may lead to muscle atrophy, arthritis, and other neurological problems.

Course and Prognosis

- Lyme disease is rarely associated with fatalities. Those that do occur are usually the result of coinfection with another pathogen that is also carried by ticks.
- Death can occur from neurologic manifestations, if they are not diagnosed with the disease early and treated promptly.
- Prognosis of those with early treatment is excellent. However, careful follow-up monitoring is essential to ensure that the patient has responded to treatment, and does not develop extra-cutaneous signs and symptoms.

Treatment

- The medical treatment for Lyme disease depends on the stage of the disease and whether or not there are simply cutaneous symptoms or if there is more serious neurological manifestations.
- Tick removal and prevention is the first line of treatment.
- Cutaneous manifestations can be treated simply with the use of oral antibiotics like doxycycline or amoxicillin and progress of

the disease should be kept in check. If the patient shows severe manifestations, quick referral should be made to a medical physician. However, in most cases, cutaneous manifestations are the prime presenting symptom and no further consult is needed but the condition must be monitored by the treating physician.

- Thiamin supplementation has been shown to treat associated hypersensitive hearing and hypersensitive nervous system function.
- In conjunction with manual therapies, other modalities such as massage, heat, and ultrasound may also aid in the rehabilitation of these patients. Resistance weight training is the type of exercises that the patient would benefit from the most, due to the atrophying skeletal muscles.
- Aerobic exercises should be avoided until stamina improves but can be implemented as a short pre-workout warm-up. The workout sessions should last one hour and should not be more often than once every other day.

Red Flags

When an individual is diagnosed with Lyme disease, they should be referred to the appropriate medical professional to receive antibiotics immediately. The faster antibiotics are administered, the likelihood of developing severe symptoms are greatly decreased.

38. Swimmer's Itch

A pruritic inflammatory condition caused by schistosomal parasites contracted from swimming in fresh water lakes.

Etiology and Pathogenesis

- Schistosomes or larvae penetrate human skin as bathing water evaporates.
- Larvae primarily found in fresh water.
- Incidence in lake areas is higher.

Signs and Symptoms

- Eruption does not occur in covered areas and the lesions could be demarcated from areas not covered by swimming suit.

- The lesions are inflammatory, discrete, red, edematous papules that erupt 5–10 days after penetration of the larvae. They are mainly confined to exposed areas.
- Intensity of the reaction depends upon sensitivity of the skin and some patients can develop urticaria or thick red plaques.
- Itching begins soon after swimming.

Diagnosis

Diagnosis is made from historical information and by clinical observation of the rash and its distribution.

Course and Prognosis

The condition is self limited and should not be confused with sea bather's eruption that is due to high chlorine content in salt water or hot tub folliculitis caused by pseudomonas.

Treatment

- Itching can be controlled by over-the-counter anti-histamines.
- Topical steroids can be used sparingly on lesions.
- Towel drying can help as most larvae penetrate when water is evaporating.

Red Flags

There are no red flags for this condition.

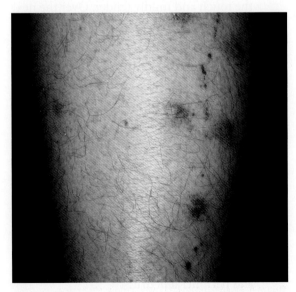

Figure 6-38 Swimmer's itch.

39. Melasma

Melasma is a hyperpigmentation of the skin that occurs mainly on the face and neck.

Etiology and Pathogenesis

- More common in females but can occur in males.
- Occurs during pregnancy and is aggravated by sunlight.
- Birth control pills are important etiological factor.

Signs and Symptoms

- Brown hyperpigmented macules that coalesce to form patches on the forehead, cheeks, upper lip and chin.
- Brown color may show darker areas with edges of the lesions showing irregularity.
- There are no symptoms of inflammation or itching and the condition is completely benign.

Diagnosis

- Typical hyperpigmentation of the rash and history of sunlight exposure.
- Use of birth control pill is a pointer that can aid in the diagnosis of melasma.

Course and Prognosis

- Melasma can regress after pregnancy but in certain cases the lesions maybe stubborn and can take a long time to resolve.

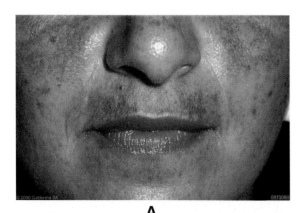

A

Figure 6-39 (A) Melasma. © *DermQuest.com. Used with permission from Galderma SA.*

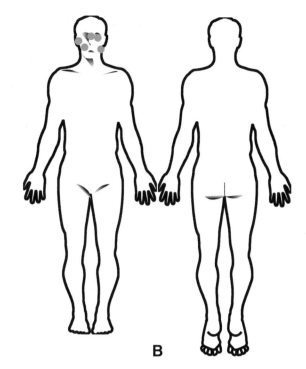

B

Figure 6-39 (B) Melasma.

Treatment

- Sun protection is very necessary and sunblock creams and lotion with SPF factor greater than 30 help subside the condition. Hydroquinone cream application from 4–6 months is required.
- Azelaic acid cream.
- Glycolic acid peeling are used in combination with other treatments.

Red Flags

Melasma is not contagious and is a benign condition with no systemic symptoms.

40. Acanthosis Nigricans

Acanthosis nigricans is a velvety hyperpigmentation of the skin that occurs mainly in the skin folds.

Etiology and Pathogenesis

- Mostly in diabetics and obese patients.
- Family history.
- Endocrine disorders, gastric cancer and pineal gland tumors. The best example is HAIR-AN syndrome comprising of

hyperandrogenism, insulin resistance and acanthosis nigricans.
- Presents when body cells become resistant to insulin.
- Estrogen and nicotinic acid are known causes.
- Malignant tumors can lead to acanthosis nigricans.

Signs and Symptoms

- Symmetric, brown hyperpigmented velvety skin with thick, warty surface.
- The axillae, neck, popliteal fossae, umbilicus, mouth, areolas of breast, fingers, or any flexural skin can be involved.
- There are no symptoms of inflammation or itching although the thick skin can extend to many areas.
- Excessive washing or scrubbing that does not help can lead to superimposed dermatitis and infection.

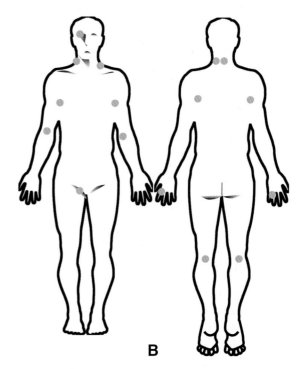

Figure 6-40 (B)   Acanthosis nigricans.

Diagnosis

- Diagnosis is made by clinical observation and historical information that may include insulin resistance and Type II Diabetes.

Course and Prognosis

- Acanthosis nigricans is usually asymptomatic and does not require aggressive treatment.

Treatment

- Retinoic acid cream.
- Lactic acid cream.
- Glycolic acid peeling can be used in combination with other treatment.

Red Flags

Acanthosis nigricans is a benign condition but sudden onset may suggest an underlying malignancy.

41. Vitiligo

Vitiligo is a pigmentation disorder in which melanocytes in the skin, the mucous membranes, and the retina are destroyed. This causes white patches of skin to appear on different parts of the body.

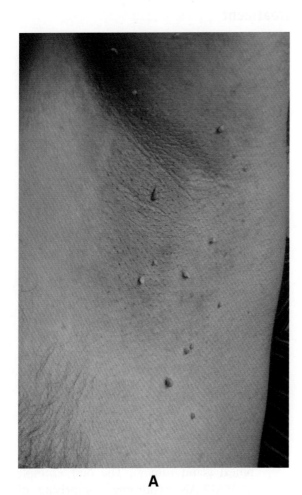

A

Figure 6-40 (A)   Acanthosis nigricans.

Etiology and Pathogenesis

There are several different theories on the cause of vitiligo.

- Autoimmune destruction of melanocytes.
- Autodestruction of melanocytes.
- Spontaneous generation of vitiligo following a single trigger event such as sunburn or emotional distress.
- Hypopigmentation may be preceded several months by a rash, sunburn, or other skin trauma.
- Vitiligo can be hereditary and patients could have a family history of the disorder.

Signs and Symptoms

- Changes in skin color develop often before the age of 20. The white patches appear anywhere on the body, but generally on the hands, knees, feet, face and hair.
- Patches often occur symmetrically across both sides on the body. The location of vitiligo affected skin changes over time,

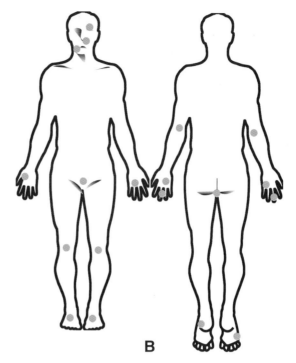

Figure 6-41 (B)   Vitiligo.

with some patches re-pigmenting and others losing pigmentation. Vitiligo on the scalp may affect the color of the hair, leaving white patches or streaks.
- Premature (before age 35) graying of the hair.

Diagnosis

- Diagnosis is made on the basis of a family history of autoimmune diseases, history of triggering factors such as high exposure to sunlight, trauma, and stress, as well as the characteristic appearence.
- A small sample (biopsy) of the affected skin will confirm diagnosis.
- Blood test to look for the presence of antinuclear antibodies may be performed.

Course and Prognosis

- Vitiligo is an autoimmune disease that typically runs in families. Most people demonstrate a slow progression of the disease. If the symptoms of the autoimmune disease increase substantially, medical attention should be sought.
- Vitiligo is usually self-limiting.

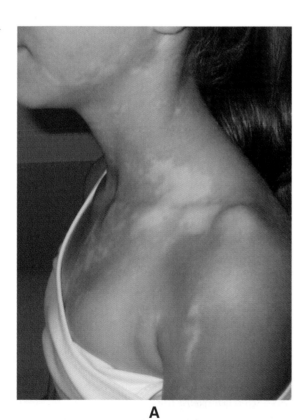

A

Figure 6-41 (A)   Vitiligo.

- Vitiligo is not considered a disease that requires immediate treatment.

Treatment

- Reassure the patient that the disease is non communicable.
- Topical corticosteroid cream must be applied to the white patches on the skin for at least 3 months before seeing any results.
- Psoralen photochemotherapy (psoralen and ultraviolet A therapy, or PUVA) has been shown to be a very beneficial. The goal of PUVA therapy is to repigment the white patches. Psoralens are drugs that contain chemicals that react with ultraviolet light to cause darkening of the skin. The treatment involves taking psoralen by mouth or applying it to the skin. This is followed by carefully timed exposure to ultraviolet A (UVA) light from a special lamp or to sunlight.
- In cases of limited depigmented patches, topical psoralen photochemotherapy is used. It may be used for children who are 2 years old and older who have localized patches of vitiligo.
- Depigmentation is another form of treatment that involves fading the rest of the skin on the body to match the white areas. For people who have vitiligo on more than 50 percent of their bodies, depigmentation may be the best treatment option.
- Counseling should be suggested to treat underlying depression associated with the disease.
- Patients with vitiligo should take a B-complex multivitamin each day, in addition to taking folic acid 1 mg, Vitamin E 600–800 IU, and Vitamin C 1000 mg a day.
- Vitamin D ointment by prescription is of some benefit to patients with vitiligo.

Red Flags

The disease is not contagious and is a benign condition that could be familial. It bears a social stigma that may lead to depression.

42. Urticaria

Urticaria, also known as "hives," consists of localized red wheals on the skin that may be prurutis or tender.

Etiology and Pathogenesis

- Wheals occur as a result of allergic reactions that as much as 20% of the population will encounter at least once in their lives.
- Hives are a result of an allergic reaction from stress, food or drugs and diagnosis will revolve around the causative agent. These allergic reactions cause the body to release chemicals that cause swelling under the skin resulting in wheals or raised areas of red skin.

Signs and Symptoms

- Well demarcated violet or white plaques with lichenification will last from 4 to 36 hours and will reoccur until the trigger is eliminated. The hives can go on and off for months or years.
- Due to scratching the condition can present with pustules and crusting.
- Nodules and lesions can appear behind the scalp, lower legs, wrists, ankles, upper eyelids, ear folds, scrotum or anal skin. The majority of the areas are accessible for pleasurable scratching.
- Usually asymptomatic but some itching can occur with a red flare.

Diagnosis

- Diagnosis is based on historical information and clinical observation. Allergy tests may be ordered to assess for allergen sensitivities.

Course and Prognosis

- Hives pose no risk of being spread to others.
- Angioedema will occur in about 40% of patients affected by hives. This is a condition in which the allergic reaction causes swelling of the airways, making it hard to breathe and, if untreated, can result in death from asphyxia. These symptoms constitute a medical emergency and require emergency treatment.

Treatment

- Reassure the patient and recommend the sparing use of moisturizers.
- Affected areas can be soaked with warm water followed by use of steroid creams.

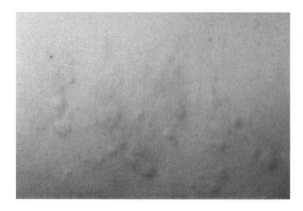

Figure 6-42   Urticaria (hives).

- An intake diary can be kept to correlate symptoms with intake of certain substances.
- Intralesional steroid injections can be used for chronic and nodular plaques.
- Antihistamines can be given to break the itch scratch cycle.
- Reduce stress.
- The goal of alternative treatment is simply removal of the allergen. By keeping a daily intake/contact diary to match up symptoms with intake/contact, the causative agent can be found and eliminated to prevent future occurrences.
- These substances can be foods, drinks or physical irritants to the skin (clothing material, soap/detergents, plants etc.) and even stress can play a role.
- Superficial X-ray therapy has helped in some cases.

Red Flags

The condition can be chronic and may be difficult to treat. Allergic urticaria is not contagious. Respiratory reaction leading to anaphylactic shock must be considered.

▨ 43. Cutaneous Lupus Erythematosus

Cutaneous lupus erythematosus is a skin presentation that can occur with or without systemic lupus erythematosus. Systemic lupus Erythematosus (SLE) is a chronic, multisystem, inflammatory disorder of probable autoimmune etiology, which occurs predominantly (70–90%) in young women of child bearing age.

Etiology and Pathogenesis

- The mechanism or cause of autoimmune disease is not fully known, but it is theorized that it occurs following infection with an organism that looks similar to particular proteins in the body which are later mistaken for the organism and wrongly targeted for attack.
- SLE is more common in African Americans, and can affect a large range of patients from middle age females to neonates. Cutaneous lupus erythematous (cutaneous LE) is a skin manifestation of this disease.
- Drug induced.

Signs and Symptoms

- Common exacerbations, or flare ups, include the dermatologic presentation called a malar, or butterfly, rash. It commonly affects the cheeks and upon inspection reveals erythema that may be flat or raised.
- This condition usually doesn't affect the nasolabial folds, and the absence of papules and pustules help distinguish this from rosacea. There are a variety of other erythematosus, firm, maculopapular lesions that can occur on the face, neck, upper chest and elbows.
- SLE may develop abruptly with a fever or insidiously over months with episodes of arthralgias and malaise. Vascular headaches, epilepsy, or psychoses may be some of the initial findings.
- Systemic presentation of lupus has a tricky presentation and can mimic other connective tissue disorders such as rheumatoid arthritis, systemic sclerosis, polymyositis, dermatomyositis and/or infections that develop as a result of treatment caused by immunosuppression.

Diagnosis

- Diagnosis requires clinical and serologic testing. These tests include an antinuclear antibody panel (ANA) which includes antiDNA and antiSmith antibodies. When the antiDNA and antiSmith antibody tests are positive, SLE is a highly likely diagnosis.
- Other identifying factors that aid in the diagnosis include the characteristic malar

butterfly rash that is located around the eyes and on the cheeks.

- Chest X-rays may also indicate pleuritis or pericarditis in certain stages of SLE. This can also be assessed using auscultation of the heart and lungs to aid in the identification of a heart or pleural friction rub.
- Urinalysis may indicate blood, casts or proteinuria. If SLE has affected or involved the CNS a neurologic exam may be utilized to rule out nervous system involvement.
- In order to properly diagnosis SLE, there must be at least four of the following to make a clinical diagnosis. These include but are not limited to: malar rash, discoid rash, photosensitivity, oral ulcers, arthritis, serositis, renal disorder, leucopenia, lymphopenia, hemolytic anemia, thrombocytopenia, neurologic disorder, positive antiDNA/antiSmith antibody, positive antiphospholipid antibodies and anti-nuclear antibodies.

Course and Prognosis

- The effects that are rendered from drug induced SLE is usually reversible when the particular medication is stopped.
- Overall, SLE varies all the way from a mild episodic illness to a severe fatal disease. Complications may include pleuritis or pericarditis; renal or CNS involvement; and hematologic cytopenia. These manifestations typically occur with periodic exacerbations or "flare ups".

Treatment

It is important to note that there is no permanent cure for SLE; however, it can be managed using several types of medications. The ultimate goal of these medications is to minimize symptoms, and protect organs by decreasing the level of autoimmune activity in the body.

- NSAIDs are the primary agent for reducing inflammation and pain in muscles and joints.
- For cutaneous rash topical steroids are effective.
- Corticosteroids are the next step in the fight against reducing inflammation and restoring function.

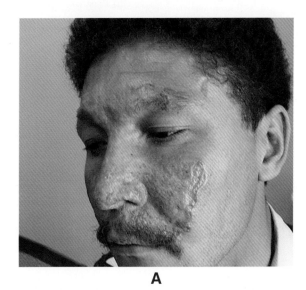

Figure 6-43 (A)   Cutaneous lupus erythematosus.

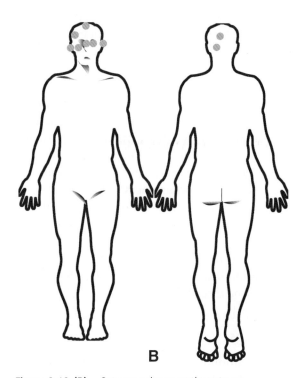

Figure 6-43 (B)   Cutaneous lupus erythematosus.

- Hydroxychloroquine is an antimalarial drug that has been found to be effective with patients that have SLE and associated joint disease.
- Cytotoxic drugs, immunosuppressive drugs, are limited to SLE patients with damage to internal organs.
- Plasmapheresis is yet another treatment rendered for SLE patients who have serious brain or kidney disease. This process re-

moves antibodies from the plasma to suppress the immune response that the body is generating.

- Dapsone and retinoic acid have been found to be effective for an uncommon wart like form of SLE skin disease.
- The battle with SLE can be draining physically and mentally, a support group from fellow SLE suffers may be beneficial to the patient's psyche and well being.
- Patient should be encouraged to avoid any high impact activities that include running. Instead, a low impact exercise such as swimming would be more beneficial.

Red Flags

There are several manifestations that may indicate immediate care. They include renal involvement that may be progressive and fatal, severe neurological symptoms that affect the CNS/PNS, obstetric manifestations that may result in fetus fatality and/or GI complications may include bowel perforation

■ 44. Purpura/Cutaneous Vasculitis

Cutaneous vasculitis can be classified as a group of small blood vessel disease of the skin caused by circulating immunoglobulins (IgG, IgM, IgA) that deposit in the small blood vessels like post capillary venules. They present on the skin as palpable purpura.

Etiology and Pathogenesis

- *Streptococcus; candida albicans.*
- Hepatitis A, B and C, Influenza and Herpes Simplex.
- Drugs such as insulin and penicillin.
- Insecticides.
- Milk proteins and gluten.
- Henoch Schonlein purpura is the most common form of childhood dermatitis with characteristic red macules that evolve into purpuric papules, mainly on the buttocks and lower extremities. Joint and abdominal pain with glomerulonephritis with the characteristic rash is the hallmark of this disease. The condition is caused by circulating IgA antibody deposited in small venules.

Signs and Symptoms

- Asymptomatic purpuric macules that coalesce to form large nodular purpuras.
- Lesions occur in crops on any area of the body and can be itchy and painful.
- The purpuras most commonly present on the legs, buttocks, thighs and back.
- The skin rash can be accompanied by fever, malaise, joint pains.

Diagnosis:

- Physical examination.
- Testing for circulating immunoglobulins.

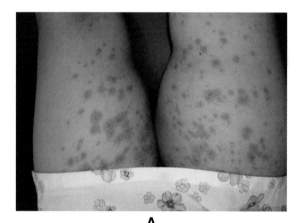

A

Figure 6-44 (A) Vasculitis.

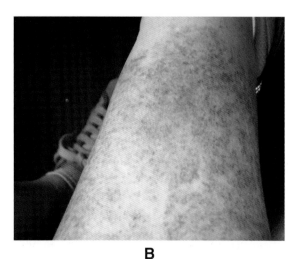

B

Figure 6-44 (B) Asymptomatic vasculitis in a female patient.

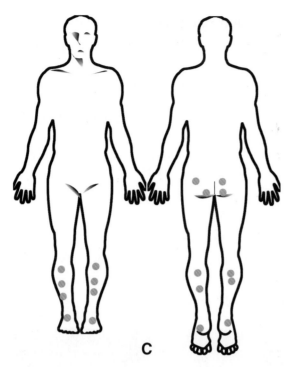

Figure 6-44 (C)   Vasculitis.

Course and Prognosis

- The condition subsides in one month but may be triggered by further exposure. In some forms the immune complexes deposit in the eyes, joints, kidneys, lungs, heart and nervous system resulting in end organ damage.

Treatment

- Removal of the causative agent.
- Topical steroids and antibiotics.
- Oral antihistamines and NSAIDs can help control fever and pain.
- Systemic corticosteroids are helpful for managing chronic relapses.
- Immunosuppressive agents like cyclophasphamide, methotrexate and azathioprine are second line drugs used to treat vasculitis when systemic steroids fail.

Red flags

There are no red flags for vasculitis.

▇ 45. Herpes Simplex and Herpes Zoster

Herpes simplex (HSV) is of dermatologic importance as it affects the mucous lining of the mouth as well as the genitalia during outbreaks. Herpes simplex is a common viral infection of the skin or mucous membranes. Herpes zoster is caused by varicella zoster virus, more commonly known as shingles, the same virus that causes chicken pox.

The lesions caused by these infections are often painful, burning, or pruritic, and tend to recur in most patients.

Etiology and Pathogenesis

Herpes simplex

- Estimates suggest that 20–40% of Americans have recurrent HSV infections.
- Most new cases are diagnosed among young teens. Both women and men are equally affected with herpes type 2 virus.

Herpes zoster

- A person must have been exposed to chicken pox (naturally or by the vaccine). It then remains dormant in the dorsal root ganglion of the spinal cord until becoming activated, usually during a period of weakened immunity.
- It is more common in people over 60, but can be seen in people of any age.

Signs and Symptoms

Herpes simplex

- Symptoms of herpes usually develop within 2 to 20 days after exposure, although it could take longer. Some people do not experience outbreaks where a rash like appearance is present.
- When an outbreak is occurring, the skin becomes red and sensitive, and soon afterward, one or more blisters or bumps appear.
- Lesions can appear as clear fluid filled vesicles anywhere on the body but are typically found around the mouth, lips, cornea, conjunctiva, and genitals. A cluster may be 0.5–1.5 cm in diameter.
- The vesicles persist for a few days, and then begin to dry, forming a thin yellowish crust. An outbreak generally lasts 8–12 days.

Herpes zoster

- Pain from shingles is very intense and follows a dermatomal pattern. It causes such intense pain that it may be mistaken for pleurisy, kidney stones, gallstones, appendicitis, or even a heart attack.

- The rash appears along a dermatome in a band-like distribution a couple days after the pain starts.
- The rash of shingles begins as red bumps, and progresses into blisters. The blisters crust over and turn into scabs. The rash and bumps are more painful than itchy. The scabs eventually fall, and pain begins to subside. However, the pain may last long after the skin is healed. The process may span three to five weeks.
- Shingles may show up in a variety of locations. The trunk is the area affected in 50% to 60% of cases. The next most common site is one side of the face, which may even involve the tongue, the eye, or the ear.
- Usually a single nerve is involved, so the rash and blisters appear only on one side of the body, in a specific location (following a dermatome).
- Locally, the main symptoms are pain and a rash along the dermatome, but sometimes a person may experience systemic symptoms, such as fever, headache, visual or hearing disturbances, and other flu-like symptoms.

Diagnosis

Herpes Simplex

- Diagnosis is by history of presentation and characteristic clinical observation.
- Antibody testing for the virus is currently available.

Herpes Zoster

- History and characteristic dermatomal rash appearance is usually diagnostic.
- If uncertainty still remains, a Tzanck test may be performed. In this procedure, the skin lesion is scraped and the cells are examined microscopically for multinucleated giant cells (Tzanck cells).

Course and Prognosis

Herpes simplex

- Herpes simplex is contagious, more so during outbreaks.
- Transmission is primarily through sexual contact or direct contact. It has a transmis-

sion rate of 75% following intercourse. Herpes simplex alone does not influence mortality.

Herpes zoster

- Shingles is contagious, but only in certain circumstances. If the person has not been exposed to chicken pox, and comes in direct contact with the shingles rash, they may contract chicken pox, but not shingles. A person who has had chicken pox and comes in contact with the shingles rash will most likely not get shingles. Shingles is usually only on the skin, and does not travel in the bloodstream or to the lungs, so it cannot be spread via air or bodily fluids.
- Shingles is not life-threatening to healthy individuals, but may pose a serious threat to immuno-compromised patients. Their weakened state may lead to spread of the virus to vital organs, causing death by viral pneumonia or secondary bacterial infection.

Treatment

Herpes simplex

- Short-term treatment with acyclovir (Zovirax), available as an ointment and pill, can accelerate the healing of an acute outbreak, and continuous acyclovir therapy is often prescribed for people with frequent recurrences. While this drug can reduce the recurrence rate by 60–90 percent, it can also cause a wide array of side effects, including renal failure, hepatitis, and anaphylaxis.
- Other treatments include famciclovir, usually used to treat a recurrent outbreak of genital herpes and to prevent recurrence. Most recently valacyclovir has been prescribed due to a new study indicating its efficiency in reducing the transmission of the virus. It is usually used to treat recurrent outbreaks of genital herpes. A vaccine may be ready in 3–5 years to treat new cases of HSV-2 but will not affect those already infected with HSV-2.

Herpes zoster

- The chicken pox vaccine is believed to decrease the incidence of shingles. However, the FDA has not evaluated the effects of the vaccine on shingles.

- Prescription medication includes Acyclovir to combat the actual virus.
- Prednisone or other corticosteroids to reduce pain and inflammation.
- Antidepressants may be needed in cases of postherpetic neuralgia, which is pain from shingles that persists for months after the rash has resolved. Over-the-counter medications such as acetaminophen for fever and pain reduction, and antihistamines for itching.
- Nutritional treatments include lysine, vitamin C, zinc, thymus extract, lemon balm (Melissa officinalis), deglycyrrhizinated licorice (DGL).
- L-lysine taken orally at a dose of six grams at first onset of mouth ulcer, followed by

four grams daily, until symptoms reduce, in divided doses with meals. Maintenance dose of 500–3000 mg daily may have added benefit including reduction of occurrence, severity and healing time for recurrent HSV infection.
- Vitamin C can be taken at 2000 mg per day which is generally coupled with 1000 mg of bioflavonoids.
- Zinc can be taken orally at 25 mg per day. Thymus extract can be taken orally at 500 mg crude polypeptide fraction.
- Deglycyrrhizinated licorice (DGL) can be used topically twice daily or orally. Zinc sulphate solution of 0.025% can be used topically three times per day. Lemon balm is very effective when applied thickly twice daily during an outbreak.
- Cayenne pepper can be beneficial in controlling the pain associated with shingles. Capsaicin is extracted from cayenne pepper, put into cream form and used topically.
- Applied relaxation has been shown in a small study to be effective in reducing frequency of outbreaks. Stress is the best predictor of recurrence.
- Common clinical practice suggests that manipulative therapy directed to the spinal segments associated with the involved dermatome(s) may influence the recovery period and possibly reduce the likelihood of postherpetic neuralgia.

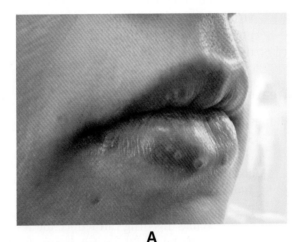

A

Figure 6-45 (A)   Herpes simplex.

Red Flags

Patients should be made aware of the potential for transmission both during outbreak and between outbreaks. However, HSV does not pose an imminent threat to health at any time. Shingles is usually self-limiting and will completely resolve after 3–5 weeks. Only rarely do shingles cause more serious problems. If a small patch of blisters appears on the tip of the nose, it is an ominous sign (Hutchinson's sign), meaning the ophthalmic nerve and eye are affected, which may cause temporary or permanent blindness.

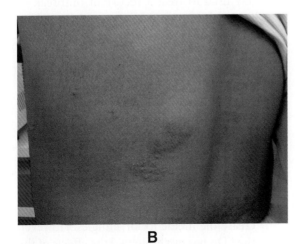

B

Figure 6-45 (B)   Herpes zoster (note pattern of lesions).

▨ 46. Viral Warts

Warts are benign epidermal proliferations caused by human papilloma virus. The lesions are sometimes confused with corns.

Etiology and Pathogenesis

- Transmission is by local contact through skin breaks or trauma.
- Can happen at any age, but peak incidence is from 12–16 years.
- Incubation can be from 1–6 months.
- Epidermodysplasia verruciformis is a hereditary form.

Signs and Symptoms

- Warts are found on hands, chin , neck, legs and even the face.
- The lesions are flesh colored papules that contain dead blood vessels.
- They develop into brown hyperkeratotic or form finger like flesh colored projections on a narrow broad base.
- Flat warts are pink, light brown or yellow papules.
- Warts can present as multiple reddish brown macules in epidermodysplasia verruciformis.

Diagnosis

- Physical examination of the characteristic warty like lesions.
- Rarely a biopsy is performed.
- Polymerase chain reaction linked with ELISA.

Course and Prognosis

- Warts can undergo spontaneous remission or could be widespread if the patient is immunocompromised.
- Warts can spread into an injured area, a reaction known as Koebner's phenomenon, that can also present in skin conditions like psoriasis, lichen planus and keloids.

Treatment

- Many warts regress without treatment.
- 30–40% topical salicylic acid application daily, Mediplast, Duofilm all contain high concentration of salicylic acid.
- Imiquod 5% cream can be effective when combined with cryotherapy.
- Liquid nitrogen cryotherapy. Retreatment is required every 2–3 weeks.

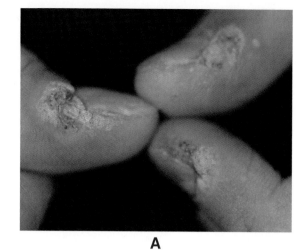

A

Figure 6-46 (A) Verruca vulgaris on fingers.

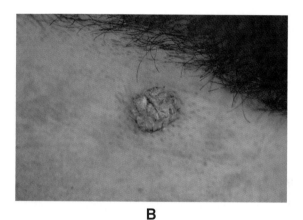

B

Figure 6-46 (B) Single nodular wart.

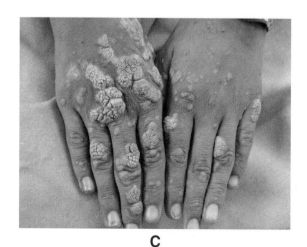

C

Figure 6-46 (C) Bilateral warts.

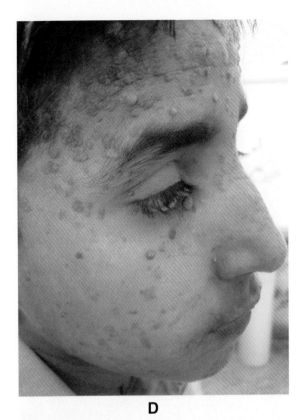

D

Figure 6-46 (D)   Plane warts on the face of a child.

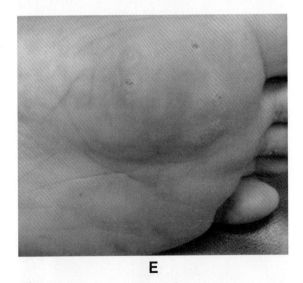

E

Figure 6-46 (E)   Warty lesions on the sole.

- Triretinonin cream can be used for flat warts.
- Intralesional bleomycin is helpful.
- Laser surgery is an alternative but an expensive treatment.
- Electrocautery or cryotherapy to snip off small pedunculated warts.

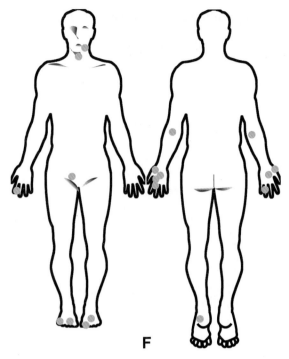

F

Figure 6-46 (F)   Viral Warts.

- Surgical dissection can be advised that produces minimal scarring.

Red Flags

Warts can spread from one area to another, so care should be advised to patients not to pick at the warty skin (autoinoculation). Warts are contagious.

47. Molluscum Contagiosum

Molluscum contagiosum (MCV) is a cutaneous and mucosal eruption caused by the Mollusc pox virus. It is one of the most common primary viral skin diseases that occur without systemic problems.

Etiology and Pathogenesis

- Molluscum contagiosum is the largest known virus and is classified as a DNA poxvirus. It was first described by Bateman in the early nineteenth century and has since been described as intracytoplasmic inclusion bodies known as Henderson-Paterson bodies.
- The virus is confined to the skin and mucous membranes. It is a relatively common viral infection of the skin that most com-

monly infects children, although it can also affect adults. In adults, it may appear on the genitals as an STD, and is more common in the immunosuppressed.

■ This condition is spread through direct contact with either an infected person or a contaminated object.

■ This disease is found worldwide but is most commonly found in tropical areas, with a higher incidence of the virus occurring in institutions or communities that are overcrowded, have poor hygiene, or in areas of poverty. There are four main types of molluscum contagiosum and they are named the following:

• MCV I is the most common type of molluscum contagiosum with the exception of those with a decreased immune system.

• MCV II, MCV III, and MCV IV. They all present with similar lesions throughout the body including genital areas.

Signs and Symptoms

■ Molluscum contagiosum presents as firm bumps that are painless and can disappear in a year without treatment.

■ The papules of molluscum contagiosum can occur anywhere on the body except the palms and soles. The face, trunk, extremities, and genitalia are the most common location for the papules to appear.

■ They present as clusters of smooth, waxy, or pearly umbilicated papules which are 1 to 5 mm in diameter. The lesions are flesh-colored, white, translucent, or yellow in color and can range from one papule up to hundreds of papules. There is a central depression within the lesions which contains a white, waxy core.

■ Molluscum contagiosum is a contagious virus that is spread by direct contact by autoinoculation and can be spread by scratching or rubbing papules causing the virus to

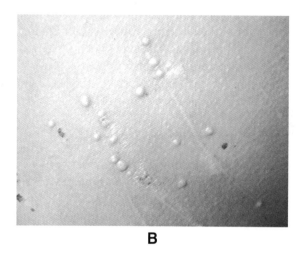

B

Figure 6-47 (B) Umbilicated lesions of molluscum contagiosum.

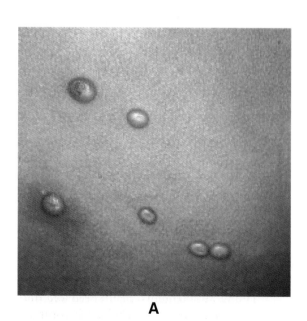

A

Figure 6-47 (A) Molluscum contagiosum.

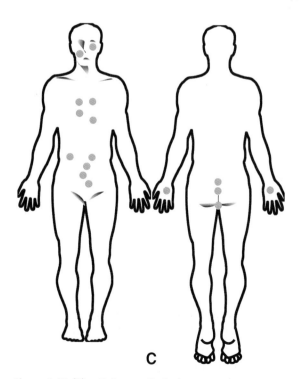

C

Figure 6-47 (C) Molluscum Contagiosum.

extend to nearby skin. It has been noted that fomites can be another source of infection acquired from bath towels, tattoo instruments, and beauty parlors.

- In people with HIV, or similar patients, the lesions may be as large as 15 mm in diameter. While most patients are asymptomatic, some symptoms include pruritus, tenderness, and pain.

Diagnosis

- Diagnosis of MCV is typically made with visual appearance.
- Histological examination can be done to aid in the diagnosis with the use of hematoxylin and eosin stains, Giemsa, Gram, Wright, or Papanicolaou stains.
- Fluorescent antibody test for the MCV antigen can also be performed.

Course and Prognosis

- Incubation time is typically between two and seven weeks but may be up to six months.
- The bumps may remain for 2 to 3 years and treatment is primarily cosmetic or to prevent the spread of the condition.

Treatment

The need for medical treatment of molluscum contagiosum depends on the needs of the patient. The common goal of the various treatment methods is destruction of the lesions.

- The goal for treatment in children is to use treatments that produce minimal pain first such as: tretinoin, imiquimod, and cantharidin.
- Curettage is very effective in adults; however it is also very painful. Many times, dermatologists will use combination therapy with liquid nitrogen or cantharidin in the office, and imiquimod cream at home. Combination therapy is successful in most patients after 1 to 2 months of treatment.
- Other treatments include podophyllin and podofilox, iodine solution and salicylic acid plaster, cimetidine, potassium hydroxide, and cidofovir.
- Tape stripping is a method where adhesive tape is repeatedly applied and removed from the lesion for 10–20 cycles to remove

the superficial epidermis from top of the lesion. The patient must be cautious when using this form of treatment because repeated use of the same strip of tape may spread the virus to nearby skin.

- Fish oils may also be useful for inflammatory conditions associated with the disease.
- Vitamin E is beneficial.
- Other supplements that may aid in the treatment of MCV are Vitamin C, zinc, Echinacea, and Goldenseal.
- Laser therapy has been shown to be beneficial in the treatment of molluscum contagiosum. The use of pulsed dye laser is well tolerated by the patient, is quick and efficient, and does not leave scars or pigment anomalies.

Red Flags

Although molluscum contagiosum is usually self-resolving, it is contagious. Removal of the papules is recommended to prevent scarring for cosmetic reasons; however, they are more likely to be removed in immunocompromised patients or to prevent them from being spread sexually.

48. Measles, Chicken Pox, and Viral Exanthemas

Numerous viral infections present with a skin rash. Almost all viral infections are communicable. This section discusses the most common viral exanthemas that chiropractors can come across in a clinic. Table 6-1 outlines the features of the most common viral exanthemas.

Treatment

- Bed rest is very helpful, and if the child is in school, they need to stay out of school for at least 7–10 days.
- Eating bland foods and adequate fluid intake is necessary.
- Advise not to scratch lesions. Calamine lotion can be applied to relieve itching.
- Oral antihistamines can be prescribed in small quantities.
- Lysine supplements may speed recovery time and reduce the chance of recurrent breakouts.

Table 6-1   Common Viral Exanthemas

Viral Infection	Etiology and Pathogenesis	Signs and Symptoms	Course and Prognosis
Measles	Paramyxovirus Young and old Occurs once in a lifetime	A red blotchy macular and papular rash begins on the head or behind the ears and spreads down to cover the rest of your body. Koplik spots will usually develop inside the mouth of a person with measles, and they consist of red spots with bluish-white centers opposite the second molars. Fever, cough, conjunctivitis and itching accompany the skin rash.	Highly contagious Can result in complications such as pneumonia, laryngitis
Chicken Pox	Winter and Spring Any age but can be severe in the immuno-compromised	Papular rash on the face, scalp, abdomen and back, that quickly turns into small vesicles that break open and crust. New spots continue to appear for several days and may number in the hundreds. Fever, abdominal pain, loss of appetite, conjunctivitis, runny nose and mild to moderate itching presents with the rash.	Highly contagious Secondary bacterial infection can precede after chicken pox vesicles rupture Scarring can be permanent
Rubella (German measles)	Any age	Red rash beginning from the face and affecting the entire body. This is accompanied by low fever, malaise, runny nose, joint pains and swollen glands.	Contagious Encephalitis, blindness can occur as a complication Can cause birth defects in women
Hand Foot and Mouth Disease	Young children Coxsackie virus	Tiny, painful red blisters on the soles of the feet, palms of the hands, in the throat and on the tongue, gums, hard palate, and inside of the cheeks. Other signs and symptoms include fever, sore throat, headache, fatigue, irritability and loss of appetite.	Can develop into viral meningitis, encephalitis, myocarditis, cardiopulmonary distress
Fifth Disease	Young children Also known as erythema infectiosum or slapped cheek syndrome Parvovirus B19	A red lacy rash especially on the on cheeks (slapped cheek), arms, legs, and trunk, but not palms or soles. Mouth and nose are spared. The rash is warm to touch. Fever and malaise are associated symptoms. Symmetric polyarthritis is most common in adults.	Self limiting and resolves in 5–10 days

- Ensure vaccinations are current and up to date for children.
- Acetaminophen may be helpful in treating fevers, and antibiotics will help with bacterial complications like pneumonia or ear infection.
- Immune compromised people, infants, and pregnant women may be given protein injections that will help to fight off infections.
- Oral acyclovir is recommended in severe cases.
- Good personal hygiene is always recommended.
- Colloidal oatmeal baths are soothing.
- Probiotics are beneficial.

- Capsaicin cream made from cayenne pepper has powerful pain-relieving properties when applied to the skin.
- German chamomile, peppermint oil, aloe, burdock root, lemon balm, licorice root, and the Madonna lily are other herbs that have been used traditionally for skin lesions.
- Avoid contact with infected people.
- Increase vitamin A intake.

Red Flags

All viral infections may develop secondary complications such as encephalitis, meningitis or myocarditis and are contagious.

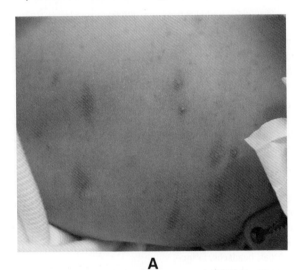

A

Figure 6-48 (A) Chicken pox.

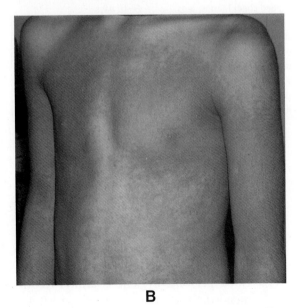

B

Figure 6-48 (B) Viral exanthems like measles can present as a generalized rash.

49. Polymorphous Light Eruption

Polymorphous light eruption (PLE) is a recurrent dermatitis that occurs upon exposure to the sun. The condition is also known as sun poisoning or sun allergy.

Etiology and Pathogenesis

- All races, especially in young women.
- Sunlight exposure in spring, mainly ultraviolet A.
- Can be hereditary in Native Americans.

Signs and Symptoms

- Burning, itching and papules on sun exposed areas appearing after 2 hours to 5 days of exposure such as the dorsum of hands, chest, extensors of the forearms and lower legs.
- Papules can coalesce to form plaques.
- Erythema is patchy with areas of sparing.
- Pruritus, chills, headache can accompany the skin lesions.

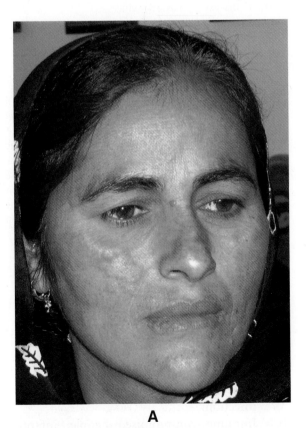

A

Figure 6-49 (A) Polymorphous light eruption.

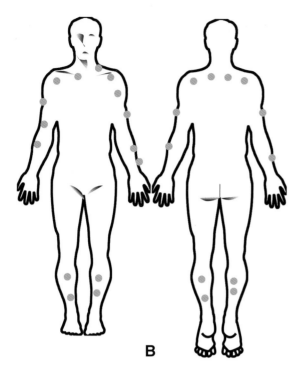

Figure 6-49 (B)   Polymorphous light eruption.

Diagnosis

- Characteristic rash and history of sunlight exposure.

Course and Prognosis

- PLE can persist for 7–10 days and can recur every season upon sun exposure for many years.

Treatment

- Use sun block screens containing titanium oxide or sun protective clothing.
- Minimize sun exposure between 10:00am and 3:00pm.
- Topical steroids can be applied for two weeks or until the lesions disappear.
- Antihistamines can be given to control pruritus.
- Hydroxychloroquine 400mg/day can be used in severe cases.

Red Flags

Polymorphous light eruptions are noncontagious but the rash can be embarrassing. To prevent seasonal flare, long term monitoring of patients is required.

▨ 50. Hyperhidrosis

Hyperhidrosis is defined as a condition leading to excessive localized or widespread sweating.

Etiology and Pathogenesis

- Emotional or neural in origin.
- Drugs such as insulin and caffeine can cause hyperhidrosis.
- Mercury and arsenic ingestion can lead to hyperhidrosis.
- Hyperhidrosis at night can be caused by conditions such as tuberculosis and Hodgkin's lymphoma.
- Obesity.
- Metabolic disorders such as hyperthyroidism, diabetes mellitus, carcinoid syndrome, pheochromocytoma.
- Exercise is a physiological cause.

Signs and Symptoms

- Palmar, plantar and axillary areas are most common.
- Excess moisture results in flaky skin with cracks and fissures, which lead to bacterial or fungal overgrowth.
- Pitted keratolysis is a condition resulting in small pits mainly on the soles of the feet associated with intense odor.

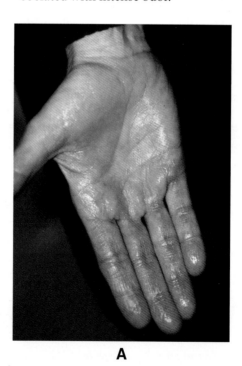

Figure 6-50 (A)   Hyperhidrosis. © *DermQuest.com. Used with permission from Galderma SA.*

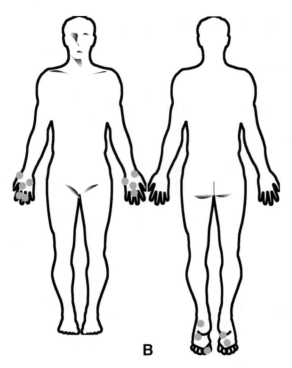

B

Figure 6-50 (B) Hyperhidrosis.

Diagnosis

- Typical symptoms of excessive sweating especially in hands, feet and armpits are classical.

Course and Prognosis

- Hyperhidrosis can be socially debilitating and at times the patients may use napkins in office to dry skin when writing on paper or may just be embarrassed in shaking hands, leading to social debilitation.

Treatment

- 6–20% aluminum chloride solutions under occlusion.
- 30 minutes daily ion water ionotophoresis.
- Oral glycopyrrolate and botulinus toxin can be beneficial to suppress sweating by anti-cholinergic effects.
- Topical antibiotics and antibacterial soaps for treatment of pitted keratolysis.
- Topical anesthetics.
- Cervical, thoracic, lumbar sympathectomy are some more aggressive options.
- Local surgical ablation can be used to treat axillary hyperhidrosis.

Red Flags

Hyperhidrosis is a benign condition and is not contagious unless superseded by bacterial infection. Treating underlying systemic conditions such as obesity, diabetes, tuberculosis improves hyperhidrosis.

Cross-reference of conditions and treatment

For the convenience of readers, **Table 6–2** cross references the therapeutic approaches listed in Chapter 7 with the appropriate conditions described in this chapter.

Table 6-2

	Condition	Therapeutics
1	Psoriasis vulgaris	6, 7, 8, 9, 10, 11, 14, 15, 20, 21, 22, 24,25, 26, 27, 31, 33, 34, 37, 40, 44, 47, 50
2	Seborrheic dermatitis	7, 8, 9, 10, 22, 23, 24, 34, 38, 40, 44
3	Atopic dermatitis	6, 7, 9, 10, 11, 12, 16, 18, 20, 21, 24, 26, 27, 31, 34, 35, 37, 41, 43, 44, 47, 49
4	Lichen planus	14
5	Lichen simplex chronicus	14, 50
6	Pompholyx	6, 49
7	Keratosis pilaris	14, 50
8	Contact dermatitis - allergic or irritant	1, 4, 6, 7, 9, 10, 11, 12, 16, 18, 20, 21, 25, 31, 34 , 35, 37, 43, 44, 49

Table 6-2   (continued)

	Condition	Therapeutics
9	Pityriasis alba	44
10	Pityriasis rosea	6, 14, 21, 43
11	Ichthyosis	2, 7, 11, 12, 14, 22, 25, 37, 40, 47, 50
12	Seborrheic keratosis	9, 12, 14, 50
13	Xanthoma	
14	Keloid	1, 12
15	Hemangioma	1, 21, 44
16	Epidermal cyst and pilar cyst	
17	Skin tags	1
18	Neurofibromatosis	
19	Squamous cell carcinoma	10
20	Basal cell carcinoma	
21	Melanoma	
22	Acne vulgaris	2, 4, 6, 7, 12, 14, 16, 17, 18, 22, 24, 25, 27, 28, 31, 32, 34, 36, 42, 43
23	Rosacea	2, 7, 10, 14
24	Perioral dermatitis	12, 22, 28, 31, 34, 36, 45
25	Hidradenitis suppurativa	1, 4
26	Eosinophilic folliculitis	4, 44
27	Carbuncle	4, 12, 23, 25, 26, 27, 32, 34, 38, 47
28	Impetigo	17, 23, 27, 32, 38, 47
29	Skin abscess	4, 17, 23, 26, 27, 32, 38, 47
30	Lymphangitis	19, 32
31	Pyogenic granuloma	1, 19
32	Candidiasis	12, 32, 39, 40, 47
33	Tinea infections	12, 22, 23, 24, 32, 33, 34, 39, 40, 45, 48
34	Pediculosis	9, 12, 13, 23, 28
35	Flea bites	1, 12, 13, 18, 23, 26, 28, 29, 43, 47
36	Scabies	18, 23, 28, 44, 50
37	Lyme disease	
38	Swimmer's itch	9, 23, 28, 44
39	Melasma	
40	Acanthosis nigricans	14
41	Vitiligo	6, 44
42	Urticaria	11, 30, 35, 37, 43, 48
43	Cutaneous lupus erythematosus	
44	Cutaneous vasculitis (purpura)	42, 44
45	Herpes simplex and Herpes zoster	1, 6, 22, 23, 32, 34, 36, 39, 44, 47
46	Viral warts	1, 5, 23, 24, 25, 38, 40, 46
47	Molluscum contagiosum	16, 19, 40, 46
48	Viral exanthemas (incl. measles, chicken pox)	21, 22, 25, 27, 30, 31, 36, 37, 43, 48
49	Polymorphous light eruption	44
50	Hyperhidrosis	5, 18, 42

General References

Arnold L Harry. *Diseases of the Skin Clinical Dermatology*, 8th ed. Philadelphia, PA: W.B Saunders Company, 1990.

Bickley LS. *Bates Guide to Physical Examination and History Taking*, 9th ed. Chicago, IL Lippincott Williams and Wilkins, 2007.

Burns DA, Breathnach SM, Cox N, Griffiths CE. *Rook's Textbook of Dermatology*, 7th ed. Oxford, UK. Blackwell Publishing, 2004.

Fitzpatrick JE, Morelli JG. *Dermatology Secrets*. 3rd ed. Philadelphia, PA. Mosby. 2006.

Habif TP. *Skin Disease: Diagnosis and Treatment*. 2nd ed. Philadelphia, PA, Elsevier Mosby; 2005.

Kumar Vinay et. al. (ED) *Robins Pathologic Basis of Disease* 7th ed Philadelphia, PA Elsevier 2005.

Mackie RM. *Clinical Dermatology* 4th ed. New York, NY, Oxford Press 2004.

Oyelowo Tolu. *Mosby's Guide to Women's Health: A Handbook for Health Professionals*, 1st ed. St. Louis, MO, Mosby Elsevier, 2007.

Wolff Klaus, et al. *Fitzpatrick's Color Atlas &Synopsis of Clinical Dermatology*. New York, NY, McGraw-Hill, 2005.

Further Reading

Psoriasis

Behnam SM, et al. "Smoking and psoriasis." *SKINmed*. 2005 May-June;4(3):174–176.

Eriksson MO, et al. "Palmoplantar pustulosis: A clinical and immunohistological study." *Br J Dermatol*. 1998. March;138(3):390–398.

Fortes C, et al. "Relationship between Smoking and the Clinical Severity of Psoriasis." *Arch Dermatol*. 2005. Dec;141(12):1580–1584.

Herron MD, et al. "Impact of Obesity and Smoking on Psoriasis Presentation and Management." *Arch Dermatol*. 2005. Dec;141(12):1527–1533.

Mease PJ, et al. "Quality-of-life issues in psoriasis and psoriatic arthritis: Outcome measure and therapies from a dermatologic perspective." *J Am Acad Dermatol*. 2006. April;54(4):685–704.

Seborrheic Dermatitis

Johnson B. Treatment of seborrheic dermatitis. *Am Fam Physician* 2000, 61: 9.

Schwartz MA, Janusz CA, Janniger CK. Seborrheic Dermatitis: An Overview. *Am Fam Physician*. 2006; 74: 125–130.

Atopic Dermatitis

Brown S, Reynolds NJ. Atopic and non-atopic eczema. *BMJ*. 2006, 332: 584–8.

Buys LM. Treatment options for atopic dermatitis. *Am Fam Physician* 2007, 75: 523–8.

Faergemann J. Atopic Dermatitis and Fungi. *Clin Microbiol Rev*. Oct 2002; 15(4): 545–563.

Moro G, Arslanoglu S, Stahl B, Jelinek J, Wahn U, Boehm G. A mixture of prebiotic oligosaccharides reduces the incidence of atopic dermatitis during the first six months of age. *Arch Dis Child*. 2006; 91:814–9.

Williams H. Evening primrose oil for atopic dermatitis. *BMJ*. Dec 2003; 327: 1358–1359.

Wollina U. The Role of Topical Calcineurin Inhibitors for Skin Diseases Other Than Atopic Dermatitis. *Am J Dermatol*. 2007; 8(3):157–173.

Lichen Planus

Katta Rajani. Lichen Planus. Am Fam Physician. 2000 June;(61):3319–3324,3327–3328. http://www.aafp.org/afp/20000601/3319.html. Accessed March 17, 2009.

Pompholyx

Kostantopoulou M, et al. Azathioprine—induced pancytopenia in a patient with pompholyx and deficiency of erythrocyte thiopurine methyltransferase. *BMJ*. 2005 Feb; 330(7487): 350–351.

Morris ME. An adolescent boy with blistered feet. *West J Med*. 2001 Dec; 175(6): 375–376.

Keratosis Pilaris

Zouboulis C, Stratakis C, Gollnick H, Orfanos C. Keratosis pilaris / ulerythema ophryogenes and 18p deletion: is it possible that the LAMA1 gene is involved?. *J Med Genet*. 2001 Feb; 38(2): 127–128.

Contact Dermatitis—Allergic or Irritant

Allergic contact dermatitis. New Zealand Dermatological Society, Inc. [DermNet NZ Web site] Available at http://www.dermnetnz.org/dermatitis/contact-allergy.html. Accessed March 16, 2009.

Ngan V. Irritant contact dermatitis. New Zealand Dermatological Society, Inc.[DermNet NZ Web site]. Available at http://www.dermnetnz.org/dermatitis/ contact-irritant.html. Accessed March 16, 2009.

Pityriasis Alba

duToit MJ, Jordaan HF. Pigmenting Pityriasis Alba. *Pediatr Dermatol*. 1993 Mar; 10(1): 1–5. [PubMed website]. Available at http://www.ncbi.nlm.nih.gov/sites/entrez?Db=pubmed&Cmd=ShowDetailView&TermToSearch=8493158&ordinalpos=1&itool=EntrezSystem2.PEntrez.Pubmed.Pubmed_ResultsPanel.Pubmed_RVAbstractPlus. Accessed March 14, 2009.

Fujita WH, McCormick CL, Parneix-Spake A. An exploratory study to evaluate the efficacy of pimecrolimus cream 1% for the treatment of pityriasis alba. *Int J Dermatol.* 2007 July; 46(7): 700–705. [PubMed website]. Available at http://www.ncbi.nlm.nih.gov/sites/entrez?Db=pubmed&Cmd=ShowDetailView&TermToSearch=17614797&ordinalpos=4&itool=EntrezSystem2.PEntrez.Pubmed.Pubmed_ResultsPanel.Pubmed_RVDocSum. Accessed March 16, 2009.

Pityriasis Rosea

Stulberg W, Daniel J. "Pityriasis Rosacea." *Am Fam Physician.* 2004;69.

Ichthyosis

DiGiovanna J, & Robinson-Bostom, L Ichthyosis, Etiology, Diagnosis and Mangement. *Am J Clin Dermatol.* 2003. 4(2). 81–95.

Seborrheic Keratosis

Bryant J. Conservative Clinical Diagnosis in Seborrheic Keratosis. *Arch Dermatol.* 1998;134:752–753.

Gill D, Dorevitch A, Marks R. The Prevalence of Seborrheic Keratosis in People Aged 15 to 30 Years. *Arch Dermatol.* 2000; 136:759–762.

Izikson L, et.al. Prevalence of Melanoma Clinically Resembling Seborrheic Keratosis. *Arch Dermatol.* 2002; 138:1562–1566.

Keloid

Ogunbiyi A, George A. Acne keloidalis in females: case report and review of the literature. *J Natl Med Assoc.* 2005 May; 97(5):736–738.

Roseborough IE, Grevious MA, Lee RC. Prevention and treatment of excessive dermal scarring. *J Natl Med Assoc.* 2004 Jan; 96(1):108–116.

Hemangioma

Barrio R, Victoria. Treatment of Hemangiomas of Infancy, *Dermatol Ther* 2005;(5):151–159.

Bruckner A, Frieden, I. Hemangiomas of Infancy. *J Am Acad Dermatol.* 2003;48(4).

Haggstrom AN, et al. Patterns of Infantile Hemangiomas: New Clues to Hemangioma Pathogenesis and Embryonic Facial Development, *Pediatrics* 2006;117:698–703.

Worth AF, Lowitt MH. Diagnosis and Treatment of Cutaneous Vascular Lesions. *Am Fam Physician.* 1998 Feb. Available at http://www.aafp.org/afp/980215ap/wirth.html Accessed. March 16, 2009.

Epidermal Cyst and Pilar Cyst

Polychronidis A, Perente S, et al. Giant Multilocular Epidermoid Cyst on the Left Buttock. *Dermatol Surg.* 2005;31:1323–1324.

Zuber TJ. Minimal Excision Technique for Epidermoid (Sebaceous) Cysts. *Am Fam Physician.* 2002; 65: 1–6.

Neurofibromatosis

Gajeski BL, Kettner N W & Boesch R J. Neurofibromatosis Type 1: Clinical and Imaging Features of Von Recklinghausen's Disease. *J Manipulative Physiol Ther.* 2003; 26: 116–127.

Squamous Cell Carcinoma

Chak A, Das A, Zablotska L. Increased Risk of Squamous Cell Esophageal Cancer after Adjuvant Radiation Therapy for Primary Breast Cancer. *Am J Epidemiol.* 2005; 161: 330–337.

Basal Cell Carcinoma

Crandell B, Fawcett S, Stulberg D. Diagnosis and Treatment of Basal Cell and Squamous Cell Carcinomas. *Am Fam Physician* 2004; 70: 1481–1488.

Crowson AN. Basal cell carcinoma: biology, morphology, and clinical implications. *Mod Pathol.* 2006; 19: 127–147.

Harris CC. Molecular epidemiology of basal cell carcinoma. *J Natl Cancer Inst.* March 1996; 88(6): 315–316.

Melanoma

Schneider J, Gilford S, The chiropractor's role in pain management for oncology patients. *J Manipulative Physiol Ther.* 2001;24:52–57.

Swerdlow AJ. Melanocyutic naevi and melanoma: an epidemiological perspective. *Br J Dermatol.* 1986; 117:137.

Xia S, Lu Y, Wang J, et al. Melanoma growth is reduced in fat-1 transgenic mice: Impact of omega-6/omega-3 essential fatty acids. *Proc Natl Acad Sci USA.* 2006;103:12499–12504.

Acne Vulgaris

Chiu A Chon, S Alexa K. The Response of Skin Disease to Stress. *Arch Dermatol.* 2003; 139(7): 897–900.

Katzmam M and Logan A. Acne Vulgaris: Nutritional Factors May Be Influencing Psychological Sequelae. *Med Hypotheses.* 2007 Feb;69(5):1080–1084.

Leyden James. "Therapy for Acne Vulgaris." *N Engl J Med.* 1997; 336;16: 1156–1165.

Magin P, Adams J, Heading G, Pond D, Smith W. Complementary and Alternative Medicine Therapies in Acne, Psoriasis, and Atopic Eczema: Results of a Qualitative Study of Patient' Experiences and Perceptions. *J Altern Complement Med.* 2006; 12: 451–457.

Qa'dan F, Thewaini A, Ali D, Afifi R, Elkhawad A, Matalka K. The Antimicrobial Activities of Psidium guajava and Juglans regia Leaf Extracts to Acne-Developing Organisms. *Am J Chinese Med.* 2005; 33: 197–204.

Smith R, Mann N, Braue A, Makelainen H, Varigos G. The effect of a high-protein, low glycemic load diet versus a conventional, high glycemic load diet on biochemical parameters associated with acne vulgaris: A randomized, investigator-masked, controlled trial. *J Am Acad Dermatol.* 2007; 57: 247–256.

Strauss J, Krowchuk D, Leyden J, et al. Guidelines of care for acne vulgaris management. *J Am Acad Dermatol.* 2007; 56: 651–663.

Rosacea

Gupta AK, Chaudhry MM. Rosacea and its management: an overview. *JEADV.* 2005; 19:273–285.

Laube S, Lanigan SW. Laser treatment for Rosacea. *J Cosmet Dermatol.* 2002; 1:188–195.

Sharquie KE, Najim RA, Al-Salman HN. Oral zinc sulfate in the treatment of Rosacea: A double-blind, placebo-controlled study. *Int Soc Dermatol.* 2006; 45:857–861.

Perioral Dermatitis

Watt CJ, Chih-ho Hong H. Dermacase. Lip licker's dermatitis. *Can Fam Physician.* 2002 June; 48: 1051–1059.

Hidradenitis Suppurativa

Adams DR, et al. Severe hidradenitis suppurativa treated with infliximab infusion. *Arch Dermatol.* 2003 Dec;139:1540–1542. Available at http://archderm.ama-assn.org/cgi/content/full/139/12/1540. Accessed March 16, 2009.

Mortimer PS, Lunniss PJ. Hidradentitis suppurativa. *J R Soc Med.* 2000; 93:420–422.

Moul DK, Korman NJ. Severe hidradenitis suppurativa treated with adalimumab. *Arch Dermatol.* September, 2006;142:1110–1112. Available at http://archderm.ama-assn.org/cgi/content/full/142/9/1110?maxtoshow=&HITS=10&hits=10&RESULTFORMAT=1&andorexacttitle=and&andorexacttitleabs=and&andorexactfulltext=and&searchid=1&FIRSTINDEX=0&sortspec=relevance&volume=142&firstpage=1110&resourcetype=HWCIT. Accessed March 16, 2009.

Shah N. Hidradenitis Suppurativa: a treatment challenge. *Am Fam Physician.* 2005 Oct;72:1547–1552. Available at http://www.aafp.org/afp/20051015/1547.html. Accessed March 16, 2009.

Ting PT, Barankin B. Brown macules on the checks. *Can Fam Physician.* 2005 March;51(3):353–355.

Eosinophilic Folliculitis

Barker S, Oakley A. Eosinophilic Folliculitis [DermNet NZ—Website]. Updated Dec. 2008, Available at, http://dermnetnz.org/acne/eosinophilic-folliculitis.html. Accessed March 17, 2009.

Eiland Gordon, Ridley David, "Dermatological Problems in the Athlete," *J Orthop Sports Phys Ther.* 1996 June;23(6):388–402.

Hayes BB, et al. Eosinophilic Folliculitis in 2 HIV-Positive Women. *Arch Dermatol.* 2004;140:463–465.

Rajendran PM, et al. Eosinophilic Folliculitis Before and After the Introduction of Antiretroviral Therapy. *Arch Dermatol.* 2005;141:1227–1231.

Carbuncle

Kabir OA. Olukayode O. Chidi EO. Ibe, CC. Kehinde AF. "Screening of crude extracts of six medicinal plants used in South-West Nigerian unorthodox medicine for anti-methicillin resistant *Staphylococcus aureus* activity," *BMC Complement Alt Med.* 2005 March; 5(6) Available at http://www.biomedcentral.com/content/pdf/ 1472–6882–5–6.pdf Accessed March 17, 2009.

Impetigo

Ernst E, Martin K. Herbal medicines for treatment of bacterial infections: a review of controlled clinical trials. *J Antimicrob Chemother.* 2003; 51:241–246.

George A, Rubin G. A systematic review and meta-analysis of treatments for impetigo. *B J Gen Pract.* 2003; 53:480–487.

Hawkins A. Mupirocin in the treatment of impetigo. *CMAJ.* 1990; 142:543–544.

Sladden MJ, Johnston GA. Clinical Review: Common skin infections in children. *BMJ Journal.* 2004; 329:95–99.

Taylor J. Interventions for Impetigo. *Am Fam Physician.* 2004; 70:1–3.

Skin Abscess

Okeniyi JAO, Olubanjo OO, Ogunlesi TA, Oyelami OA. Comparison of Healing of Incised Abscess Wounds with Honey and EUSOL Dressing. *J Alt Comp Med.* 2005; 11: 511–513.

Candidiasis

Clancy CJ, et al (ED). Immunoglobulin G Responses to a Panel of Candida albicans Antigens as Accurate and Early Markers for the Presence of Systemic Candidiasis. *J Clin Microbiol.* 2008 May; 46(5)1647–1654.

Tinea Infections

Noble SL, Forbes RC, Stamm PL. Diagnosis and Management of Common Tinea Infections. *Am Fam Physician.* 1998 July; 58(1):163–174 & 177–178.

Satchell AC, Saurajen A, Bell C, Barnetson RS. Treatment of interdigital tinea pedis with 25% and 50% tea tree oil solution: a randomized, placebo-controlled, blinded study. *Australas J Dermatol.* 43.3 (2002): 175–178.

Tan JS, Joseph WS. Common fungal infections of the feet in patients with diabetes mellitus. *Drugs Aging.* 2004;21(2):101–112.

Pediculosis

Burgess IF, Brown CM, Lee PN. Treatment of head louse infestation with 4% dimethicone lotion: randomized control equivalence trial. *BMJ.* 2005 June 18;330(7505):1423.

Vander Stichele RH, et al. Wet combing for head lice: feasibility in mass screening, treatment preference and outcome. *J R Soc Med.* 2002 July;95(7):348–352.

Flea Bites

Brown K, Bennett, M., Begon, M. Flea-Borne Bartonella grahamii and Bartonella taylorii in Bank Voles. *Emerg Infect Dis.* 2004 April;10 (4).

Scabies

Elston DM. Prevention of arthropod-related disease. *J Am Acad Dermatol.* 2004;51:947–54.

Freiman A, Barankin B, Elpern DJ. Sports dermatology part 2: swimming and other aquatic sports. *CMAJ.* 2004 November;171(11):1339–1341.

Naimer SA, Cohen AD, Mumcuoglu KY, Vardy DA. Household Papular Urticaria. *IMAJ.* 2002;4:911–913.

Steen CJ, Carbonaro PA. Arthropods in dermatology. *J Am Acad Dermatol.* 2004; 50:819–42.

Ting PT, Barankin B. Dermacase—Perioral Dermatitis. *Can Fam Physician.* 2006 Jan; 52: 35–36.

Acanthosis Nigricans

Kong AS, et al. Acanthosis Nigricans and diabetic risk factors: Prevalence in young persons seen in southwest US primary care practices. *Ann Fam Med.* 2007 May;5(3):202–208.

Vitiligo

Lepe V, Moncada B, Castanedo-Cazares JP, Torres-Alverez MB, Ortiz CA, Torres-Rubalcava AB. Double-blind Randomized Trial of 0.1% Tacroli-mus vs 0.05% Clobetasol for the Treatment of Childhood Vitiligo. *Arch Dermatol* 2003;139.

Szczurko O and Boon H. A systematic review of natural health product treatment for vitiligo. *BMC Dermatology* 2008;8:2.

Urticaria

Guldbakke K & Khachemoune A. Etiology, classification, and treatment of urticaria. *Cutis.* 2007;79: 41–49.

Iraji F, Sanghayi M, Mokhtari H, Siadat AH. Acupuncture in the treatment of urticaria: A double blind study. *Internet journal of dermatology.* 2006; 3(2): 5.

Mlynek A, et al. Update on chronic urticaria: focusing on mechanisms. *Curr Opin Allergy Clin Immunol.* 2008;8: 433–437.

Cutaneous Lupus Erythematosus

Current Treatment of Cutaneous Lupus Erythematosus. *Victoria Werth MDDermatology Online Journal* 7(1):2 Available at. http://dermatology.cdlib.org/DOJvol7num1/transactions/lupus/werth.html. Accessed March 17, 2009.

Mittal RR, Walia R.Clinico-histopathological study of subacute cutaneous lupus erythematous *Indian J Dermatol Venereol Leprol.* 2001 Jul-Aug; 67(4): 183–4.

Werth VP. Cutaneous lupus: insights into pathogenesis and disease classification. *Bull NYU Hosp Jt Dis.* 2007;65(3):200–4.

Cutaneous Vasculitis (Purpura)

Guillevin L, Domer T. Vasculitis: mechanisms involved and clinical manifestations. *Arthritis Res Ther.* 2007 August 15;9(suppl2):S9.

Herpes Simplex and Herpes Zoster

Gaby AR. Natural Remedies for Herpes Simplex. *Altern Med Rev.* 2006 Jun;11(2):93–101.

Nossaman N. "A Case of Herpes Zoster." *Am J Homeopathic Med.* 2006;99(3); 225–226.

Thomas S, et al. Micronutrient intake and the risk of herpes zoster: a case-control study. *Int J Epidemiol.* 2006;35(2):307–314. Available at http://ije.oxfordjournals.org/cgi/-content/abstract/35/2/307 Accessed. March 17, 2009.

Tyring Stephen K. Management of herpes zoster and postherpetic neuralgia. *J Am Dermatol.* 2007;57: S136–S142.

Weinberg Jeffrey M. Herpes zoster: Epidemiology, natural history, and common complications. *J Am Acad Dermatol.* 2007;57:S130–S135.

Viral Warts

Bohlooli S, et al. Comparative Study of Fig Tree Efficacy in the Treatment of Common Warts (Verruca Vulgaris) vs. cryotherapy. *Int J Dermatol.* 2007 April; 46: 524–526.

Focht D, Spicer C, and Fairchok M. The Efficacy of Duct Tape vs Cryotherapy in the Treatment of Verruca Vulgaris (the Common Wart). *Arch Ped Adol Med.* 2002 Oct:156.

Rahimi AR, Emad M and Rezaian G. Smoke from Leaves of Populus Euphratica Olivier vs. Conventional Cryotherapy for the Treatment of Cutaneous Warts: a Pilot, Randomized, Single-Blind, Prospective Study, *Int J Dermatol.* 2008 March;47: 393–397.

Molluscum Contagiosum

Grichnick J. Ed. Dermascopy of Molluscum Contagiosum. *Arch Dermatol.* 2005 Dec; 141: 1644.

Hanson D, Diven D. Molluscum Contagiosum. *Dermatology Online Journal.* Vol9, Number2. Available at http://dermatology.cdlib.org/92/reviews/molluscum/diven.html. Accessed March 17, 2009.

Viral Exanthemas (Incl. Measles, Chicken Pox)

Chang Luan-Yin, King Chwan-Chuen, et al. Risk Factors of Enterovirus 71 Infection and Associated Hand, Foot, and Mouth Disease/Herpangina in Children During an Epidemic in Taiwan. *Pediatrics.* 2002;109:e88.

Chang Luan-Yin, Huang Li-Min, et al. Neurodevelopment and Cognition in Children after Enterovirus 71 Infection. *N Engl J Med.* 2007 March; 356(12): 1226–1234.

Chen Kow-Tong, Chang Hasiao-Ling, et al. Epidemiologic Features of Hand-Foot-Mouth Disease and Herpangina Caused by Enterovirus 71 in Taiwan, 1998 2005. *Pediatrics.* 2007; 120:244–252.

Hussey GD, Klein M. A Randomized, Controlled Trial of Vitamin A in Children with Severe Measles. *N Engl J Med.* 1990, July; 323:160–16.

Robertson SE, Cochi SL. Preventing Rubella: Assessing Missed Opportunities for Immunization. *Am J Pub Health.* 2006;77:1347–1349.

Servey JT, Reamy BV, Hodge J. Clinical presentations of parvovirus B19 infection. *Am Fam Physician.* 2007 Feb;75(3):373–376.

Sharan S, Sharma S. Congenital rubella cataract: a timely reminder in the new millennium? *Clin Exper Ophthalmol.* 2006;34:83–84.

Weir E. Parvovirus B19 infection: fifth disease and more. *CMAJ.* 2005 Mar; 172(6):743.

Wilkins J, Leedom LM. Clinical Rubella with Arthritis Resulting from Reinfection. *Ann Int Med.* 2006; 77:930.

Hyperhidrosis

Chang Y, et al. Treatment of Palmar Hyperhidrosis. *Ann Surg.* 2007, August. 246(2):330–336.

Haider A, Solish N. Focal hyperhidrosis: diagnosis and management. *CMAJ.* 2005, January 4;172(1): 69–75.

Robertson SE, Cochi SL. Preventing Rubella: Assessing Missed Opportunities for Immunization. *Am J Pub Health.* 2006;77:1347–1349.

Stolman, LP. Hyperhidrosis Medical and surgical treatment. *Eplasty.* 2008 April 18;8:e22.

Therapeutics and Formulary

The various therapeutic methods or agents discussed in this chapter are shown in the following chart:

Category	Therapeutic Method or Agent
Procedures	1. Cryotherapy
	2. Dermabrasion and exfoliation
	3. Hair removal
	4. Hydrotherapy—hot water therapy
	5. Iontophoresis with salicylic acid
	6. Ultraviolet light
Natural oils	7. Almond oil
	8. Lanolin
	9. Mineral oil
	10. Olive oil
	11. Evening primrose oil
	12. Tea tree oil
	13. Vaseline—white petroleum jelly
Vitamins	14. Vitamin A
	15. Vitamin D
	16. Vitamin E
Minerals	17. Colloidal silver
	18. Epsom salt
	19. Iodine/Potassium iodide
	20. Sodium bicarbonate
	21. Zinc oxide
Natural Products	22. Aloe vera
	23. Apple cider vinegar
	24. Black walnut
	25. Burdock
	26. Calendula
	27. Chamomile
	28. Chaparral
	29. Comfrey
	30. Cornstarch
	31. Elderberry
	32. Garlic
	33. Ginger
	34. Goldenseal
	35. Green tea
	36. Lemon
	37. Oatmeal
	38. Onion
	39. Undecycline
	40. White willow bark
	41. Witch hazel

Category	Therapeutic Method or Agent
Over-the-counter products	42. Antibiotics
	43. Calamine
	44. Hydrocortisone
	45. Hydrogen peroxide
Miscellaneous	46. Dimethysulfoxide
	47. Menthol
	48. Talc
	49. Normal saline and water
	50. Urea

Part 1: Procedures

1. Cryotherapy

History: Cryotherapy, the use of cold, to treat conditions primarily of the skin, dates back to the Egyptians who used it to treat the effects of inflammation. Cold and ice have been used to aid in the amputation of limbs and slow the growth of surface tumors. In the early 1900s, as science developed, the use of agents such as solid carbon dioxide which freezes at −78.5° C became the primary agent. Oxygen which is liquid at −182.9° C was first used in approximately 1920, but due to its combustibility was not used long. Then in 1950 liquid nitrogen, which is a liquid at −196° C, became the primary cryotherapeutic agent.

Cryosurgery is the technique used to effectively freeze an area to cause irreversible tissue destruction leading to the removal of a skin lesion.

Dermatological Application: Medically cryotherapy / cryosurgery is used for the following:
- Actinic keratosis.
- Cherry angioma.
- Common warts.
- Dermafibroma.
- Hypertrophic scars.
- Ingrown nails.
- Keloids.
- Keratosis.
- Myxoid cysts.
- Pyogenic granulomas.

- Removal of tattoos.
- Sebaceous hyperplasia.
- Skin tags.
- Solar lentigo.
- Headaches.
- Relief from Herpes zoster pain.
- Common warts.
- Reduce pain of local infections.
- Reduce effects of allergic reactions such as Poison Ivy or Poison Oak.

Toxicity: Cryotherapy stings and may be painful at the time of application, as well as for a variable period afterwards. There may be immediate swelling and redness. This may be reduced by applying a topical steroid on a single occasion directly after freezing. Complications can be divided into acute, delayed, prolonged-temporary, and permanent. Acute complications include headache, pain, and blister formation. Delayed complications include hemorrhage, infection, and excessive granulation formation. Prolonged-temporary complications include milia, hyperpigmentation, and change in sensation. Permanent complications include alopecia, atrophy, keloids, scarring, hypopigmentation, and ectropion formation.

Directions for Therapeutic Use: Cryotherapy for headaches, muscle pain and inflammation includes ice packs and cold packs. These can be placed over the affected area for ten to twenty minutes until a slight numbing is noticed. Excessive lengths of time can lead to freezing the area.

Cryotherapy for Herpes zoster, allergic reactions and local infections is the use of ice. Rubbing ice over the area is very cooling, numbing and slows the inflammatory process. When dealing with Herpes zoster prevent the water from running onto cloths, bedding or other areas of the body in order to prevent spread.

Cryotherapy for common warts is over-the-counter (OTC) liquid nitrogen products. Since these products will cause some local tissue damage, dress the area to prevent further damage to the skin and prevent infection. After the blister ruptures apply some Vaseline to keep the skin moist and prevent infection until the area is healed.

2. Dermabrasion and Exfoliation

History: Dermabrasion has been used as a treatment for the skin for more than 100 years. The technique has changed greatly over time; however the basic sanding or planing concept has remained consistent. This technique fell out of favor for some time in the early 1900s due to some of the side effects. However, in the 1960s, dermabrasion experienced a large resurgence. Because of this increase in popularity, the resurfacing techniques have been continuously improved upon over the last several decades.

Microdermabrasion was introduced into medical offices several years ago. Basically a form of sandblasting the skin, these machines contain either aluminum or salt crystals that hit the skin at high speeds and are simultaneously vacuumed away along with the cellular debris that they remove.

Exfoliation is the means of removing dry dead cells from the surface of the skin by either a mechanical or chemical means. Mechanical exfoliation includes such things as a body rub with salt, sugar or coffee grounds. Another mechanical way is dry skin brushing. Dry skin brushing is not only very effective at removing dead skin cells, but is also effective in stimulating the circulatory and lymphatic systems. Stimulation of the lymphatic system is important for developing a strong immune system. Chemical exfoliation uses enzymes, and alpha or beta hydroxyl acids. This type of exfoliation process may be very mild and performed at home using a Loofa brush, while others are very aggressive and need to be performed by a dermatologist.

Dermatological Applications

- Scarring (from acne, smallpox, or trauma).
- Liver spots.
- Wrinkles.
- Moles.
- Tattoos.
- Blackheads.
- Dry skin.
- Calluses.
- Corns.

Toxicity: The procedure is not toxic. However, there are several side effects that need to be considered. The procedure can lead to uneven changes in the skin, which may be temporary or permanent. There may be darkening of the skin on either a temporary or permanent basis. These changes can often be avoided by carefully following patient instructions regarding sun exposure and aftercare. Additionally, there is a small risk of scar formation and there is potential for infection.

Directions for Therapeutic Use: For two weeks preceding the treatment, the patient will be required to apply a topical cream that will help to prevent postprocedural infection. It is also the patient's responsibility to inform the doctor of any changes in the skin that is to be treated. Specifically, the patient must report the occurrence of any cold sores. With surgical microdermabrasion, do not drink alcohol for 48 hours after the surgery, do not take aspirin or any products that contain aspirin or ibuprofen for one week after the surgery, avoid smoking, as advised by your doctor, and attend your follow-up appointments.

Microdermabrasion causes skin to look pink, feel dry and tight (like sunburn or windburn), for about 24 hours. Moisturizers and sun block (SPF 15) should be applied after the procedure. Avoidance of direct sunlight for several days is advised.

Skin brushing is best done before showering or bathing when the skin is completely dry. Brush the entire body, except the face. Brush always moving toward the heart to assist lymphatic drainage. Start with the feet, moving from the bottom of the legs toward the heart. Then do the hands, and move up the arms. Use the long handle, and brush the low back up through the spine, over the shoulders to the heart. Then brush the abdomen starting in the lower abdominal area and brush up toward the chest and heart. A special face brush may be used on the face.

3. Hair Removal

History: Hair removal is performed for many reasons, the most common for cosmetic appearances.

Hair can be removed by shaving which cuts the hair shaft at the level of the skin. This is not permanent and will need to be repeated frequently. Bleaching does not remove the hair but makes it much less noticeable. Plucking pulls each hair shaft out of its follicle.

Waxing removes hairs from a larger area. As the wax cools the hairs are embedded into it and when cooled completely the wax is quickly pulled off pulling the hairs out of the follicles at the same time.

Electrolysis is the use of a small amount of electricity gently applied to the base of the hair follicle which destroys the tissue at the base of the hair follicle and thus disables its regenerative capability. Electrolysis was invented in 1875 when Dr. Charles Michel, an ophthalmologist, tried to

identify a new way to remove in-grown eyelashes. He developed this technique by inserting a small gauge wire connected to a battery into the skin surrounding the follicle and disseminated a small amount of electricity, destroying the regenerative cells. Electrolysis of today is nearly the same process using modern day equipment.

Pulsed-light systems work with high intensity light being emitted in pulses. This high intensity light is absorbed by the pigment in hair follicles and turned to heat which then destroys the follicular cell inhibiting hair growth.

Laser hair removal uses laser energy to heat the shaft of the hair which in turn heats the hair follicle. The heat is intense enough to force the follicle into the telogen or resting phase of hair growth, thus reducing the rate of hair growth temporarily or permanently.

Dermatological Application
- Hirsuitism.
- Medical (micro-organisms, ingrown hairs, body odor).
- Cosmetic.
- Surgical (e.g. hairy warts).

Toxicity: The most common side effects of hair removal are redness, swelling, scabs and crusts resulting from cuts or abrasions, ingrown hair, folliculitis, dryness, flaking and itching due to not moisturizing the area afterwards, skin infections, discoloration of skin and scarring.

Directions for Therapeutic Use: Any method of hair removal disrupts the integrity of the skin to some degree. In preparation, have the area clean, dry and free of any fragrances, lotions or cosmetics, unless prescribed by the practitioner. Following the procedure, follow the prescribed directions of the clinic. In general, keep the area clean and dry and protected with a moisturizer. With some of the procedures, such as laser and electrolysis, limit sun exposure for 2–4 days and when outside use at least a UV 15 sunblock.

4. Hydrotherapy—Hot Water Therapy

History: Hydrotherapy is the generic term indicating the use of hot water, steam or cold water in treating a patient. The use of hot water as a therapeutic modality goes back to ancient Chinese civilization. It is primarily used now as a physical therapy modality. Modalities include general baths, regional baths (such as sitz baths), showers, steam baths, whirlpools, compresses, wraps or hot fomentations. Hot water therapy has been used effectively for back pain, respiratory conditions, hypertension, muscle spasm, arthritic pain, stress management, weight loss and detoxifying the body.

It is effective in soothing nerves, stimulating the immune system and calming and relaxing the body. Heat stimulates the dilation of capillaries and increases blood flow through the area.

Dermatological Application

- Acne.
- Carbuncles.
- Folliculitis.
- Abscess.
- Local infections.
- Poison Ivy.
- Hordeolum.
- Dry skin.
- Splinter or other small imbedded object.

Toxicity: Hot compresses and hot water therapies are considered safe but caution must be used to prevent burns and scalding the patient.

Directions for Therapeutic Use: A hot compress is made by taking a standard wash cloth and soaking it in hot water, then applying it to the target area. Hold the wash cloth in place until cooled, re-warm the cloth and reapply. Apply the compress several times throughout the day until the acne pustule, carbuncle, hordeolum or abscess comes to a head, ruptures and drains.

A sitz bath is a bath used to soak an area of the body or the whole body in order to bring about relief from pain or itch. For pain and calming, an Epsom salt bath is made by adding 2 cups to a warm bath. For control of itch, 2 cups of oatmeal or corn starch may be added to the bath.

An alternating hot and cold shower may be used to stimulate the immune system and thyroid function. It is performed by first warming the body with a warm water shower followed by cold water for 30 seconds to a minute then return to warm water. This may be repeated a number of times but always start and finish with warm water.

5. Iontophoresis with salicylic acid

History: Iontophoresis uses a galvanic current to transmit chemical ions into and through the skin. Like electrical charges repel each other, and a low volt DC current is used to repel or drive electrically charged ions into the skin and underlying soft tissues. The negative pole repels acids, such as salicylic acid, driving it into the skin while attracting alkaline substances, hydrogen and water causing a relaxation of the softens tissues, and dilation of the local blood vessels. The most common medications delivered by iontophoresis are anesthetics, analgesics, and anti-inflammatory agents.

Salicylic acid has primarily been studied as a treatment for plantar warts, which are often more difficult to treat because of the thickness of skin on the soles of the feet. Treatment of warts is often aimed at eliciting an inflammatory response by applying an irritant, such as salicylic acid. A liquid or cream of salicylic acid is applied to the wart then a galvanic current is applied causing a deeper penetration, decreasing treatment time and number of applications necessary.

Dermatological Application

- Acute and chronic skin inflammation.
- Arthritis.
- Hyperhidrosis.
- Warts.

Toxicity: Iontophoresis comes with very few side effects. Erythema of the skin may result after the treatment where the pads were placed. Burns are possible below the delivery and/or the return electrode if the amperage is set too high. The medication being delivered may cause local or systemic adverse reactions.

The most common adverse reaction to salicylic acid is a local chemical burning.

Directions for Therapeutic Use: A dispersal pad is placed 8–10 inches away from the treatment pad and, in the case of plantar warts of the foot, on the ipsilateral gastrocnemius muscle. The active or treating electrode soaked with 2% sodium salicylate solution is applied over the plantar wart or cluster of warts. Patients are instructed that they might feel an itchy or prickly sensation with treatment and to notify the doctor if they feel a burning sensation, which might indicate skin burning. The current is then slowly adjusted to the maximum tolerable current for the patient, with a recommended treatment time of 25 minutes. Patients generally show significant improvement in 3 weeks with weekly treatment.

6. Ultraviolet Light

History: Ultraviolet (UV) light is a form of radiation that is not visible to the human eye, making up part of the electromagnetic spectrum that is invisible. These are emitted naturally from the sun or can be administered artificially via special

UV lamps. There are three forms of ultra violet light UVA, UVB, and UVC. Short wavelength UVC is absorbed by the ozone and does not harm people. The UV light which affects the skin is the long wave UVA, and intermediate wave UVB. UV light helps to power some of the chemical reactions in the skin cells such as the formation of Vitamin D. However, overexposure of UVB and UVA can cause burns and lead to skin disease. Burning the skin can cause premature aging and predispose patients to skin cancer. Patients need to take precautions to protect their skin at all times with sun block and UV blocking clothing when outdoors.

Narrowband UVB is the latest Ultraviolet Light therapy. Narrow-band UVB refers to a specific wavelength of ultraviolet (UV) radiation, 311 to 312 nm. This range has proved to be the most beneficial wavelength of natural sunlight.

Dermatological Applications

- Psoriasis.
- Dry, itchy, scaly skin.
- Atopic dermatitis.
- Allergic dermatitis.
- Acne.
- Cutaneous T-cell lymphoma.
- Vitiligo.
- Herpes zoster or Shingles.

Toxicity: Acute overexposure of ultraviolet light can lead to burns and skin damage. The severity of the burn is directly related to both the intensity and length of exposure. Chronic overexposure of UV light may eventually cause squamous or basal cell carcinoma.

Directions for Therapeutic Use: Patient should be advised to completely expose the area that needs to be treated throughout the prescribed treatment time. Failure to expose the area for an adequate amount of time will diminish the results, and overexposure of the area will lead to skin damage

▓ Part 2: Natural Oils

7. Almond Oil

History: Almond oil is derived from the pressed ripe seeds of the almond tree. There are two types of almonds, sweet almond which does not contain amygdaline and bitter almond which does. Amygdaline is a naturally occurring compound containing protein-bound cyanide which causes a bitter taste. Each of these is different in their composition and use. Historically, sweet almond oil was used on smallpox infections to prevent scarring. The main dermatological use for almond oil today is for moisturizing, pruritis and inflammation of the skin. Almond oil, being a carrier oil, is one that can be mixed with other essential oils or compounds in order to provide multiple benefits. It is a nourishing, smooth and silky, easy to apply oil. Many moisturizers today contain sweet almond oil for added benefits.

Sweet almond traditionally has been used as an antibacterial, for chapped lips, an emollient, a moisturizer while bitter almond traditionally has been used as an antibacterial, an antiinflammatory agent, antipruritic, a local anesthetic, a muscle relaxant, and in the treatment of psoriasis. Bitter almond oil contains a compound that when hydrolyzed releases cyanide, therefore, this compound must be removed from the oil before it is used on the skin.

External use of the oil has many benefits for the skin and can be especially useful in the treatment of conditions that are characteristically dry and scaly. Almonds are a major source of natural vitamin E in the alpha-tocopherol form and contain such essential oils as Palmitic Acid, Stearic Acid, Oleic Acid, and Linoleic Acid.

Dermatological Applications

- Atopic dermatitis.
- Eczema.
- Acne.
- Sunburn.
- Psoriasis.
- Ichthyosis.
- Xerosis (dry skin).
- Rosacea.

Toxicity: Sweet almond (from trees with solid pink flowers) ingestion has shown no adverse effects except for those associated with an allergic response. Topical use also may result in allergic responses of swelling and may in severe cases of almond nut allergy, cause anaphylactic reaction. The bitter almonds (from trees whose flowers are red or pink at the base and white at the tip of the pedal) contain amygdalin, which when hydrolyzed releases hydrocyanic acid which is highly toxic.

Directions for Therapeutic Use: Pure almond oil can be applied directly to the skin as a moisturizing agent after bathing or washing.

Ground almonds may be added to almond oil, soaps or creams and rubbed on the skin to act as an exfoliant. After the application rinse the area with warm water, pat dry and apply moisturizer or almond oil to the area.

Pure almond oil may be added to other moisturizers to enhance the action effect due to the natural oils it contains.

Almond oil may also be used as carrier oil. It provides the base for the addition of other essential oils. Many essential oils may be too strong and irritating to the skin. By diluting them, the active components are carried into the skin and the irritating effect is diminished.

8. Lanolin

History: Lanolin, a waste product in wool processing known also as wool wax, wool fat, or wool grease, is a greasy, yellow substance extracted from the fibers of sheep's wool. This substance is secreted from the skin of sheep and gets trapped in the sheep's wool, giving the sheep protection from rain and moisture. This natural secretion is very similar to the oils that secrete from our own skin. Lanolin's chemical composition is chiefly a mixture of cholesterol and the esters of several fatty acids. If water is added to lanolin, it forms an emulsion which will enhance the moisturizing properties. Lanolin is thick, similar to petroleum jelly. When it is applied to the skin, lanolin seals the body's moisture in and protects it from dry air. There are two forms of lanolin used as treatment. Hydrous lanolin contains 25% to 30% water, while the anhydrous form will contain no more than 0.25% water. Lanolin has multiple uses, and in health care it is used as a cream to soothe dry scaly skin conditions. Lanolin is considered a heavy duty moisturizer and emollient that can be used on dry, rough, and chapped skin. It is also used as a lubricant, and it is found in some hair conditioners to lock in moisture and soften hair.

Dermatological Application
- Xerosis (dry, red, flaky skin).
- Chapped lips.
- Diaper rash.
- Psoriasis.
- Eczema.
- Rough dry skin on the feet.
- Minor cuts and abrasions.
- Breast nipples during nursing.
- Barrier against secondary infections.

Toxicity: Lanolin is for external, topical use only. When use topically, there are no known contrain-

dications or adverse effects recorded. There have been rare complaints of allergic contact dermatitis reactions to lanolin. Ingestion of lanolin may cause gastrointestinal irritation. Mothers who use lanolin for breast feeding should wipe off the lanolin before nursing.

Directions for Therapeutic Use: For nursing mothers, a pea-sized amount may be applied to the nipple to prevent chapping, cracking and drying. Lanolin does not need to be removed during feeding but the infant will feed better when it is removed. Lanolin should be re-applied after each feeding.

For dry chapped, cracked hands, application of anhydrous lanolin twice a day reduces the dryness, cracking, redness, and itching. For diaper rash, the area should be cleaned well and allowed to dry before application of lanolin or a lanolin-based product.

9. Mineral Oil

History: Mineral oil is a clear, odorless liquid. It is a derivative of petroleum and is known as baby oil or white oil. Mineral oil has been used in the manufacture of soaps, moisturizing creams, and lotions to create a protective barrier on the skin to reduce water loss to the environment.

The uses of mineral oil are quite varied. It can be used in cleaning ears by softening the ear wax in preparation for removal. Mineral oil is used as an ingredient in many dermatological products, including baby lotions and oil, cold creams, ointments, and some cosmetics. Mineral oil is used as an ingredient in various eye drops. Mineral oil is used as a cathartic to treat constipation. It also has industrial uses as a lubricant for metal working, the textile industry and acts as a base and thinning agent in the paint industry.

Dermatological Applications
- Eczema, including seborrheic.
- Psoriasis.
- Pediculosis.
- Myiasis (infestation by the larvae of *Diptera*).
- Xerosis.
- Swimmers itch.
- Ear wax.
- Dry, brittle hair.

Toxicity: Mineral oil can be used safely and effectively with no side effects. Burning, stinging, redness, or irritation may occur if the patient is sensitive. However, allergic reactions to mineral oil are rare. Fragrances added to the oil are the primary cause of an allergic reaction.

Mineral oil may cause irritation to the respiratory tract if inhaled. It is a cathartic and may cause nausea, vomiting or diarrhea if ingested.

Mineral oil may also be photoallergic meaning that atopic dermatitis may result with extended exposure to heat or the sun. This may result from the oil film on the skin that prevents the body form absorbing oxygen and from eliminating toxins and other waste products.

Directions for Therapeutic Use: Clean the area of skin before applying mineral oil to avoid trapping anything that may be harmful against the skin. Areas to avoid include eyes, inside the mouth and nose, as well as the groin unless directed by a physician. Avoid using mineral oil on broken skin like cuts, scrapes, and skin that has been recently shaved.

Dry, scaly skin may either by treated by applying the mineral oil directly to the skin or by adding the oil to bath water during bathing. If bathing results are not satisfactory, the patient should try applying the mineral oil directly to the skin immediately following a bath or shower.

For infestation of lice, mineral oil can be applied to hair after washing the hair. The oil should entirely coat the hair. With lice and other parasitic infestations mineral oil should completely coat the area at all times.

For ear wax removal, place 2 to 3 drops of mineral oil into the ear canal with the patient lying on their side. Let it disperse in the ear for 5 minutes then put a small wad of cotton in the outer canal to prevent oil from draining onto the clothes. Typically the wax can easily be syringed from the ear after an overnight use of oil.

10. Olive Oil

History: Olive oil is extracted from crushed olives and has been used since the ancient times, when the Hebrews used it in religious ceremonies.

Olive oil has historically been used for fuel in oil lamps, as a cleanser for athletes, as a symbol relating to health and strength and, of special note, it has been used as a medicinal agent. It is very curious to note that even in ancient time olive oil was useful for its overall health benefits. Today the known benefits relating to health range from improving cardiovascular disease, decreasing blood pressure, enhancing the appearance of the skin, as well as its excellent antioxidant prop-

erties. Olive oil has been used for many years as a moisturizing agent and is added to soaps, cosmetics, shampoos and conditioners due to its rich, moisturizing properties.

Olive oil can be used topically, ingested as part of the diet or used for cooking.

Dermatological Applications
- Wound healing and dressing.
- Eczema, including seborrheic and atopic.
- Xerosis.
- Rosacea.
- Psoriasis.
- Thermal radiation and minor burns.
- Ear wax.
- Stretch marks (prevention and reduction of).
- Protection from UV light damage.

Toxicity: There is no known toxicity associated with olive oil. However, if skin irritation arises discontinue use. An allergy to olives can cause an allergic contact dermatitis with the presence of dry scaly skin, fissures and occasional vesicular eczema. These patients will have a positive patch test to olives and olive oil.

Directions for Therapeutic Use: Ear wax can be removed by placing 2 to 3 drops of olive oil into the ear canal with the patient lying on their side. Let it disperse in the ear for 5 minutes, then put a small wad of cotton in the outer canal to prevent oil from draining onto the clothes. After overnight application, the wax may be removed by syringing the ear.

Stretch marks are treated by rubbing the oil into the skin as a moisturizer.

For minor burns of all types, put a thin film of oil over the surface with a soft cloth or cotton applicator.

For wound healing, saturate a piece of gauze, cover the wound then cover with an occlusive bandage.

Skin conditions such as eczema, psoriasis and seborrhea gently rub the oil into the area this will soften any scales and crusts.

11. Evening Primrose Oil

History: Evening Primrose, also known as Oenothera biennis, was named by the Greek physician Theophrastus and is a native plant of North America. It has yellow flowers that bloom only in the evening, hence its name, and the seeds of the plant are used as the source of the Evening Primrose Oil (EPO). All parts of the plant can be used and its young leaves, fruit and root can be eaten raw or steamed as a food source. EPO is a source of Gamma-Linolenic Acid (GLA) a long chain fatty acid.

Dermatological Applications

- Eczema.
- Atopic dermatitis.
- Allergic dermatitis.
- Ichthyosis vulgaris.
- Psoriasis.
- Hives.

Toxicity: The oil is generally well-tolerated when taken orally, with occasional reports of headache, gastrointestinal upset and decreased blood pressure. Topically, the oil rarely causes an allergic reaction. Patients taking anti-epileptic medication should explore other treatment options, as there have been reports of increased seizure activity with EPO.

Directions for Therapeutic Uses. Topically Evening Primrose Oil can be applied directly to the skin. It acts to moisturize and soften the skin.

Orally, for adults 4 to 8 grams per day can be taken and for children 3 grams per day in divided doses.

12. Tea Tree Oil

History: Tea tree oil (TTO) is a volatile essential oil that is obtained by steam distillation of the leaves of Melaleuca alternifolia, a plant native to Australia. The indigenous Bundjalung people used the crushed leaves of the plant to treat coughs and upper respiratory infections and skin wounds. Use of the extracted oil began in the 1920s after Penfold published papers on the antibacterial effects of the oil which he described as 11 times more active than phenol, a common disinfectant at the time. There is good evidence for the use of tea tree oil as an antibacterial, antiviral, and acaricidal agent. TTO is composed of terpene hydrocarbons and their associated alcohols. Terpenes are volatile, aromatic hydrocarbons. TTO is regulated and defined by international standards which specify the levels of 14 components which are needed to define the oil as tea tree oil.

Dermatological Applications

- Tinea pedis (athlete's foot).
- Dandruff.
- Oral candidiasis.
- Acne.
- Eczema.

- Local infections and sores on mucous membranes (canker sores, boils, abscesses).
- Scabies.
- Staphylococcus aureus infections.
- Dandruff.
- Onychomycosis.

Toxicity: Topical use of Tea Tree Oil is generally safe but may cause mild contact dermatitis, blisters or rashes are self-limiting and can be avoided by lowering the concentration. Tea tree oil should not be taken internally, even in small quantities. It can cause impaired immune function, diarrhea, and potentially fatal central nervous system depression (excessive drowsiness, sleepiness, confusion, and coma).

Directions for Therapeutic Use: Tea Tree Oil should be stored in a dark, cool place, preferably in a dark colored bottle and best purchased in 1 or 2 ounce quantities. Light, heat, exposure to air, and moisture will affect TTO's stability.

Patients with a staphylococcus aureus infection should use a 4% tea tree oil body wash in the shower followed by a 10% tea tree oil cream after the skin has dried. A bandage may be applied over the sore.

The treatment for acne, a tea tree oil gel should be applied once or twice a day for three months.

For the treatment of Scabies, the patient should be advised to take off their contaminated clothing, apply the ointment and wait at least three hours before contact with others. Scabies mites are usually killed by the Tea Tree Oil within 3 hours. The family members of the patient should also be treated with the ointment simultaneously due to the highly contagious nature. All clothing and sheets should be washed and the house should be thoroughly cleaned.

13. Vaseline—White Petroleum

History: Robert Chesebrough discovered the substance in 1859. Petroleum jelly is a mixture of saturated petroleum hydrocarbons and is predominantly branched chain hydrocarbons. Petroleum jelly, or petrolatum, is a byproduct of refining petroleum, made from the residue of petroleum distillation left in the still after all the oil has been vaporized. It is thick and greasy, translucent in color, and odorless.

Historically petroleum jelly was used on cuts and burns that the refinery workers experienced. Chesebrough's patent includes stuffing, currying, and oiling of all kinds of leathers. New mothers use it as an absorbent shield for diaper rash. Professionals working in an extremely cold temperature use it to relieve their dry chapped skin. Even Commander Robert Perry, the first man to reach the north-pole, took Vaseline because it wouldn't freeze. Soldiers carried the substance in WWI to treat cuts and bruises, and to prevent sunburn. During WWII, it was used to produce a sterile antiseptic wound dressing. Some of the finest quality petroleum jelly was used as pomade for styling hair.

Dermatological Application

- Eczemas, including pityriasis alba, lichen simplex chronicus.
- Psoriasis.
- Ichthyosis.
- Prevent skin drying from sun exposure or UV treatment.
- Protect skin of premature infants.
- Xerosis.
- Minor burns, cuts and bruises.

Toxicity: Petroleum jelly is a very safe, nontoxic substance that, when used alone, has no known side effects. It is petroleum based and is very flammable. It also interacts with latex causing gloves and condoms to fail. When used on the mucous membranes of the nose to prevent drying and bleeding use only a thin coat so as not to limit the ability of the nasal cilia from cleaning the air that is breathed.

Directions for Therapeutic Use: The substance can be applied topically to any surface of the body except the surface of the eye. It is applied on an as needed basis to the skin or lips as a protective barrier or moisturizer.

Part 3: Vitamins

14. Vitamin A

History: Vitamin A is an antioxidant used in the treatment of a variety of dermatological conditions. Vitamin A (Retinol) is one of the fifteen different twenty-carbon molecules with various groups on the 15th carbon that collectively make up the family of chemical compounds called *retinoids*. They are used systemically and topically and contain properties that benefit the skin on a structural level. Vitamin A protects cells from oxidative damage and acts as a hormone to activate genes which inhibit lipid peroxidation, increase vitamin E levels, and activate growth factors.

Dermatological Applications

- Acne.
- Eczema, including seborrheic.
- Psoriasis.
- Herpes simplex.
- Wounds, sunburn, sunspots.
- Grover's disease.
- Ichthyosis.
- Lichen planus.
- Keratosis pilaris.
- Wrinkles.
- Lentigo.

Toxicity: Vitamin A toxicity, or hypervitaminosis A, is rare in the general population and the toxicity level varies from person to person. It can occur with excessive amounts of vitamin A taken over short or long periods of time. Consequently, toxicity can be acute or chronic. An infant with acute toxicity can develop a bulging fontanelle and symptoms similar to a brain tumor. Adults experience less specific symptoms such as headache, dizziness, fatigue, malaise, blurry vision, bone pain and swelling, nausea, and/or vomiting. Severe toxicity can lead to eye damage, high levels of calcium, and liver damage. People with liver disease and high alcohol intake may be at risk for hepatotoxicity from vitamin A supplementation.

Topical Vitamin A toxicity is much less severe. It increases sensitivity to sun and may lead to skin irritation resulting in redness, dryness and peeling.

Directions for Therapeutic Use: When beginning Vitamin A (retinoid) skin treatment, use it on alternate nights. Approximately 30 minutes after washing the area apply the oil or cream and rub into the skin as a moisturizer. Apply less often, or remove after one hour if irritation results. The skin gradually accommodates to the vitamin allowing more frequent usage. Use sunscreen on the treated areas as the skin is more sensitive to the UV waves of the sun.

15. Vitamin D

History: Vitamin D is a chemical that is produced in the skin or consumed in food that has systemic effects on the rest of the body. Vitamin D is actually a group of fat-soluble prohormones. The two major forms are D2 (ergocalciferol) and D3 (cholecalciferol). Vitamin D is unique in that it is the only vitamin that is a biologically active hormone. Vitamin D is responsible for absorbing calcium and phosphorus from food and re-absorption of calcium in the kidneys. It also promotes bone formation and mineralization and promotes immunosuppression, phagocytosis, and has anti-tumor activity.

Until recent studies, vitamin D was used primarily to influence the calcium-phosphorus absorption and balance. Currently, vitamin D is being used to aid in the control of dermatological conditions as well.

Dermatological Applications

- Antiproliferative agent for keratinocytes.
- Stimulator of epidermal cell differentiation.
- Psoriasis.

Toxicity: When Vitamin D is applied topically and taken in high doses orally, toxic levels may be attained. Patients diagnosed with hypercalcemia or hypervitaminosis D should not use Vitamin D topically or orally. Hypercalcemia may elicit symptoms such as nausea, vomiting, weakness, headache, dry mouth, constipation, metallic taste, muscle pain, and bone pain.

Directions for Therapeutic Use: Vitamin D is available for topical use in oil, cream and lotion formulas. It can be applied to the area of skin that is of concern as a moisturizer. Calcium and phosphorous levels should be checked periodically to prevent any adverse effects.

16. Vitamin E

History: Vitamin E is one of the best known antioxidants and is used in foods including vegetable oils, cereal grains, animal fats, meat, poultry, eggs, fruits and vegetables to slow spoiling. Its biological function is to protect fats, a major part of cell membranes, from free radical damage. Vitamin E is not a single compound, but a group of eight isomers: alpha, beta, gamma, and delta tocopherols and alpha, beta, gamma tocotrienols. Although vitamin E exists in these different forms, supplemental vitamin E usually consists of the alpha-tocopherol form due to it being the most active in the body. Biochemically, vitamin E can be further classified by the D/L-system. The D isomer is the most active form of Vitamin E.

Dermatological Application

- Burns.
- Scars, both surgical and traumatic.
- Acne.
- Aging skin.
- Bee stings and other insect bites.
- Cutaneous candidiasis.

- Alopecia.
- Frost bite.
- Lentigo.
- Oral leukoplakia.
- Xerosis.

Toxicity: Topical administration of vitamin E does not have an upper tolerable limit and does not cause any side effects when used within the recommended dose. Side effects associated with excessive use of topical vitamin E may include dryness of the skin, contact dermatitis, an inflammatory reaction and eczematous lesions. Use should be discontinued if these or any other reactions occur.

Directions for Therapeutic Use: It is recommended the patient applies vitamin E oil as a moisturizer after bathing to seal in moisture and after sun exposure. For scar and wound healing apply regularly to keep the skin supple.

◼ Part 4: Minerals

17. Colloidal Silver

History: The first recorded use of silver medicinally was in the year 980 by Avicenna. However, he noted that too much caused a bluish grayish discoloration of the eyes, later termed ocular argyrosis. Since then, silver has been used as silver nitrate in the Middle Ages for epilepsy and tabes dorsalis, a silver foil under gauze prevented infection and promoted healing of wounds. Silver proteinate was added to nasal drops for sinusitis and common colds and silver arsphenamine was used to treat syphilis.

Currently silver sulfadiazine (Silvadene) is used in topical creams for burns. In 2006 it was reported that silver embedded medical dressings were effective in treating atopic dermatitis, hyperhidrosis and skin conditions related to diabetes mellitus and aging. These bioactive textiles appear to be antibacterial. The silver acts as a catalyst and disables bacteria and fungal enzymes necessary for oxygen metabolism.

Dermatological Applications

- Cutaneous lupus.
- Scarlet fever.
- Herpes zoster or shingles.
- Cuts, abrasions, open wounds, burns.
- Diabetic ulcerations and pressure sores.
- Skin/tissue grafts.
- Acne.
- Eczemas, including atopic dermatitis.

Toxicity: The National Institute for Health discusses argyria as a possible complication from a colloidal silver toxicity. Argyria is a bluish grey discoloration of the skin that is irreversible. Chronic long term use of topical silver products may lead to skin discoloration. Silver products have been known to rarely cause allergic skin reactions and contact dermatitis.

Directions for Therapeutic Use: Colloidal silver may be administrated as a nasal or topical spray for areas of skin irritation or infection, sore throat, eyes, or burns. It can be used as an underarm deodorant, since most underarm odor is caused by bacteria.

When applying topically, use 2–3 drops of solution on the affected area or on the dressing to prevent infection and promote healing. For eye and ear infections, apply 2–3 drops in each eye or ear. Unlike other antibiotics and antiseptics, silver colloids do not sting.

18. Epsom Salt

History: Epsom salt, magnesium sulfate, has been used for centuries, since its discovery in Epsom, England, in the 17th Century. Since then, it has been used to treat myriad conditions from ingrown nails, to constipation, to the seizures of eclampsia. Historically, it has been used in hot baths to ease pain due to stiff and sore joints and muscles, and it is still an effective therapy for arthritic joints. The strongest research is in preventing seizures in patients with eclampsia.

The two components of Epsom salt, magnesium and sulfate, each have their own health applications. Magnesium is a cofactor in the function or regulation of more than 325 enzymes; it helps to reduce inflammation, eases stress, and improves oxygen use. Sulfate has been used in the treatment of migraine headaches, it is a component of joint proteins, and it works with chelating compounds to eliminate heavy metals and other toxins, and improves the absorption of some nutrients. These facts, together with the research show these two compounds can be absorbed through the skin, make Epsom salts a popular bath-time therapy.

Dermatological Application

- Flea bites.
- Bruising.
- Cleansing and exfoliating agent.
- Acne.
- Xerosis.
- Minor skin irritations.
- Splinter removal.
- Hyperhidrosis (Epsom salt foot soaks).
- Pitted Keratolysis.

Toxicity: Toxicity is low and an allergic reaction may present as a mild contact dermatitis or hives. Patients with diabetes, high blood pressure, kidney disease, or who may be pregnant should be cautious with their use of Epsom salts in hot baths due to an increased possibility of adverse events.

Directions for Therapeutic Use: As an additive to a bath, dissolve 2 cups of Epsom salts in an average size bathtub filled with warm water. Soak in the bathtub for at least 12 minutes three times a week for best results.

As a compress for bruises, sprains, insect bites and splinters; dissolve 2 tablespoons of Epsom salt in 2 cups of warm water, soak a towel or gauze squares in it. Apply directly to the affected area, may be held in place with an occlusive wrap.

As a facial cleanser, add ½ teaspoon of Epsom salt to a cleansing cream and wash.

For exfoliation, gently rub handfuls of Epsom salts on wet skin, rinse the area with warm water and apply a moisturizer.

19. Iodine / Potassium iodide

History: Iodine was first identified in the early 1800s. Clinicians spent years experimenting with iodine in almost every condition that did not respond to routine treatment from syphilis to psoriasis. Potassium Iodide is wcightcd 23% alkali metal potassium and 76% halogen iodine. The compound is prepared by reacting iodine with a hot solution of potassium hydroxide. The final step consists of heating the dry reaction mixture with carbon for the reduction to iodide. One of the earliest uses of potassium iodide was to treat sporotrichosis, a fungal disease sometimes acquired by people who handle certain plants. Patients typically present with a small, painless nodule on the finger or wrist where the fungus entered the body. Untreated the infection progresses to bumps that resemble boils and finally to open sores that are very slow to heal. The mechanism by which potassium iodide functions is uncertain, however, it is thought it primarily affects neutrophil activity.

Dermatological Applications

- Erythema nodosum.
- Sweet syndrome.
- Cutaneous fungal infections.
- Pyoderma gangrenosum.
- Molluscum contagiosum.
- Cuts and abrasions.

Toxicity: Toxicity is rare when taken orally in low doses and short courses. Common side effects include nausea and vomiting, abdominal pain and diarrhea. Less common side effects include hives, swelling of the arms, hands, legs, lips, tongue, and lymph nodes.

When used topically side effects include allergic responses such as hives and contact dermatitis.

Symptoms of iodine toxicity include burning sensation in the mouth or throat, a metallic taste, increased salivation, sore teeth and gums and headaches.

Symptoms of potassium toxicity include confusion, lethargy, irregular heartbeat (typically tachycardia), and tingling, numbness or weakness in the extremities.

Directions for Therapeutic Use: Topically, iodine and potassium iodide are used as a wash. Clean the area with warm water and soap or other cleansing agent. Rinse the area with the iodine or potassium iodide solution and cover. The gauze used for covering may be saturated with a dilute iodine solution to prevent infection.

20. Sodium Bicarbonate

History: Sodium bicarbonate occupies the shelves of nearly every household pantry in the United States. Sodium bicarbonate is a cooking ingredient known as baking soda. Aside from its use in the kitchen, baking soda, which is alkaline in nature, has many other uses, including a general deodorizer and a detergent for clothes and dishes.

Historically, sodium bicarbonate has also been used as a home remedy to treat many dermatological conditions. The use of this chemical as a treatment for psoriasis is gaining in popularity. Many commercial types of toothpaste advertise the use of baking soda as a main ingredient, implying that it may be beneficial in preventing tooth decay or whitening the teeth.

It has also been known as a home remedy to lessen the pain associated with contact dermatitis and insect stings.

Dermatological Application

- Psoriasis.

- Bees, wasps and hornet stings or fire ant bites.
- Poisonous plants (Poison Ivy or Oak).

Toxicity: Prolonged use of baking soda may dry out the skin, so always rinse the area with warm water and follow with a moisturizer.

Directions for Therapeutic Use: For a bath to alleviate the symptoms of psoriasis, add 2 cups of sodium bicarbonate to a tub of warm water, then soak for a minimum of 12 minutes, rinse with warm water.

As a tooth paste, use 1 teaspoon of sodium bicarbonate mixed with a few drops of water and a small pinch of salt, make a paste and apply to the toothbrush.

As a paste for insect bites or stings, make a paste with 1 teaspoon or more of sodium bicarbonate and water, apply to the sting or bite and cover.

As a paste for contact with poisonous plants such as Poison Ivy or Oak, mix sodium bicarbonate with water until the mixture is thin enough to paint the area of contact.

21. Zinc Oxide

History: Zinc oxide is the primary active ingredient in many topical products and is used when the skin needs to be covered and protected from bacterial infection. It has been used throughout the years as a topical medication that helps soothe irritated skin due to its analgesic properties. The lotion has a cooling soothing effect which relieves itching preventing excessive scratching.

Dermatological Applications

- Sunburn.
- Eczema.
- Poison Ivy / Oak dermatitis.
- Chicken pox.
- Insect bites.
- Candidiasis.
- Psoriasis.

Toxicity: Topically, there are rare side effects and the incidence of toxicity is very low. Chronic topical exposure to zinc oxide may result in skin irritation of a papular-pustular skin eruption generally in the axilla, inner thigh, inner arm, scrotal, pubic, rectal, and perineal areas.

Directions for Therapeutic Use: Wash and completely dry the affected area before applying the lotion, ointment or cream. Apply this medication to the affected area of skin, three to four times daily or as directed.

Part 5: Natural Products

22. Aloe Vera

History: The Aloe vera is a stemless plant with very thick fleshy leaves that originated in North Africa and is now used and grown around the world. Historically, Aloe vera was first used by Egyptians, Greeks and Romans for typical treatment of cuts, burns, and skin irritations. The gel which is found in the central parts of the leaves contains active phytonutrients. When collecting the gel, care should be taken to remove the green colored gel close to the skin, because this contains the bitter substance aloin, which is a strong laxative. Aloe vera contains water, minerals such as sodium, potassium, manganese, copper, zinc, chromium, and iron. It also contains trace minerals, vitamins A, C, E , B12, niacin and folic acid, amino acids and enzymes. Aloe vera has active plant compounds such as carboxypepsidase (which breaks down bradykinin), triterpenes, glycoproteins, mono and polysaccharides, lignan, salicylic acid and sterols.

Dermatological Application

- Minor burns, wounds.
- Bed and canker sores.
- Herpes simplex.
- Psoriasis.
- Seborrheic dermatitis.
- Skin ulcers.
- Acne.
- Tinea pedis.
- Candidiasis.

Toxicity: Aloe vera can cause allergic reactions resulting in rashes, contact dermatitis, hives or blisters in those with known allergies to garlic, onion, tulips, or other plants of the *Liliaceae* family.

Deep penetrating wounds and surgical wounds should not be treated with Aloe vera due to its ability to inhibit healing in deep tissues.

Oral use of Aloe vera may lead to abdominal cramps and diarrhea when there is a high concentration of aloin.

Directions for Therapeutic Use: Wash and completely dry the affected area before applying the aloe vera gel. Rub the gel over the affected area of the skin then massage it into the skin as a moisturizer. For treating sensitive areas such as burns or abrasions apply a coating of the gel and allow it to air dry or apply a gauze bandage over the area for protection.

23. Apple Cider Vinegar

History: Vinegar is the product of fermented alcohol. The alcohol is commonly derived from wine, cider, fermented fruit juice or beer. The ethyl alcohol is oxidized to acetaldehyde then converted to acetic acid through the action of the *Acetobacter*, an aerobic bacterium. The acetic acid concentration is regulated in the United States. All vinegars must contain at least four percent acetic acid. However, depending upon the initial source, vinegar may contain additional micronutrients including vitamins, mineral salts, amino acids, catechins, and other organic acids.

Historically, vinegar was the cure-all for many disorders. Hippocrates recommended vinegar as a disinfectant for wounds and used it in a mixture to fight gastrointestinal and respiratory illnesses. The Samurai warriors drank it for strength and power.

Dermatological Application

- Acne.
- Skin toning.
- Seborrheic dermatitis.
- Viral warts.
- Pediculosis.
- Sunburn.
- Herpes zoster.
- Insect bites.
- Impetigo.
- Carbuncle.
- Folliculitis.
- Tinea pedis.
- Jellyfish and Portuguese man-of-war stings.

Toxicity: Vinegar does contain acetic acid. The pH of a 5% acetic acid solution is 2.4, which is less acidic than lemon juice but more acidic than tomato juice. Because of its acidity vinegar can cause irritation of the skin.

Patients that have allergies to the base juice (e.g. apple juice) should avoid its vinegar.

Directions for Therapeutic Use: To treat bug bites, bee stings, jellyfish stings, skin conditions, sunburn, and dandruff, apply liberally with cloth or rag to affected areas.

To treat warts, use apple cider vinegar and soak a cotton ball, wring out excess vinegar, place over top of wart, and secure in place with a band-aid.

Treatment for sunburn, tinea infections, and shingles would be a vinegar bath. Put 2–3 cups of vinegar into a bath tub of warm water, and soak in the bath for 20 to 30 minutes then rinse and apply a moisturizer.

24. Black Walnut

History: Black walnut (*Juglans nigra*), also known as the American Walnut tree, is a native hardwood that grows in small natural groves in the central and eastern parts of the United States. Black walnut has two main active chemicals: juglone and astringents called tannins. Juglone is known for its antibiotic and antifungal effects while tannins are responsible for its antihelmintic effect. Tannins have an astringent effect which is to dehydrate mucosal tissue, tighten the epidermis, mucous membranes, decrease secretions, relieve irritation, and re-establish tissue firmness.

Historically, the nuts from black walnut trees have served both nutritional and medicinal purposes. Black walnut as a food source is used as a flavoring in baked goods and candy. Whole black walnuts are an important nutrition source since they are 20% protein and are high in essential fatty acids. They are also rich in manganese.

Dermatological Applications

- Xerosis.
- Tinea pedis, cruris, corporis.
- Poison Ivy and Oak dermatitis.
- Viral warts.
- Psoriasis.
- Eczema.
- Acne.

Toxicity: There are few potential side effects with Black Walnut when applied topically for skin conditions. The astringent action of Black Walnut causes dehydration of the top layers of skin, forming a thickened layer of dense tissue similar to a callus. An allergic reaction to Black Walnut may occur in patients with nut allergies resulting in hives, rashes, itchy swollen skin and possibly breathing problems or chest pain.

Directions for Therapeutic Use: A wash or compress can be made by adding 2 tablespoons of finely chopped walnut to 1 liter of water, bringing it to a boil and letting it steep for 5 minutes. Soak a cloth or cotton gauze in the solution and apply to the area affected daily.

25. Burdock

History: Burdock has been used throughout history. English herbalists in the Middle Ages and the Native Americans have used burdock for a variety of ailments such as diabetes, scurvy, boils, and even rheumatism. The Burdock root has been used as a food source as well as medicinally. The root, the leaf and the seeds of the Burdock plant have medicinal uses. The scientific name for burdock is *Arctium lappa* and it is native to Europe, Northern Asia and now commonly found in the United States. It is a member of the daisy family and in many areas is considered a common weed with burrs and grows to a height of 3–4 feet. The medicinal and food value consists in the combination of carbohydrates, volatile oils, plant sterols, tannins, and fatty oils contained in the various parts of the plant.

Dermatological Application

- Skin Abscesses.
- Acne.
- Psoriasis.
- Snake bite.
- Promotion of hair growth.
- Viral warts.
- Contact eczema.
- Ichthyosis.

Toxicity: Toxicity is low; however, precaution should be taken in relation to prescription drugs and dietary supplements. An allergic reaction may occur in individuals with allergy to members of the Asteraceae/Composita family, including ragweed, chrysanthemums, marigolds, and daises. Such manifestations include skin irritations, hives and dermatitis. Other side effects include dry mouth and slow heart rate. Burdock contains tannins, which can cause upset stomach, kidney, or even liver damage when ingested

Directions for Therapeutic Use: When making a compress use the dried roots. Steep 2–6 grams in 150 ml of boiling water for 10–15 minutes, then soak a cloth in the liquid and, once cooled, wrap the cloth around affected skin area. Do not use on open sores.

A tincture is a solution in which the active components are extracted into an alcohol solution. 2–8 ml may be applied to a cloth and wrapped around affected skin area or wound. If the alcohol content is irritating dilute the tincture in 2–4 oz of water.

26. Calendula

History: Calendula officinalis, also known as the pot marigold, is an ancient herb, having been used since the 12th century in Europe and earlier in Egypt, where it was used to ward off illness. The dried bright yellow flower petals were used to give cheese its yellow color and it has been used as a dye for fabrics and foods. Many varieties of calendula exist, and one of the varieties is the marigold referred to as garden marigold, golden flower of Mary, and Mary-bud. The chemical and nutrient content of the calendula flower petals is carotene, calenduline, lycopine, saponin, resin and essential oil. It is high in carotenoids that assist in the repair of damaged skin.

Dermatological Application
- Burns, bruises and minor cuts.
- Frostbite.
- Skin ulcers.
- Skin abscesses.

Toxicity: Calendula has no known side effects or interactions; however, those patients with pre-existing allergies to ragweed or daisies may also be allergic to calendula.

Calendula when taken orally is suspected to interact with anti-hypertensive, sedative, and hypoglycemic medications.

Directions for Therapeutic Use: For sore or bleeding gums, add 15 drops of calendula tincture to 2 ounces of water, swish around the mouth for 30 to 60 seconds and spit out.

For bruises, burns, minor cuts and abrasions, and sore muscles calendula may be applied topically in a gel or cream form 2 to 4 times per day.

27. Chamomile

History: Chamomile (*Matricaria recutita, Maticaria chamomilla*) is an herb whose flower is daisy-like and apple-scented. The flower has been used medicinally for thousands of years. The name is derived from the Greek *Chamos* (ground) and *Melos* (apple). It is a low-growing plant and is indigenous to Europe and Northwest Asia. Roman and German chamomile are the major types used in health care. Both are thought to have similar effects on the body, although German chamomile may be slightly stronger. German chamomile was an important ancient Egyptian, Greek and Roman medicine.

One of the active ingredients in chamomile is levomenol, which has antiinflammatory properties, it promotes granulation and epithelialization, and it has antibacterial and antifungal properties. Other active components are the flavonoids which have anti-inflammation and antispasmodic actions.

Dermatological Application
- Wound healing.
- Carbuncle, furuncles, folliculitis.
- Skin abscesses.
- Acne.
- Eczemas.

Toxicity: Currently, there is no known toxicity for the topical use of chamomile. Chamomile may cause hypersensitivity or allergic reactions in people with allergies to ragweed, sunflowers or plants of the aster family such as Feverfew, Echinacea, or Milk Thistle. There have been a few studies identifying people with severe allergies to the herb reporting skin rashes, throat swelling, shortness of breath, and anaphylaxis. Chamomile is contraindicated in treating pregnant women as it can act as a uterine stimulant leading to abortion of the fetus.

Directions for Therapeutic Use: A chamomile compress is made by mixing 2 teaspoons of chamomile into 12 oz of boiling water, covering and steeping for 15 minutes. Soak a clean cloth or gauze in the mixture and cover the affected area.

For a Chamomile bath, add 50 grams of chamomile to 1 liter of water, boil, steep for 15 minutes, then add to bath water. Soak in the bath for 20 to 30 minutes.

28. Chaparral

History: This plant was commonly used by the Native Americans for a wide variety of purposes. Chaparral is a plant found in arid regions of North and South America, it is very abundant in the American southwest. The common name for Chaparral is the creosote bush. This name arose from the odor the bush gives off during times of rain and when the oily leaves are crushed. The entire plant that is above the soil is harvested for use in herbal forms. It is one of the most abundant desert plants, but many of these plants are well over a hundred years old. Due to the harsh conditions, many of the spores do not take hold and die.

Nordihdroguaiaretic acid (NDGA) was isolated in the 1940's. NDGA is considered the most active component of the plant. It is considered a strong antioxidant as well as having antibacterial and antiviral actions. The food industry used NDGA until 1973 as a means to keep oils and fats from becoming rancid.

Dermatological Application
- Skin parasites (swimmer's itch).
- Molluscum contagiosum.
- Acne.
- Herpes simplex.
- Minor cuts, bruises and abrasions.

Toxicity: Topically Chaparral may cause contact dermatitis, rashes or swelling in those patients who are sensitive to the plant.

Directions for Therapeutic Use: For a bath, steep 4 tablespoons of the dried herb in a liter of boiling water, then add this mixture to the bath water and soak for 20 minutes.

A therapeutic compress can be made by soaking 1 tablespoon of the herb in 1 cup of warm oil. Then, soak a clean cloth in the warm oil and apply to the skin until the cloth cools.

Chaparral powder can be sprinkled directly over minor cuts, scrapes and abrasions or mixed with water to make a paste. The paste is then applied to the minor wound and covered with a gauze bandage.

29. Comfrey

History: Comfrey (*Symphytum officinale, S. asperum, S. tuberosum*) is also known commonly as knitbone, bruisewort, slippery root, boneset, blackwort and woundwort. Russian comfrey is a hybrid of *S. officinale* and *S. asperum*.

Comfrey is a perennial plant that grows predominantly in moist grasslands of Western Asia, North America and Australia. It is a low dense shrub that grows to a height of 3–5 feet. The flowers grow in clusters of 15–20 and are lavender, white or pale yellow. The leaves and roots are normally used for making a poultice for topical application.

The naturally occurring substances that appear to aid in skin and tissue regeneration and healing effects are allatonin, tannins and rosmarinic acid.

Dermatological Application
- Bruises.
- Lymphangitis.
- Cutaneous vasculitis.

Toxicity: Topically, Comfrey may cause contact dermatitis, rashes or swelling in those patients who are sensitive to the plant. However, the pyrrolizidine alkaloids (PA) that are present in Comfrey are hepatotoxic substances. These substances can pass through the skin and over time may accumulate in the liver. It is recommended that Comfrey not be used on open wounds and not be used for more than 6 weeks.

Directions for Therapeutic Use: Comfrey can be applied topically or externally as a poultice. The poultice is made by taking the powdered herb and mixing it into warm water to make a paste.

Apply the paste to the affected area and cover with gauze.

A therapeutic compress can be made by soaking 1 tablespoon of the herb in 1 cup of warm oil. Then soak a clean cloth in the warm oil and apply to the skin until the cloth cools.

30. Cornstarch

History: Cornstarch is an ordinary cooking starch found in many households. Cornstarch is a fine white powdery starch used to thicken liquids such as puddings, pie fillings, and sauces. It can also be used alone or as an ingredient as a deodorant, facial mask, shampoo, skin softener, anti-perspirant and a deodorizer for shoes.

Dermatological Applications
- Intertrigo.
- Candidiasis.
- Chicken pox.
- Measles.
- Insect bites.
- Urticaria.
- Sunburns.

Toxicity: Topically Cornstarch may cause contact dermatitis, rashes or swelling in those patients who are sensitive the corn or have known corn allergies.

Directions for Therapeutic Use: For intertrigo, the patients should clean and pat dry the affected area. They should then apply a light dusting of cornstarch, try to keep the infected area clean and dry. Exposing the affected skin folds to air can help eliminate heat and moisture. Patients should wear loose fitting clothing to eliminate friction.

For diaper rash, clean and dry the diaper area then sprinkle the cornstarch over the area and cover with a diaper.

For Measles and Chicken pox, add 1 cup of cornstarch to a warm bath and soak for 15 to 20 minutes.

For sunburn add enough corn starch to water to make a soft loose paste and apply the paste directly to the burn.

31. Elderberry

History: *Sambucus nigra*, commonly known as Elderberry, is a tall tree-like shrub brought to the United States from Europe, Asia, and North Africa. The entire shrub including the bark, leaves, flowers, and berries are used. Historically, the Choctaw people, of central and Southern Mississippi, would mix elderberry juice with boiled honey for treatment of skin eruptions and first degree or minor burns. The Elderberry tree has been appreciated for its constituents, dating back to 400 BC.

Elderberry contains anthocyanins, which are powerful antioxidant phytochemicals that also have demonstrated antiviral activity. Additionally elderberry has shown to stimulate cytokines which then act as immune stimulants.

Dermatological Applications

- Acne.
- Eczema.
- Psoriasis.
- Burns, cuts, scrapes.
- Chafing.
- Herpes simplex.
- Measles.

Toxicity: Patients who have an allergy to the honeysuckle family should avoid Elderberry products. There is a risk of abdominal cramps, diarrhea, gastrointestinal distress, vomiting, and weakness when taken internally. Topically, an allergic reaction would present as a rash, skin irritation or contact dermatitis. Elderberry has a diuretic effect when taken orally thus should be used with caution when a patient is taking prescription medication that cause diuresis.

Directions for Therapeutic Use: The historic Choctaw salve requires one teaspoon of honey with two tablespoons of elderberry juice, then heating the mixture until the juices are nicely blended. Cool the mixture before applying to the affected burn or eruptive sore.

32. Garlic

History: Garlic has been used for centuries for treating various conditions and illnesses. Cultures that never had contact with one another came to the same conclusions about garlic and its role in the treatment of disease. Garlic was classified as a "hot food" and was to be consumed in the winter months to limit the development of pulmonary and breathing disorders.

In ancient Rome and Greece, people used garlic for strength and endurance. Hippocrates, the father of medicine, advocated its use for an array of problems. He also used it as a cleansing or purgative agent. The Bible mentions that the Egyptians fed garlic to the slaves in order to give them strength as well as to increase productivity. In ancient China and Japan, garlic was used as a food preservative, to aid in digestion and respiration, to provide energy, to decrease depression, and to improve male potency. In ancient India garlic was used to treat heart disease and arthritis.

Allicin, the best known active component of garlic, is an oxygenated sulphur compound, formed when garlic cloves are crushed, and is recognizable by its very strong garlic odor.

Dermatological Applications

- Warts.
- Acne.
- Cutaneous fungal infections.
- Cutaneous viral and bacterial infections.

Toxicity: Patients who are allergic to garlic should avoid contact with all garlic and allicin products. Topically garlic may cause contact dermatitis, blistering, redness, burning, and hyperpigmentation. These side effects usually disappear within one to two weeks once garlic has been discontinued.

Directions for Therapeutic Use: Garlic powder may be sprinkled over areas of minor bacterial or fungal infections and then covered with a gauze bandage.

Garlic oil may be poured on to a gauze pad and then applied to the wound or infected area.

33. Ginger

History: Ginger, *Zingiber Officinale*, has been used in Asia medicinally for 2500 years. This herb has a wide variety of health-related claims. Ginger is a perennial herb that is structurally composed of a rhizome, an underground root, and an above ground stem that can grow to one meter tall. The rhizome of the plant is used medicinally and as a spice. Ginger has been used for such things as stomach aches, diarrhea, nausea, cholera, stomach ulcers, baldness, toothaches, rheumatoid and osteoarthritis. As a spice, ginger is found in everything from cookies to meats, alcoholic beverages, ginger ale, and in perfumes. Originally ginger was native to southern Asia but the leading growers today include India, Australia, Nigeria, Jamaica, and Sierra Leone.

Pungent vallinoids and oils present in ginger have been found to have anticancer properties, antioxidant activities, as well as antiinflammatory effects.

Dermatological Application

- Burns.
- Minor skin irritation.
- Tinea pedis.
- Snake bites.
- Insect bites.

- Psoriasis.
- Antiseptic.

Toxicity: Ginger is generally recognized as safe by the FDA. Ginger is a member of the Zingiberacae family and those with allergies to this family have an increased risk of rashes associated with topical ginger applications. Other herbs that are in the Zingiberacae family are Tumeric and Cardamon. Ginger is associated with clot prevention so any patient taking blood-thinning medications should consult a doctor before starting ginger therapy.

Directions for Therapeutic Use: For topical application, ginger is to be mashed in order for the oils and juices to be released. To treat a burn, rash, minor wound or psoriasis a cotton ball should be saturated in the oil and juice and applied directly to the area.

Powdered ginger is an alternative to the oils and may be added to a full bath for more widespread complaints. The powder should be added one tablespoon at a time and gradually increased to reduce the risk of skin sensitivity.

For more focal complaints, a ginger compress may be used. The compress is prepared by combining 2–3 teaspoons of ginger oil or ginger powder with hot water, saturate a sterile dressing and apply the compress directly to the area.

34. Goldenseal

History: Goldenseal (*Hydrastis canadensis*) is a perennial plant that grows in the rich woodlands of North America. The Cherokee and Iroquois used these roots to treat a variety of conditions including indigestion, diarrhea, whooping cough, fever, wounds, snake bites and local inflammation. Eclectic physicians in the United States saw goldenseal as an antiseptic, astringent and antiinflammatory for the mucous membranes.

The action of Goldenseal is attributed to the alkaloids hydrastine and berberine. These compounds provide the antibacterial, disinfectant, antiseptic and astringent qualities that Goldenseal is used both topically and internally.

Dermatological Application

- Psoriasis.
- Eczema.
- Tinea pedis, corporis.
- Herpes simplex.
- Cuts and scrapes.
- Skin abscesses.
- Acne.

Toxicity: Patients who are allergic to Goldenseal should avoid contact with all Goldenseal products. Topically, Goldenseal may cause contact dermatitis, redness, burning, and purities, however, these side effects usually disappear within a week once it has been discontinued. When applied topically, goldenseal may increase the photosensitivity of the skin with exposure to UV rays.

Directions for Therapeutic Use: For disinfecting cuts, scrapes, boils, and acne, Goldenseal liquid extract may be applied to a gauze pad and placed on the infected area and secured into place.

For sores on gums, or sides of the mouth, a mouthwash is made by mixing 1/4 tsp salt and 1/2 tsp of Goldenseal powder in one cup of warm water, rinsing and spitting it out. This may be done three times per day.

For vaginal inflammation, a Goldenseal douche is made as follows: mix 1/4 tsp salt and 1/2 tsp of goldenseal powder to 1 cup of warm water. Strain the mixture and wash the vaginal vault, then rinse the area with warm water.

35. Green Tea

History: The Camellia sinensis is an Asian evergreen shrub whose dried leaves are used to make green tea, a popular beverage throughout the world. Green tea contains caffeine and polyphenols and epigallocatechins. It is polyphenols and epigallocatechins that have antioxidant and anticancer properties and contribute to the many health benefits green tea is recognized for.

India and Sri Lanka are the major producers of green tea in the world and produce the tea that has the most robust flavor. The use of green tea and tea in general has spread from China, where tea has been used for more than 5000 years. Green tea was first introduced to western cultures during the sixth century when trade routes were opened to the orient.

The dermatological effects of green tea have been seen with both oral and topical uses and may be used simultaneously.

Dermatological Application

- Skin cancer.
- Atopic dermatitis.
- Eczema.
- Urticaria.
- Protect skin from UV radiation, sunburn and radiation damaged skin.

Toxicity: Patients who are allergic to green or black tea should avoid contact with all tea products.

Topically green tea may cause contact dermatitis, redness, burning, and purities, however, these side effects usually disappear within a week once it has been discontinued

Directions for Therapeutic Use: Green tea is best when steeped in water at 70° C or 158° F. The tea can then be drunk as a beverage or sprayed over the affected area. Green tea may also be used to soak a dressing and placed over the affected area.

36. Lemon

History: Lemons are in the family of Rutaceae and grow on a small evergreen tree. They have been known, used and traded since approximately 600 BCE when Arab traders brought them to Asia. The lemon has been prized for its numerous medical uses, many of which are still used today. One such example is the use of lemons by the British Navy in the 1800s to fight the effects of scurvy. In today's society, lemons are not only used in the kitchen as a food flavoring but as an ingredient in stain removal products, pharmaceuticals, polishes, and facial cleansers and creams.

Dermatological Applications
- Effective natural bleach for the skin, hair, and nails.
- Age blemishes.
- Acne blemishes.

Toxicity: There are only a few undesired effects associated with lemons and they are caused by the acidic nature of the lemon. When applied to the skin a burning sensation will be noticed and may result in a mild contact dermatitis.

Directions for Therapeutic Use: For acne, a fresh cut lemon is gently applied to the face, directly over the acne lesion, hold in place for 30 to 60 seconds then pat dry. After each area is treated, rinse with warm water and apply a light moisturizer. If the lemon slice is too harsh for the skin, squeeze the juice from the lemon and dilute it in water and then apply to the acne lesions with a cotton swab.

37. Oatmeal

History: Oatmeal and its derivatives have been used for centuries for different types of skin conditions due to the exfoliating and soothing benefits from the emollient property. The oldest oats have been dated to early Egypt. Oats were brought to North America in the 1600s and have become a major part of the American diet.

Oatmeal has been used topically for the temporary relief of itching due to dry skin and rashes. In 1945 a manufacturing process was developed to extract the starch—protein fraction that is now used in many skin care products.

Dermatological Application
- Psoriasis.
- Eczema, atopic, allergic or contact.
- Chicken pox.
- Poison Ivy, Sumac and Oak dermatitis.
- Xerosis.
- Ichthyosis.
- Urticaria.
- Sunburn.

Toxicity: There is no known toxicity associated with oats, oatmeal or colloidal oatmeal.

Adverse effects with oatmeal are quite rare but may include redness of skin, hives, rash, and possibly some numbness or tingling.

Directions for Therapeutic Use: For dry itchy skin, a plaster can be made by making the oatmeal a little thicker than the recipe calls for so that it does not run, let it cool then spread over the affected area. The grain will scratch your itchy skin while the colloid properties help to soothe the skin.

For a soothing bath, prepare a bath of warm water, add 2 cups oatmeal and soak in the tub for 20 minutes.

38. Onion

History: The onion (*Allium cepa*) is known to have a global health benefit in the prevention and treatment of disease. Onions are rich in health-promoting phytochemicals. One is alkenyl cysteine sylphoxides which is a sulfur-containing compound that is responsible for the pungent odor and health-promoting effects. Additionally, onions are a rich source of chromium, a trace mineral that helps cells respond to insulin. Onion is also a good source of Vitamin C, and flavonoids, most notably, *quercitin*.

Dermatological Applications
- Cutaneous bacterial infections.
- Keloids.
- Insect repellant.
- Insect bites.
- Skin abscesses.
- Viral warts.
- Seborrheic dermatitis.

Toxicity: When applied topically onions produce redness, dilation of the capillaries, and an increase in blood circulation.

Directions for Therapeutic Use: Onion juice is an aromatic substance and patients may be hesitant to use it topically. However, it has several therapeutic benefits that may outweigh this concern.

For seborrheic dermatitis (dandruff), onion juice should be rubbed on the scalp area twice a week.

To clean and remove skin spots, blemishes, and prevent bacterial and fungal infections, fresh onion juice should be rubbed on the skin in the affected area.

To age, or mature, abscesses, a raw onion as a poultice should be applied over the affected area. The poultice may be made in 3 ways. First, chopped onion is pressed and applied to the affected area covered with gauze and held in place. Second, the onion is sliced then slow cooked in water until soft then the mixture is cooled and applied to the area. Third, the onion is sliced and slow cooked in olive oil until soft then cooled and placed over the affected area.

39. Undecycline

History: Undecylenic acid is an eleven—carbon mono-unsaturated fatty acid derived commercially from Castor Oil by vacuum distillation and found in the human perspiration. Most organic fatty acids are antifungal and antimicrobial. Undecyclenic acid is now used in cosmetics, antimicrobial powders, anti-dandruff shampoos and antifungals.

Dermatological Applications
- Tinea pedis.
- Tinea cruris.
- Eczemas.
- Candidiasis (diaper rash).
- Herpes simplex.

Toxicity: Topical use rarely has adverse effects. However, in a sensitive patient, blisters, itching, dryness and dermatitis may result.

Directions for Therapeutic Use: Undecylenic acid is available in creams, powders and ointments. Wash and dry the affected area. When using a cream or ointment apply to the affected area and rub it in, in the same manner as a moisturizer. For powders, sprinkle or spray the area so that it is well covered, then apply light gauze covering to protect the clothing but allow air to circulate over the area.

40. White Willow Bark
History: White Willow (*Salix Alba*) tree bark contains phenolic glycoside and salicortin which is hy-drolyzed to salicin. Salicin is the substance from which salicylic acid is derived. White Willow tree bark itself has been used for 2000 years. The first century Greek physician, Discoides, recommended a poultice made from the willow bark. The bark was valued for its anthelmintic (destruction of parasitic organisms), antiinflammatory, antipyretic (fever reduction), and hemostatic (hemorrhage control) properties. In 1853, aspirin was made commercially available. Salicylic acid today is used in many different products.

Dermatological Application
- Seborrheic dermatitis.
- Ichthyosis.
- Psoriasis.
- Viral warts.
- Cutaneous fungal and parasitic infections.

Toxicity: White Willow may cause dryness, peeling, flushing and redness of the skin in those patients with known aspirin allergies.

Directions for Therapeutic Use: For warts and fungal infections soak a cotton swab or gauze in tincture and apply to the affected area. Test in a small area to determine the concentration that can be tolerated.

41. Witch Hazel

History: Witch Hazel, *Hamamelis virginiana*, is a deciduous shrub or small tree that flowers in the fall, native to damp woods in eastern North America. The extract is produced from the leaves and bark of the shrub. It has been used by Native Americans as a poultice of witch hazel leaves and bark to treat hemorrhoids, wounds, painful tumors, insect bites, backaches and sore muscles, and skin ulcers. All aspects of the witch hazel shrub, the bark, leaves, and twigs are high in tannins. Tannins are vasoconstrictive and tighten capillaries and venules beneath the skin's surface. They are what give the extract its astringent properties. Astringents aid in drying and tightening tissues. Commonly, astringents are used to tighten skin pores and eliminate excess oil. Additionally, witch hazel contains procyanadins, resin, and flavonoids which have anti-inflammatory properties.

Dermatological Application
- Bruises and lacerations.
- Skin abscess.
- Burns.
- Insect bites.
- Removal of eye makeup.

- Reduction of edematous swelling under the eyes.
- Eczemas including atopic dermatitis.

Toxicity: There are no known side effects when used topically. Commercial preparations of witch hazel should not be used internally because they contain isopropyl alcohol. Some minor skin irritations have been noted by individuals with sensitive skin.

Directions for Therapeutic Use: A witch hazel solution to be used as a compress to treat skin conditions requires 1 tablespoon of finely ground bark and/or leaves boiled in 1 cup of water for 20 minutes. Strain the grounds and let the solution cool. Soak a cotton swab or gauze in the solution and apply to the affected area. The herbal tinctures produced commercially may be used to form the compress; however, they may need to be diluted due to the higher concentration of tannins.

Commercial products containing isopropyl alcohol may be used as well but cannot be taken internally.

Part 6: Over-The-Counter Products

42. Antibiotics

History: Antibiotic ointments are viscous, petroleum based substances used to prevent topical infections caused by bacteria. Penicillin was discovered in 1928 by Sir Alexander Fleming. The most common antibiotic ointments are a combination of neomycin, bacitracin, and polymyxin which were first used more than 50 years ago. Neomycin and polymyxin are effective against Gram negative bacteria while bacitracin is used for Gram positive infections. However, various other kinds of antibiotic ointments are now available.

Dermatological Application
- Cuts, scrapes.
- Burns.
- Acne.

Toxicity: The most common side effects of antibiotic ointments include itching and burning. Signs of allergic or toxic reactions include: rash, swelling, sweating, tightness and discomfort in the chest, breathing problems, fainting or dizziness, low blood pressure, nausea, diarrhea and hearing loss or ringing in the ears.

Directions for Therapeutic Use: Wash and dry the wound and the surrounding area, apply a small amount of the antibiotic ointment, enough to cover the area. Clean and reapply the ointment one to three times per day, or as instructed by a doctor. Once the ointment is applied cover with a sterile bandage.

43. Calamine

History: Calamine is a mixture of zinc oxide with about 0.5% iron oxide. Calamine is a topical cream or lotion that is used to treat minor skin irritations that cause itching and discomfort. It has a cooling and soothing effect on the skin for symptomatic relief of the itching. Also, the active ingredient zinc oxide has antiseptic properties that help prevent infection from scratching.

Dermatological Application
- Sunburn.
- Eczema.
- Poison Ivy / Poison Oak dermatitis.
- Chickenpox.
- Insect bites.
- Frostbite.
- Urticaria.
- Pityriasis rosea.
- Acne.

Toxicity: The toxicity of calamine when used topically is very low and side effects of calamine use are rare. However, an allergic reaction can present as a rash, itching, swelling, severe dizziness, and in severe reactions trouble breathing.

Directions for Therapeutic Use: Calamine is typically applied to the skin with a cotton ball by dabbing or wiping it across the affected area or with a brush. Allow it to dry and wrap the area with sterile gauze, especially if the patient is a child. Calamine is applied directly 3–4 times per day.

44. Hydrocortisone

History: Hydrocortisone is the man made analog to the naturally occurring corticosteroid cortisol which is produced by the adrenal gland. Hydrocortisone was first introduced as an effective treatment for eczematous dermatitis in 1952. It remained a prescription drug until FDA approval was granted for over-the-counter sale in 1979. It is available in a wide variety of creams, sprays, and pastes. Hydrocortisone continues to be used to treat inflammatory conditions of skin and other medical conditions such as mycosis fungoides and rheumatoid arthritis.

Dermatological Applications
- Atopic and contact dermatitis.
- Psoriasis.

- Ano-genital itching.
- Insect bites.
- Poison Oak / Ivy / Sumac dermatitis.

Toxicity: Side effects of hydrocortisone application include skin atrophy, striae, steroid induced rosacea, burning, itching or dryness at the site of application. The long term use of hydrocortisone in children can cause altered hormonal function as a result of the body down-regulating the production of endogenous cortisol.

Directions for Therapeutic Use: Wash and dry the area to be treated with the hydrocortisone before each application. Apply a small amount and rub it gently into the skin. Avoid using this medication on the face, near the eyes, mouth or on body areas where skin folds or thin skin is present. Do not cover treated skin areas with a bandage or other covering unless so directed.

For diaper rash do not use plastic pants or tight-fitting diapers. Covering the skin which is treated with topical hydrocortisone can increase the amount of the drug absorbed increasing the chance of unwanted side effects.

45. Hydrogen Peroxide

History: Hydrogen peroxide, a clear liquid at room temperature, is produced by the white blood cells in the body. The hydrogen peroxide used for the treatment of skin conditions is a dilute aqueous solution of 3 to 10%. However, it is used at higher concentrations in industry, where it is used as a bleach for textiles, paper and art restoration.

Hydrogen peroxide is used as a wound cleanser because of the antibacterial action caused by the abundant release of oxygen that occurs when hydrogen peroxide is added to an open wound. The release of oxygen increases oxidation which causes the antibacterial effects of hydrogen peroxide. The effervescence of oxygen helps loosen up dead tissue, debris and pus. Finally, hydrogen peroxide acts as a mild astringent.

In the home hydrogen peroxide is used as a disinfectant, a hair-bleaching agent, to remove excess ear wax and to whiten teeth.

Dermatological Applications
- Tinea pedis.
- Antisepsis.
- Bed sores.
- Cuts and abrasions.
- Hair bleach.

Toxicity: The ingestion of 3% hydrogen peroxide has been found to cause mild irritations to the GI tract and may cause vomiting and diarrhea. Ingestion of concentrations over 10% may cause systemic toxicity or death. 3% concentrations may irritate the skin and the eyes.

Topically, hydrogen peroxide may cause a burning, stinging, irritating sensation for a short period of time. For deep wound cleansing, hydrogen peroxide may slow the healing process.

Directions for Therapeutic Use: Wash and dry the area to be treated with a mild soap. Hydrogen peroxide is used as a rinse for fresh wounds and abrasions by directly pouring a pharmaceutical grade 3% solution over the wound. Allow the area to bubble. Then rinse with warm water, apply an antibiotic ointment and cover.

Part 7: Miscellaneous

46. Dimethylsulfoxide (DMSO)

History: Dimethylsulfoxide, or DMSO, is a natural substance derived from wood pulp. DMSO is a solvent that can mix with water and oil giving it the ability to penetrate the skin. DMSO is a carrier that rapidly introduces substances into the body. DMSO has been widely used for many years in sports medicine for a variety of problems and conditions. DMSO is also excellent for healing deep tissue, muscle injuries, burns, and other wounds.

DMSO has antiviral characteristics and has been used effectively in the treatment of the herpes virus. Since viruses lack genetic material of their own, they can only multiply within a cell. Some viruses, once in the cell, are protected by a protein coating making most antiviral drugs ineffective. Viruses tend to replicate in an anaerobic process making DMSO effective for killing them because it contains oxygen. Viruses cannot exist in a highly oxygenated environment.

Dermatological Applications
- Cutaneous lupus.
- Scleroderma.
- Cutaneous viral infections.
- Herpes simplex.

Toxicity: DMSO in elevated doses, up to 6 grams/kg (more than 3X the therapeutic dose), has shown no significant adverse effects. The most common side effect is a foul onion/garlic breath, and body odor. Due to the solvent properties, any toxic substance that is on the skin or the applicator may be transported internally with the DMSO. In order to prevent an inadvertent toxic response or infection, wash the area, hands and applicator prior to application of DMSO. Local skin irritation and focal redness may appear after application and is a common side effect, but can be easily remedied by reducing the concentration of the solution.

Directions for Therapeutic Use: DMSO should be applied topically for dermatological conditions. Wash the area thoroughly, then apply the DMSO with a sterile cotton applicator and let the area dry or cover with a sterile gauze for an hour to prevent introduction of toxic material. If using the DMSO as a carrier, cover the area with sterile gauze for an hour to prevent introduction of any toxic material.

47. Menthol

History: Menthol was first isolated from plants of the Mentha species in 1771 and contains a cyclic terpene alcohol which has been used for medicinal purposes for centuries. The peppermint plant, one of the major sources of menthol, has been grown in Japan for more than 2000 years. The primary actions are antipruritic, antiseptic, analgesic and cooling. Menthol is an organic compound now made synthetically or obtained naturally from oils of peppermint or mint leaves. Menthol triggers cold-sensitive receptors in the skin which induces a cooling sensation when inhaled, eaten, or applied to the skin without causing an actual temperature change.

Dermatological Applications
- Atopic dermatitis.
- Psoriasis.
- Insect bites and stings.
- Xerosis.
- Chapped lips.
- Cutaneous bacterial and fungal infections.
- Sunburn.
- Herpes simplex.

Toxicity: Menthol is FDA-approved for over-the-counter topical distribution in concentrations up to 16%. It is considered both safe and effective and there have not been any serious complaints filed with the FDA. However, menthol may cause allergic contact dermatitis and systemic allergic reactions especially in high concentrations.

Directions for Therapeutic Use: Topical applications include lip balms, creams, gels, lotions, patches, body sleeves, and a wide array of beauty products. First clean and dry the affected area. Apply a thin layer of the product to the clean dry skin and leave the area uncovered. Reapply the menthol as needed or prescribed.

48. Talc

History: Talc is an industrial mineral, magnesium trisilicate, that is extracted from soapstone. It has a dull to pearly luster and can be green, gray and white in color and is a very soft mineral with a soapy feel. Talcum powder produced from talc is highly absorbent and helps keeps the skin dry. Talcum powder is used to treat skin areas prone to excessive heat and moisture and is especially useful in hot and humid conditions. Talc functions by absorbing excess moisture from the skin and discouraging the fungal growth.

Talcum powder can be combined with other ingredients to aid healing. Talcum powder can be combined with aloe vera to soothe and scent the skin. Zinc oxide can be combined with talc powder to prevent diaper rash. Lavender, when combined with talc, acts as a calming agent and contains anti-bacterial properties.

Dermatological Application
- Skin areas prone to excessive heat and perspiration such as armpits, groin, buttocks, under the breasts, and between the toes.
- Remove excess oil from the skin and to reduce the shininess of skin.
- Decrease friction and chafing.
- Absorb excess moisture from the skin to discourage fungal growth.

Toxicity: Topically, talcum powder is not absorbable and is nontoxic. However, if the powder is inhaled it may cause coughing, difficulty breathing, acute respiratory distress, and potentially respiratory failure. When using talcum powder, keep the container away from the face and apply the power judiciously.

Directions for Therapeutic Use: Talcum powder is used as a drying agent especially where skin touches skin. Dust skin with talcum powder to absorb unwanted moisture and oil. Common areas of application include between the toes, armpits, groin, and under the breast.

Talcum powder can be used for newborns to prevent diaper rash, however it is important to keep the powder away from the child's face. The powder should be shaken onto one hand and then applied to the baby's diaper area.

49. Normal Saline and Water

History: Water is the mainstay for cleaning wounds and cooling first and second degree burns. Normal saline (0.9% saline solution) is an isotonic solution that neither increases nor pulls fluid from tissue that it comes into contact with. Water, however, is a hypotonic solution and may cause cellular edema and rupture when regular irrigation and washing is required. In wound care that requires regular irrigation a normal saline solution will not impede normal healing, cause further damage or alter the normal flora of the skin.

Water and normal saline may also be used in the treatment of crusts formed in contact, atopic and other dermatitis conditions that cause weeping.

Dermatological Application

- Wound cleansing.
- Ulcer irrigation and cleaning.
- First and second degree burns.
- Atopic dermatitis.
- Contact dermatitis.

Toxicity: There is no known toxicity to either water or normal saline solution but when used they should be applied at body temperature. Application of cold solutions may cause the damaged tissue to remain below normal temperature for up to 40 minutes and inhibit leukocyte activity for up to 3 hours.

Directions for Therapeutic Use: For wound care, wash hands before starting then, using warm water and a mild soap or cleansing agent, wash the wound, then pat dry. If the cleansing agent causes irritation, use normal saline solution to wash the area. Normal saline is made by adding ¼ teaspoon of non-iodized salt to 1 cup of water, bring to a boil and let cool. Cover and store in refrigerator. Normal saline is also available commercially in pharmacies.

For ulcer care, sterile water or sterile saline solution should be used to prevent contamination and infection.

For dermatitis, gauze may be soaked in the saline solution and then applied to the affected area to soften the crusts, retain moisture and calm the itch.

50. Urea

History: Urea is used in many topical, dermatological products to promote rehydration of the skin. The general consensus of studies done using urea suggest that lotions and salves containing 10% or more have more efficacy than those containing 2–5%. Urea improves the skin's barrier by supporting the lower layer of the stratum corneum, while eliminating dead and dying cells on the top layer of the stratum corneum. Urea salves can promote a pH at which healing can occur more efficiently, as well as protection against bacterial infections.

Dermatological Applications

- Psoriasis.
- Xerosis.
- Ichthyosis.
- Keratosis pilaris.
- Eczema.
- Scabies.
- Calluses.
- Ingrown nails.

Toxicity: Urea has very few side effects when used topically. If a skin rash, burning, itching, stinging or irritation is noticed at the area of application area should be discontinued. A rare severe allergic reaction would include hives, swelling of the face or hands, swelling or tingling in the mouth or throat, chest tightness, or trouble breathing.

Directions for Therapeutic Use: Urea lotions and salves are for external use only. Wash hands and the area where the urea is to be applied with soap and water and dry thoroughly. A thin layer should be applied to the affected area. The area may need to be covered by a plastic film or gauze to be kept dry.

Treatment of ingrown toenails includes allowing the urea salve to dry unbound if the patient is wearing sandals or other open-toed shoe. When wearing closed toe shoes apply the cream and cover with an adhesive gauze bandage.

▩ Cross-Reference of Treatments and Conditions

For the convenience of readers, **Table 7–1** cross references the conditions listed in Chapter 6 with the appropriate therapeutic approaches described in this chapter.

Table 7-1

	Category	Therapeutic method or agent	Conditions (reference numbers)
1	Procedures	Cryotherapy	8, 14, 15, 17, 25, 31, 35, 45, 46
2		Dermabrasion and exfoliation	11, 22, 23
3		Hair removal	
4		Hydrotherapy - hot water therapy	8, 22, 25, 26, 27, 29
5		Iontophoresis with salicylic acid	5, 50
6		Ultraviolet light	1,3, 6, 8, 10, 22, 41, 45
7	Natural oils	Almond oil	1,2, 3, 11, 22, 23
8		Lanolin	1,2
9		Mineral oil	1,2, 3, 8, 12, 34, 38,
10		Olive oil	1, 2, 3, 8, 19, 23,
11		Evening primrose oil	1, 3, 8, 11, 42
12		Tea tree oil	3, 8, 11, 12, 14, 22, 24, 27, 32, 33, 34, 35,
13		Vaseline - white petroleum jelly	34, 35
14	Vitamins	Vitamin A	1, 4, 5, 7, 10, 11, 12, 22, 23, 40
15		Vitamin D	1
16		Vitamin E	3, 8, 22, 47
17	Minerals	Colloidal silver	22, 28, 29,
18		Epsom salt	3, 8, 22, 35, 36, 50
19		Iodine/Potassium iodide	30, 31, 47
20		Sodium bicarbonate	1, 3, 8
21		Zinc oxide	1, 3, 8, 10, 15, 21
22	Natural Products	Aloe vera	1, 2, 11, 22, 24, 33, 45, 48
23		Apple cider vinegar	2, 27, 28, 29, 33, 34, 35, 36, 38, 45, 46
24		Black walnut	1, 2, 3, 22, 33, 46,
25		Burdock	1, 8, 11, 22, 27, 46, 48
26		Calendula	1, 3, 27, 29, 35,
27		Chamomile	1, 3, 22, 27, 28, 29, 48
28		Chaparral	22, 24, 34, 35, 36, 38
29		Comfrey	35
30		Cornstarch	42, 48
31		Elderberry	1, 3, 8, 22, 24, 48
32		Garlic	22, 27, 28, 29, 30, 32, 33, 45
33		Ginger	1, 33
34		Goldenseal	1, 2, 3, 8, 22, 24, 27, 33, 45
35		Green tea	3, 8, 42
36		Lemon	22, 24, 45, 48
37		Oatmeal	1, 3, 8, 11, 42, 48
38		Onion	2, 27, 28, 29, 46
39		Undecycline	32, 33, 45
40		White willow bark	1, 2, 11, 32, 33, 46, 47
41		Witch hazel	3
42	Over-the-counter products	Antibiotics	22, 44, 50
43		Calamine	3, 8, 10, 22, 35, 42, 48
44		Hydrocortisone	1, 2, 3, 8, 9, 15, 26, 36, 38, 41, 44, 45, 49

Table 7-1   (continued)

	Category	Therapeutic method or agent	Conditions (reference numbers)
45		Hydrogen peroxide	24, 33,
46	Miscellaneous	Dimethysulfoxide	46, 47
47		Menthol	1, 3, 11, 27, 28, 29, 32, 35, 45,
48		Talc	33, 42, 48
49		Normal saline and water	3, 6, 8,
50		Urea	1, 5, 7, 11, 12, 36,

General References

Arndt KA and Bowers KE. *Manual of Dermatologic Therapeutics*, 6th ed. Philadelphia, Pa: Lippincott Williams & Wilkins; 2002.

Barnes J, Anderson L, and David Phillipson. *Herbal Medicines.* A guide for healthcare professionals, 2nd edition, Pharmaceutical Press; 2002.

Basch EM, and Ulbricht CE. *Natural Standard Herb and Supplement Handbook, the bottom line.* Elsevier Mosby; 2005.

Blumenthal M, Busse WR, Goldberg A, Gruenwald J, Hall T, Riggins CW, Rister RS. *The Complete German Commission E Monographs: Therapeutic Guide to Herbal Medicines,* Austin, Texas and Boston, Massachusetts: American Botanical Council and Integrative Medicine Communications; 1998.

Blumenthal, Goldberg, Brinckmann. *Herbal Medicine.* Expanded Commission E Monographs, 1st edition, Integrative Medicine Communications; 2000.

Coulston AM, Rock CL, Monsen ER. (ED). *Nutrition in the prevention and treatment of disease.* San Diego, CA. Academic Press 2001.

Duke JA. *Handbook of Medicinal Herbs.* CRC Press, Boca Raton; 2001.

Fragakis Allison. *The Health Professional's Guide to Popular Dietary Supplements,* 2nd Edition. American Dietetic Association, 2003.

Gruenwald J, Brendler T, Jaenicke C. *PDR for Herbal Medicines.* 2nd ed. Montvale, NJ: Medical Economics Company; 2000.

Newall C, Anderson L, Phillipson J. *Herbal Medicines: A Guide for Healthcare Professionals.* London, England: Pharmaceutical Press; 1996:52–53.

Ritchason Jack ND. *The Little Herb Encyclopedia: The Handbook of Natures Remedies for a Healthier Life,* 3rd edition, Woodland Health Books; 1995.

Skidmore-Roth Linda. *Mosby's Handbook of Herbs & Natural Supplements.* 3rd edition. Elsevier Mosby; 2006.

Starky C. *Therapeutic Modalities,* 3rd ed. F.A. Davis Company, Philadelphia, PA: 2004.

The Burton Goldberg Group. *Alternative Medicine: The Definitive Guide.* Tiburon, CA, Future Medicine Publishing, Inc.:1997.

Werback MR. *Foundations of Nutritioanl Medicine.* Tarzana, CA. Third Line Press 1997.

Further Reading

Procedures

Bolanca Z, et al. Trends, habits and attitudes towards suntanning. *Coll Antropol.* 2008 October;32 Suppl 2:143–146.

Freiman A, Bouganim N. History of cryotherapy. *Dermatology Online Journal.* 2005;11(2):9. Available at. http://dermatology.cdlib.org/112/reviews/hxcryo/freiman.html. Accessed March 17, 2009.

Kaplan K. Congenital Nevi—Risk of Malignancy. *WJM;* 1989, 150:78–79.

Kempiak SJ, Uebellhoer N. Superficial chemical peels and microdermabrasion for acne vulgaris. *Semin Cutan Med Surg.* 2008 Sep;27(3):212–220.

Lipozencic J, Bukvic Mokos Z. Attention on Non-surgical cosmetic procedures. *Acta Dermatovenerol Croat.* 2008;16(4):245–246.

Plensdorf S. Martinez, J. Common pigmentation disorders. *Am Fam Physician.* 2009 Jan;79(2):109–116.

Soroko Yolunta R, Rapking MC, Clemment JA, Mitchell PL, Berg RL. Treatment of Plantar Verrucae Using 2% Sodium Salicylate Iontophoresis. *Phys Ther.* 2002; 82(12):1184–1191.

Natural Oils

Budhiraja SS, Cullu ME. Biological Activity of Tea Tree Oil Components in Human Myelocytic Cell Line. *J Manip Physiol Therap* 1999 Sept; 22: 447–453.

Budiyanto A, Ahmed N, et al. Protective effect of topically applied olive oil against photocarcinogenesis following UVB exposure in mice. *Carcinogenesis.* 2000;(21): 2085–2090.

Forrest RD. Development of wound therapy from the Dark Ages to the present. *J R Soc Med*. 1982; 75: 268–73.

Forsch RT. Essentials of skin laceration repair. *Am Fam Physician*. 2008 October;78(8):945–951.

Freiman A, Barankin B, Elpern DJ. Sports dermatology part 2: swimming and other aquatic sports. *CMAJ*. November 23, 2004;171 (11). Available at http://www.cmaj.ca/cgi/content/full/171/11/1339. Accessed March 17, 2009.

Hederos CA, Berg A. Epogam evening primrose oil treatment in atopic dermatitis and asthma. *Arch Dis Child*. 1996; 75:494–497.

Hirschmann JV. When antibiotics are unnecessary. *Dermatol Clin*. 2009 January;27(1):75–83.

Jantti J, Nikkari T, Solakivi T, Vapaatalo H, Isomaki H. Evening primrose oil in rheumatoid arthritis: changes in serum lipids and fatty acids. *Ann Rheum Dis*. 1989; 48:124–127.

Kang H, Choi J, Lee AY. Allergic Contact Dermatitis to White Petrolatum. *J Dermatol*. 2004 May. 31(5): 428–430.

Kiechl-Kohlendorfer, U, Berger, C, Inzinger, R. The effect of daily treatment with an olive oil/lanolin emollient on skin integrity in preterm infants: a randomized controlled trial: *Pediatr Dermatol*. 2008; 25(2):174–178.

Kwiecinski J, Eick S, Wojcik K. Effects of tea tree (Melaleuca alternifolia) oil on Staphylococcus aureus in biofilms and stationary growth phase. *Int J Antimicrob Agents*. 2008 December 16; [Epub ahead of print].

Malisiova F, et al. Liposomal formulations from phospholiopids of Greek almond oil. Properties and biological activity. *Z Naturforsch [C]*. 2004 May June;59(5–6):330–334.

Melli MS, Rashidi MR, Nokhoodchi A, et al. A randomized trial of peppermint gel, lanolin ointment, and placebo get to prevent nipple crack in primiparous breastfeeding women: *Med Sci Monit*. 2007;13(9): CR406–411.

Millar BC, Moore JE. Successful topical treatment of hand warts in a pediatric patient with tea tree oil (Melaleuca alternifolia). *Complement Ther Clin Pract*. 2008 November;14(4):225–227.

Mohammadzadeh A, Farhat A, Esmaeily H. The effect of breast milk and lanolin on sore nipples: *Saudi Med J*. 2004; 26(8):1231–1234.

Richert B. Parasitic infections of the nails. *DOJ*. 2003; 9 (1). Available at http://dermatology.cdlib.org/91/abstracts/nail/17C.html. Accessed March 17, 2009.

Servili M, et al. Phenolic compounds in olive oil: antioxidant, health and organoleptic activities according to their chemical structure. *Inflammopharmacology*. 2009 February 17; [Epub ahead of print].

Stamatas GN. Etal. Lipid uptake and skin occlusion following topical application of oils on adult and infant skin. *J Dermatol Sci*. 2008 May;50(2):135–142.

Williams HC. (Dec 2003). Evening Primrose Oil for Atopic Dermatitis. *BMJ*. 372, 1358–9.

Vitamins

DeLuca HF, and Zierold C. Mechanisms and functions of vitamin D. *Nutr Rev* 1998;56:S4–S10.

Reichel H, Koeffler H, Norman AW. The role of vitamin D endocrine system in health and disease. *N Engl J Med* 1989;320:980–991.

Thieltiz A, Gollnick H. Topical retinoids in acne vulgaris: update of efficacy and safety. *Am J Clin Dermatology*. 2008;9(6):369–381.

Topical retinoids. New Zealand Dermatological Society, Inc.[DermNet NZ Web Site] Available at: http://www.dermnetnz.org/treatments/topical-retinoids.html. Accessed March 17, 2009.

Van den Berg H. Bioavailability of vitamin D. *Eur J Clin Nutr* 1997;51 Suppl 1:S76–S79.

Veret WJ, et.al. A Randomized, Double-Blind Placebo-Controlled Trial Evaluating the Effects of Vitamin E and Selenium on Arsenic-Induced Skin Lesions in Bangladesh. *J Occup Environ Med*. 2005; 47: 1026–1034.

Minerals

Chakravathi A, Srinivas CR, Mathew AC. Activated charcoal and baking soda to reduce odor associated with extensive blistering disorders. *Indian J Dermatol Venereol Leprol*. 2008; 74:122–124.

Godfrey HR, Godfrey NJ, Godfrey JC, Riley D. A randomized clinical trial on the treatment of oral herpes with topical zinc oxide/glycince. *Alt Therap Health Med*. 2001; 7(3):49–56.

Haas D. Selective magnesium sulfate prophylaxis for the prevention of eclampsia in women with gestational hypertension. *Obstet Gynecol*. 2007;109(1): 201–220.

Hipler UC, Elsner P, Fluhr JW. A new silver-loaded cellulosic fiber with antifungal and antibacterial properties. *Curr Probl Dermatol*. 2006; 33:165–178.

Leaper DJ, Durani P. Topical antimicrobial therapy of chronic wound healing by secondary intention using iodine products. *Int Wounds J*. 2008 June; 5(2):361–368.

Oliveira AS, Santos VL. Use of topical iodine in acute wounds. *Rev Esc Enferm USP*. 2008 March;42(1): 193–201.

Verdolini R, Bugatti L, Filosa G, Mannello B, Lawlor F, Cerio RR. Old fashioned sodium bicarbonate baths for the treatment of psoriasis in the ear of futuristic biologics: An old ally to be rescued. *J Dermatolog Treat*. 2005; 16:26–30.

Wadhera A, Fung M. Systemic argyria associated with ingestion of colloidal silver. *Dermatology Online Journal.* 2005; 11(1):12. Avaliable at http://dermatology.cdlib.org/111/case_reports/argyria/wadhera.html. Accessed March 17, 2009.

Natural Products

An BJ, Kwak JH, Son JH, Park JM, Lee JY, Park TS, Kim SY, Kim YS, Jo C, Byun MW. Physiological Activity of Irradiated Green Tea Polyphenol on Human Skin. *Am J Chin Med.* 2005; 33: 535–546.

Brinker F. Larrea tridentata (DC) coville. (Chaparral or Creosote Bush). *Br J Phytother;* 1993; 3(1):10–31.

Cutler RR, Wilson P. Antibacterial activity of a new stable aqueous extract of allicin methicillin resilient Staphylococcus aureus. *Br J Biomed Sci.* 2004; 61(2):71–74.

Dorsch W, Schnneider E, Bayer T, Wagner H. Anti-inflammatory Effects of Onions. *Int Arch Allergy Appl Immunol.*1999; 92: 39–42.

Ehrlich SD. Ginger [University of Maryland Medical Center Web site]. Availabel at: http://www.umm.edu/altmed/ConsHerbs/Gingerch.html. Accessed on March 17, 2009.

Feily A. Namazi, MR. Aloe vera in dermatology: a brief review. *G Ital Dermatol Venereol.* 2009 February; 144(1):85–91.

Fugh-Berman A. Herbal Supplements: Indications, Clinical Concerns, and Safety. *Nutrition Today.* 2002:37(3):122–124.

Grube B, Grunwald J, KrugL, Staiger C. Efficacy of a comfrey root (Symphi offic. Radix) extract ointment in the treatment of patients with painful osteoarthritis of the knee: Results of a double-blind, randomized, bicenter, placebo-controlled trial. *Phytomedicines.* 2007 Jan; 14:1: 2–10.

Heron S, Yarnell E. The Safety of Low-Dose Larrea tridentata (DC) Coville (Creosote Bush or Chaparral): A Retrospective Clinical Study. *J Alt Comp Med.* 2001;7(2):175–185.

Kock C, Reichling J, Schneels J, Schnitzler P. Inhibitory effects of essential oils against herpes simplex virus type 2. *Phytomedicine.* 2008 January; 15 (1–2):71–78.

Korakhashville A, Kacharava T, Kilnavelidze N. Biochemical structure of Calendula officinalis. *Georgian Med News.* 2007 July August; (148–149):70–73.

Mayo Clinic Staff. Impetigo. [MayoClinic Website]. October 4, 2008. Available at: http://www.mayoclinic.com/health/impetigo/DS00464/DSECTION=9. Accessed March 17, 2009.

McLaim N, Ascanio R, Baker C, Stovhaven RA, Dolan JW. Undecylenic Acid Inhibits Morphogenesis of Candida Albicans. *Antimicrob Agents Chemother.* 2000 October; 44(10):2873–2875.

Mendelsohn Felicia A. "Wound Care After Radiation Therapy." *Adv Skin Wound Care* 15(2002): 216–224.

Miles S. Topical Antioxidants. *Alive: Canadian Journal of Health & Nutrition.* 2006 Sep; 287:146–147.

Nakachi K, Matsuyama S, Miyake S, Suganuma M & Imai K. Preventive effects of drinking green tea on cancer and cardiovascular disease: epidemiological evidence for multiple targeting prevention. *Biofactors.* 2000;134(1–4):49–54.

New Zealand Dermatological Society. Lemon [New Zealand Dermatological Society Web site]. 2002. Last updated March 2008. Available at: http://www.dermnetnz.org/dermatitis/plants/lemon.html, Accessed February 6, 2009.

O'Hara M, Kiefer D, Farrel K, Kemper K. A Review of 12 Commonly Used Medicinal Herbs. *Arch Fam Med.* 1998;7:6.

Poison Ivy, Oak and Sumac [American Academy of Dermatology Web Site]. Available at www.aad.org/public/Publications/pamphlets/Poison_IvyOakSumac.htm. Accessed March 17, 2009.

Psoriasis. AOCD Dermatologic Disease Database. [American Osteopathic College of Dermatology Web Site]. Available at www.aocd.org/skin/dermatologic_diseases/psoriasis.html. Accessed March 17, 2009.

Rajar UD, et al. Efficacy of aloe vera gel in the treatment of vulval lichen planus. *J Coll Physicians Surg Pak.* 2008 October;18(10):612–614.

Ross S. An Integrative Approach to Eczema (Atopic Dermatitis), *Holist Nurs Pract.* 2003 Jan Feb; 17(1):56–62.

Sabitha P, et al. Efficacy of garlic paste in oral candidiasis. *Trop Doct.*2005 April;35(2):99–100.

Samman S, Sandstrom B, Toft MB, Bukhave K, Jensen M, Sorensen SS & Hansen M. Green tea extract added to foods reduces nonheme-iron absorption. *Am J Clin Nutri.* 2001 Mar;73(3):607–612.

Scazzocchio F, Cometa, MF. Tomassini, L. Palmery, M. Antibacterial activity of Hydastis canadensis extract and its major isolated alkaloids. *Planta Med.* 2001 August; 67(6):561–564.

Shafran SD, et al. Topical Undecylenic Acid for Herpes Simplex Labialis: A Multicenter, Placebo-Controlled Trial. *J Inf Dis.* 1997. 176:78–83.

Smith EB, Powell RP, Graham JL, Ulrick JA. Topical undecylenic acid in tenea pedis: a new look. *Int J Dermatol.* 1977 Jan–Feb; 16(1):52–56.

Szakeil A, et al. Antibacterial and antiparasitic activity of oleanolic acid and its glycosides isolated from marigold (Calendula officinalis). *Planta Med.* 2008 November; 74(14):1709–1715.

Over-the-Counter Products

Al-Ghnaniem R, et al. 1% hydrocortisone ointment is an effective treatment of purities ani: a pilot randomized control crossover trial. *Int J Colorectal Dis.* 2007 December; 22(12):1463–1467.

Bonomo Robert A, Van Zile, Peter S, Li Qing, Shermock Kenneth M, McCormick William G, Kohut Bruce. Topical Triple-Antibiotic Ointment as a Novel Therapeutic Choice in Wound Management and Infection Prevention: A Practical Perspective. *Expert Rev Anti Infect Ther.* 2007; 5(5).

Hendley JO, Ashe KM. Eradication of Resident Bacteria of Normal Human Skin by Antimicrobial Ointment. *Am Soc Microbiol.* 2003; 47:6.

Tebruegge M, Kuruvilla M, & Margarson I. Does the use of calamine or antihistamine provide symptomatic relief from pruritis in children with varicella zoster infection? *Arch Dis Child*, 2006;91: 1035–1036.

Miscellaneous

Dulecki M, Pieper B. Irrigating Simple Acute Traumatic Wounds: A Review of the Current Literature. *J Emerg Nurs.* April 2005. 31:2 156–160.

Engel MF. Dimethyl Sulfoxide (DMSO) in Clinical Dermatology. *South Med J.* 1996;59:1318.

Fellows J. Crestodina Lea. Home–Prepared Saline: a Safe, Cost-effective Alternative for wound Cleansing in Home Care. *The J Wound Ostomy Continence Nurs.* December 2006: 33(6) 606–609.

Grether-Breck S, Muhlberg K, Brenden H, Krutmann J. Urea plus ceramides and vitamins: improving the efficacy of a topical urea preparation by adding ceramides and vitamins. *Hautarzt.* 2008 September; 59(9): 717–8, 720–723.

Hildick-Smith GY. The biology of talc. *Br J Ind Med.* 1976.33:217–229.

Hindley D, Galloway J, Gardner L. A randomized study of "wet wraps" versus conventional treatment of atopic eczema. *Arch Dis Child.* 2006; 91:163–168.

Honig PJ. Diaper dermatitis: Factors to consider in diagnosis and treatment. *Postgrad Med.*1983 December; 74(6):79–84,88.

Krug M, Oji V, Traupe H, Berneburg M. Ichthyoses—Part I: Differential diagnosis of vulgar ichthyoses and therapeutic options. *J Dtsch Dermatol Ges.* 2009 January 14.[Epub ahead of print].

Krug M, Oji V, Traupe H, Berneburg M. Ichthyoses—Part 2–Congenital Ichtyoses. *J Dtsch Dermatol Ges.* 2009 January 14. [Epub ahead of print].

Wasner G, Schattschneider J, Binder A, Baron R. Topical Menthol-a human model for cold pain activation and sensitization of C nociceptors. *Brain.* 2004 May; 127(5): 1159–71.

Witman P. Topical Therapies for Localized Psoriasis, *Mayo Clin Proc.* 2001;76:943–949.

Fifty Additional Skin Disorders You Need to Know

Chapter 6 contains the descriptions of the fifty most common skin conditions likely to be seen in a chiropractic office. Of course, there are thousands of skin diseases and disorders. Many are rare and unlikely to be seen in a chiropractic practice, let alone a specialized dermatology practice, but *any* condition *can* be seen in practice. Therefore, we have included this chapter which contains the essential diagnostic points of another fifty skin conditions. This second tier of dermatologic conditions should equip the practicing chiropractor with the knowledge to be aware of, and therefore vigilant for the possibility that any of these conditions could be found in patients attending chiropractic practices.

These conditions are presented in alphabetical order, to facilitate easy access to the information:

1. Actinic keratosis
2. Alopecia areata
3. Bee sting
4. Bowen's disease
5. Bullous pemphigoid
6. Chondrodermatitis nodularis helicis
7. Cutaneous horn
8. Cutaneous larva migrans
9. Dermatitis herpetiformis
10. Dermatomyositis
11. Epidermolysis bullosa
12. Erysipelas
13. Erythema multiforme
14. Erythema nodosum
15. Granuloma annulare
16. Grover's disease
17. Idiopathic guttate hypomelanosis
18. Kaposi's sarcoma
19. Kawasaki's disease
20. Keratoacanthoma
21. Lentigo
22. Lichen sclerosus
23. Linear IgA disease
24. Lipoma
25. Mastocytosis (urticaria pigmentosa)
26. Miliaria
27. Morphea
28. Necrobiosis lipoidica diabeticorum
29. Neurotic excoriation
30. Nevus
31. Panniculitis
32. Pemphigus vulgaris
33. Perlèche
34. Porphyria cutanea tarda
35. Prurigo nodularis
36. Pseudofolliculitis barbae
37. Pseudoxanthoma elasticum
38. Pyoderma gangrenosum
39. Rocky Mountain spotted fever
40. Scleroderma
41. Spider bite
42. Stevens Johnson syndrome
43. Sweets syndrome
44. Syringoma
45. Telangiectasia (hereditary, ataxia)
46. Telogen effluvium
47. Toxic epidermal necrolysis
48. Trichotillomania
49. Tuberous sclerosis
50. Venous leg ulcers

1. Actinic Keratosis

- Scaly or crust bumps on skin surfaces exposed to the sun; also called sunspots or solar keratosis; caused by exposure to ultraviolet light.

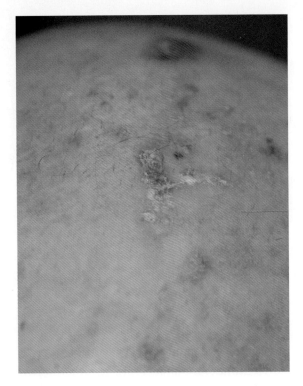

Figure 8-1   Actinic keratosis.

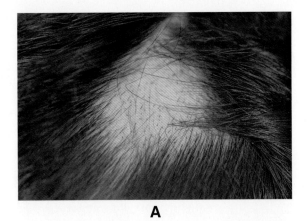

A

Figure 8-2 (A)   Alopecia areata.

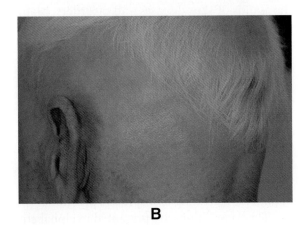

B

Figure 8-2 (B)   Alopecia areata.

- May range from asymptomatic to itching to tender lesions; most often noticed cosmetically or due to palpable elevated crusty plaque.
- More common in fair-skinned persons; some lesions (perhaps up to 10%) which appear redder and which may be tender to touch may progress to squamous cell carcinoma (3% of these carcimonas will metastasize).
- Actinic cheilitis is the most aggressive form and up to 20% of these lip lesions may progress to carcinoma.
- Treated by cryosurgery, chemical peels (skin is literally peeled off by a strong chemical agent) or curettage; early or emerging lesions may be treated using immune-active topical creams for 6-12 weeks.

2. Alopecia Areata

- Auto-immune disease (anti-hair bulb process).
- Localized loss of hair in oval or round patches, most commonly on scalp (alopecia universalis is a variant in which all body hair is lost).
- Occurs in young adults and children (and most patients regrow hair, usually within a year, but condition may be recurrent).
- Differentiate from tinea infections.
- No treatment available.

3. Bee Sting

- Technically a sting from a honey bee, but commonly used to denote stings from a wide range of species: bee, wasp, hornet, yellow jacket.
- Stinger has a barbed end that lodges in skin, tearing loose from bee and injecting apitoxin and melittin into victim; pheromones are also released by bee which attract other bees to the victim; results in painful red papule.
- Many folk remedies exist but studies show that local application of ice is better than aspirin to relieve pain and swelling (after stinger is removed as quickly as possible).
- Anaphylactic shock may occur in those allergic to bee stings (up to 2% of the population); anaphylaxis is life-threatening and must be treated promptly; allergic individuals often carry a self-injecting Epipen for such emergencies.

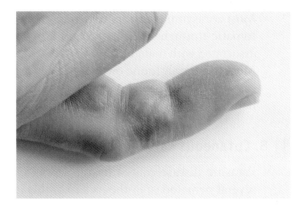

Figure 8-3 Bee sting.

- Pain and swelling may last up to a week and no specific effective treatment exists.

4. Bowen's Disease (Squamous Cell Epithelioma, or Squamous Cell Carcinoma *in situ*)

- Usually a red, scaly patch, seen on areas frequently exposed to the sun; some itch, crust or ooze, but most are asymptomatic.
- 75% of patients are female and about 75% of the lesions are on the lower extremities; most patients are older than 60 years of age.
- May be mistaken for rashes, eczema, fungus or psoriasis; mostly associated with chronic skin exposure and aging; patients may have a history of exposure to arsenic (perhaps from drinking well water).
- Lesions may grow slowly to a lesion several inches across; about 5% develop into invasive squamous cell carcinoma if untreated.
- Most commonly treated with surgical excision, curettage and electrodessication, liquid nitrogen cryotherapy, local chemotherapy or laser destruction.

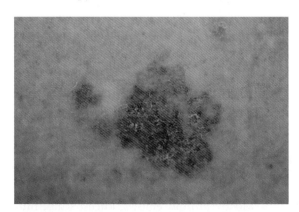

Figure 8-4 Bowen's disease.

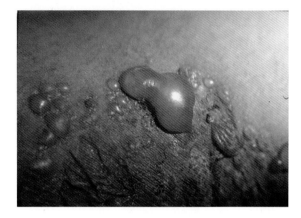

Figure 8-5 Bullous pemphigoid.

5. Bullous Pemphigoid

- Pemphigoid = like pemphigus.
- Named for the Greek word, *pemphigodes*, meaning breaking out in blisters.
- Two forms of pemphigoid: benign mucosal (produces scarring in mouth and conjunctivae; also known as cicatrical pemphigoid), and bullous.
- Causes chronic bullous eruptions in widespread distribution.
- Rarely fatal (unlike pemphigus).

6. Chondrodermatitis Nodularis Helicis (Winkler Disease)

- Typically unilateral small tender nodule on helix of ear; likely related to either sun exposure or repetitive mechanical trauma (such as the use of headphones or cellular telephones).
- Usually found on the helix (superior portion or lateral rim) or antihelix. Less commonly found on other parts of the earlobe (although pinnal lesions are extremely rare).
- Possibly due to lack of protective subcutaneous fat and/or poor vascularity, combined with sun exposure or mechanical trauma.
- Usually a small nodule covered by a crust, which when removed allows the expression of necrotic material; lesions may be mistaken for squamous cell carcinoma and biopsy is required to exclude this diagnosis.
- May be tender to touch or palpate, due to the presence of sensory nerves within the lesion; treated preventively by removing the irritating cause, or dermatologically

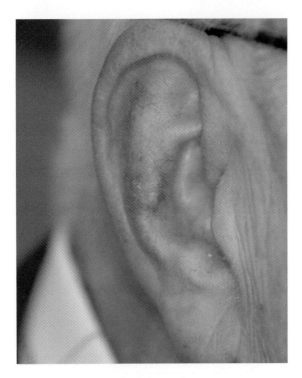

Figure 8-6   Chondrodermatitis nodularis helicis.

using a variety of methods such as cortisone injections and excision.

7. Cutaneous Horn

- Hyperkeratotic lesion (scales) associated with a horn-like projection composed of a mound of compacted keratin (usually several millimeters long, although some can be much larger).
- A wide variety of benign lesions (such as warts) and malignant lesions (such as basal cell carcinoma) may give rise to horns; a tender lesion or rapidly growing lesion suggests malignancy (up to 20% of horns have bases with malignant cells).
- About one-third of cutaneous horns on the penis are associated with squamous cell carcinoma.

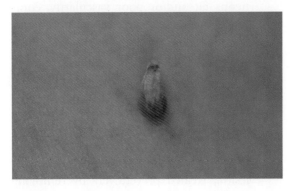

Figure 8-7   Cutaneous horn.

- Most are asymptomatic and become symptomatic through trauma or rapid growth associated with malignancy.
- Most commonly found on sun-exposed areas such as the pinnae, face, and dorsum of hands.

8. Cutaneous Larva Migrans (CLM)

- Parasitic disease caused by the larvae of several nematodes; in the Americas this is most commonly caused by *Ancylostoma Braizilense* (called sandworms in the USA) via dog and cat feces.
- Infection results in wormlike burrows visible under the skin; usually confined to the skin of the feet, buttocks, or abdomen; appear as red macular lesions.
- Hypersensitivity to the worms and their byproducts causes a red, intensely pruritic eruption which may lead to secondary infection from scratching.
- Treatment consists of anti-helminthic medications (usually oral).
- In the US, the most common location for these infections is Florida; in one study of visitors to a travel-related clinic, 6.7% of patients attended the clinic for CLM.

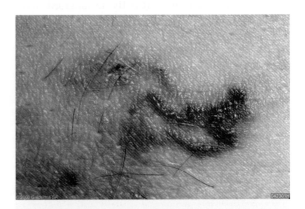

Figure 8-8   Cutaneous larva migrans. © *DermQuest.com. Used with permission from Galderma SA.*

9. Dermatitis Herpetiformis

- Small clusters of red, itchy bumps (actually tiny vesicles that are quickly scratched off, after which they scab over and heal, to be followed by new spots developing).
- Cause intense itching, burning and stinging.
- Mostly around elbows, knees, scalp, buttocks and back, in young adults.

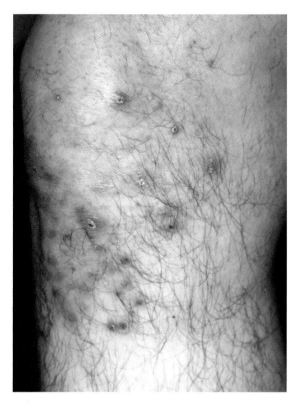

Figure 8-9 Dermatitis herpetiformis. © *DermQuest.com. Used with permission from Galderma SA.*

- Chronic, incurable; 10-20% of patients experience remission.
- Caused by allergy to gluten, therefore can be effectively treated by gluten-free diet (although this is often very difficult to achieve, therefore drug treatment is often needed concurrently); some patients also have gluten-sensitive enteropathy, or celiac disease.

10. Dermatomyositis

- Connective tissue related to polymyositis; inflammation of skin and muscle.
- Macular rash (patchy discoloration) and symmetric proximal muscle weakness with myalgia.
- Psoriasis-like rash may occur over the metacarpophalangeal and interphalangeal joints (Gottron's sign).
- Rash also commonly seen on eyelids, and may also occur on face and chest.
- Treated with drugs typically used in treatment of rheumatic disorders; most conditions respond to treatment; chiropractic care can help patients regain range of motion, strengthen affected muscles and prevent muscle atrophy.

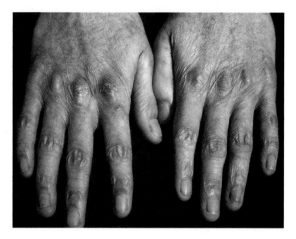

Figure 8-10 Gottron papules on the knuckles of a patient with dermatomyositis.

11. Epidermolysis Bullosa

- Hereditary disease resulting in deep-seated bullae appearing at sites of minor trauma.
- Spectrum ranges from minor annoyance to widespread life-threatening blistering disease.
- Blisters are almost always noted at birth or shortly after birth.
- Three pathologic forms—in all three cases, the epidermis separates from the dermis, causing a blister to form between the two.
- In less severe forms, blisters and bullae form quickly after minor rubbing or irritation of the skin, often leaving atrophic scars after the healing of the blisters.

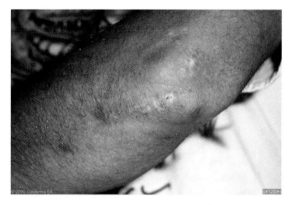

Figure 8-11   Epidermolysis bullosa. © *DermQuest.com. Used with permission from Galderma SA.*

12. Erysipelas

- Cellulitis mainly caused by Group A β-hemolytic streptococcus resulting most commonly in macular rash.
- Can affect any age group but mostly seen in children and elderly patients.

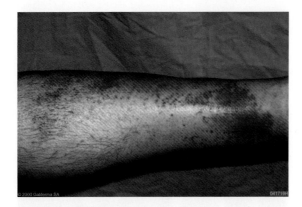

Figure 8-12   Erysipelas. © DermQuest.com. Used with permission from Galderma SA.

- Mostly seen in lower extremities, can appear on face as butterfly rash; lesions have raised edge which may help distinguish them from other forms of cellulitis; lesions are quite painful (St. Anthony's fire).
- Usually acute onset of infection with fever, chills, constitutional symptoms.
- Good prognosis if treated promptly with Penicillin (otherwise may progress into septicemia).

13. Erythema Multiforme

- Self-limited disease usually follows infection or drug treatment (most commonly follows herpes simplex infection or exposure to sulfa drugs, penicillin, phenytoin or barbiturates).
- Unknown cause but likely due to deposition of immune complexes in the microvasculature of the skin and mucous membranes.
- Mostly a mild self-limited macular rash (symmetrical and starting on extremities)

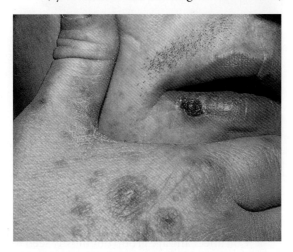

Figure 8-13   Target shaped lesions in erythema multiforme.

but may also present in a major form which resembles (and is most likely related to) Stevens-Johnson syndrome.
- Lesions may be mildly itchy and form patches, similar to target lesions with pink ring around a pale center.
- Resolves spontaneously within 7-10 days.

14. Erythema Nodosum

- Inflammation of fat cells within skin (panniculitis); usually as an immune response to a variety of conditions such as pregnancy, sarcoidosis, autoimmune disease, infections, cancer and the use of some medications, including oral contraceptives.
- Results in tender, red, smooth and shiny nodules on both shins (may occur elsewhere, wherever there is fat under the skin); lesions resolve within a few weeks and slowly progress through color changes similar to the resolution of a bruise.
- Frequently accompanied with fever, constitutional symptoms and arthralgia.
- May occur in combination with other diseases, particularly pulmonary disease such as sarcoidosis or tuberculosis.
- Symptomatic treatment by elevating legs, use of compressive dressings and wet bandages; NSAID's may be used for pain and inflammation.

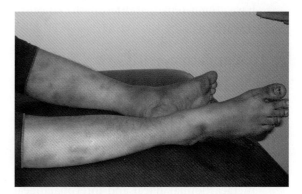

Figure 8-14   Erythema nodosum on the lower extremities.

15. Granuloma Annulare

- Chronic condition with round papules (hence, *annulare*) usually on hands and feet; lesions are small, smooth, round and slightly elevated; lesions vary in color and may be reddish, yellow, or even flesh-colored.

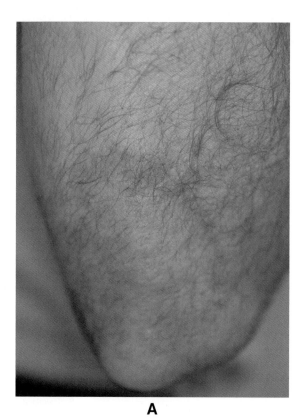

A

Figure 8-15 (A) Granuloma annulare.

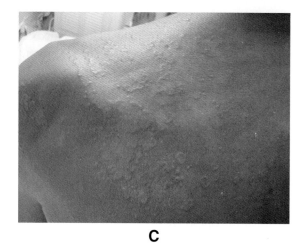

C

Figure 8-15 (C) Disseminated granuloma annulare.

- Most patients seek care for cosmetic reasons; there are usually no symptoms other than the red rings; must be differentiated from tinea corporis.
- self limited (perhaps up to 2 years).
- Unknown cause, treatment is cosmetic only.
- Most often affects children and young adults.

16. Grover's Disease (Transient Acantholytic Dyskeratosis, TAD)

- Common, with sudden onset of itching and scaly lesions on back, chest, arms and thighs.
- may persist for up to a year and recur.
- Often related to heat stress or persistent sweating; lesions usually very itchy, particularly on chest or back.

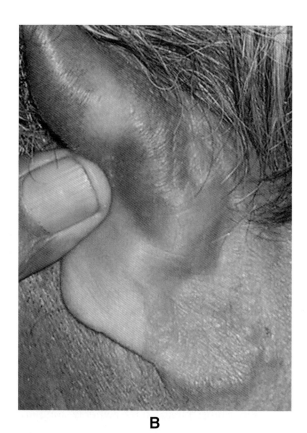

B

Figure 8-15 (B) Granuloma annulare behind the ear.

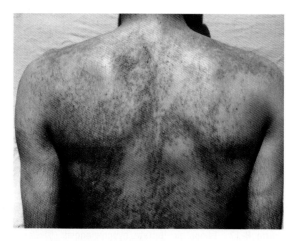

Figure 8-16 Grover's disease.

- Treated by avoiding further sweating and symptomatically treating itching; medical care consists of topical corticosteroid cream.
- Itching may be controlled with topical combination of glycerol, talc and zinc oxide.

17. Idiopathic Guttate Hypomelanosis

- Flat hypopigmented patches most commonly found on arms or shins, or other sun-exposed areas.
- Lesions are teardrop shaped or guttate, 2-5 mm.
- Very common in patients older than 40 years of age, possibly part of normal aging process; more common in females.
- Does not predispose to cancer.
- No treatment required other than elective cosmetic coloring if condition is extensive or psychologically stressful.

18. Kaposi's Sarcoma

- Opportunistic disease, once considered rare, now seen increasingly in AIDS patients.
- Caused by Human herpesvirus 8 (HHV8), also called Kaposi's sarcoma-associated herpesvirus (KSHV).

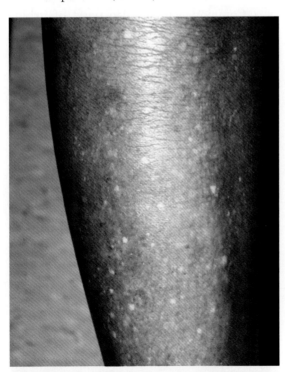

Figure 8-17 Idiopathic guttate hypomelanosis. © DermQuest.com. *Used with permission from Galderma SA.*

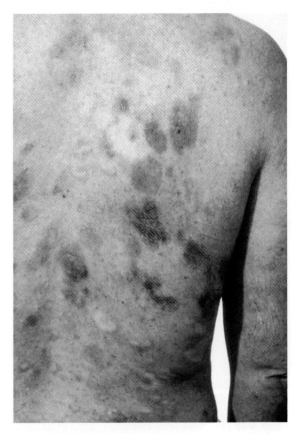

Figure 8-18   Kaposi's sarcoma.

- Begins as a pinkish-brown patch developing into a cluster of raised nodules that can be black, brown, red or purple.
- Lesions located on lower extremities, genitalia, face and mouth.
- High mortality and morbidity; incurable but may be palliated by radiation therapy or cryosurgery.

19. Kawasaki's Disease

- Lymph node syndrome or mucocutaneous lymph node disease—a form of vasculitis that affects skin, mouth and lymph nodes in children younger than age 5 (often of Japanese or Korean descent); cause unknown.
- In addition to the cutaneous and oral lesions, it may cause vasculitis affecting the heart and coronary blood vessels resulting in aneurysms and even myocardial infarction (even in young children).
- Begins as persistent fever (sometimes up to 2 weeks), followed by development of conjunctivitis, glossitis (strawberry tongue), lymph node swelling (usually in neck), arthralgia, tachycardia and other signs of

rheumatologic disease; red palms and soles often seen (which may peel later in disease); may be confused with scarlatina (scarlet fever) or Still's disease.

- Diagnosis includes 5 days of fever, plus four of the following: 1. erythema of lips, oral cavity, or cracking of lips, 2. macular rash on trunk, 3. swelling or erythema of palms or soles, 4. conjunctivitis, 5. lymph node swelling in neck of at least 15 mm.

- Requires prompt attention and hospitalization to prevent possible cardiac damage and death; treated with intravenous immunoglobulin (IVIG).

20. Keratoacanthoma

- Relatively common low grade malignancy believed to be related to squamous cell carcinoma; seen in middle-aged and elderly patients on sun-exposed skin (often the face).

- Volcano shaped, rapidly growing nodular lesions; may grow up to 1-2 cm over a few weeks; central depression of volcano becomes crusty and darkened.

- Most lesions spontaneously regress over 4-6 months; up to 2% may become non-regressive and invasive.

- Because of resemblance with squamous cell carcinoma, the lesion is usually treated aggressively with surgery.

- More common in older patients, males and persons with light skin.

21. Lentigo (plural, Lentigines)

- Also known as solar lentigo, freckles, sunspots, liver spots, lentigo simplex; observed in 90% of white skinned persons older than 60.

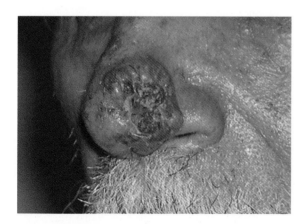

Figure 8-19   Keratoacanthoma.

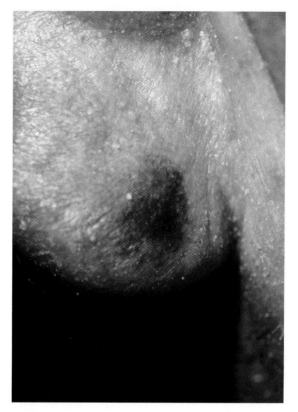

Figure 8-20   Lentigo. © *DermQuest.com. Used with permission from Galderma SA.*

- Small, sharply circumscribed, pigmented macule surrounded by normal-appearing skin.

- Lentigo simplex is the most common form and is not related to sun exposure; lesions are few and can appear anywhere on the skin.

- Solar lentigo is related to sun exposure, may serve as clinical markers of past severe sunburn and may be used to identify a population at higher risk of developing cutaneous melanoma.

- Wide variety of related forms including Peutz-Jeghers syndrome (inherited), oral and labial forms, penile and vulvar forms, and complex syndromes associated with pigmented skin (example: LEOPARD syndrome = <u>l</u>entigines, <u>e</u>lectrocardiographic conduction defects, <u>o</u>cular hypertelorism, <u>p</u>ulmonary stenosis, <u>a</u>bnormal genitalia, <u>r</u>etardation of growth, and <u>d</u>eafness).

22. Lichen Sclerosus

- Also called lichen sclerosus et atrophicus, because skin is thin; causes hypopigmented patches anywhere on body but most

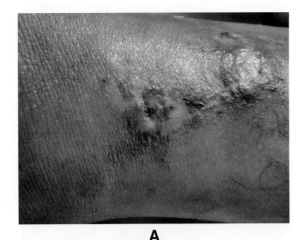

A

Figure 8-21 (A) Lichen sclerosus.

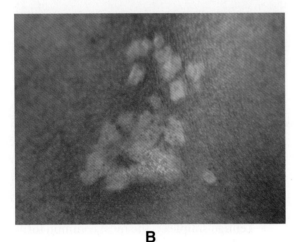

B

Figure 8-21 (B) Hypopigmented macules coalescing to patches in lichen sclerosus et atrophicus.

commonly the skin of the vulva, foreskin of the penis and perianal skin; in males it is seen almost exclusively in uncircumcised men and boys.

- More common in postmenopausal females but can also occur in prepubertal females (and may be confused with sexual abuse, since lichen sclerosus can result in itching, pain and redness in the area of the vulva); the thinning of the skin can result in bruising and signs of trauma from mild injury, such as wiping with toilet tissue.
- Differential diagnoses: psoriasis, eczema, contact dermatitis, sexual abuse, trauma, Stevens-Johnson syndrome.
- May spontaneously disappear or may be successfully treated with topical corticosteroid ointment.

- Cause is unknown; may be related to local irritation or possibly even an infection (*Borrelia*).

23. Linear IgA Disease

- A rare autoimmune disease causing blistering lesions (bullae) similar to those seen in bullous pemphigoid and dermatitis herpetiformis; cause is unknown but may be related to drug reaction (frequently vancomycin, within 1-13 days of administration).
- Occurs in children and adults, including the elderly; 50-60% remission rate within 2-6 years; in drug-induced cases, there is rapid healing without scarring once the drug is withdrawn.
- Lesions of mucous membranes are much more serious and can lead to death; ocular lesions may lead to blindness (ocular lesions begin with a feeling of grittiness in the eyes).
- May begin with itching (sometimes prolonged) and progress to discrete or herpetiform bullae; occurs on trunk and limbs (and perineally and periorally in children more commonly than adults).
- Treated using Dapsone, as well as with a variety of other drugs including corticosteroids.

24. Lipoma

- The most common benign mesenchymal tumor; composed of fat cells in discrete, easily diagnosed nodular lesions; usually small (2-3 cm.) but can also be up to 10 cm.

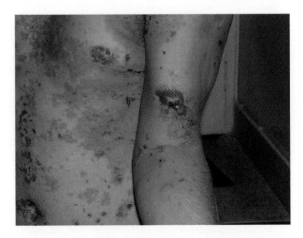

Figure 8-22 Linear IgA disease.

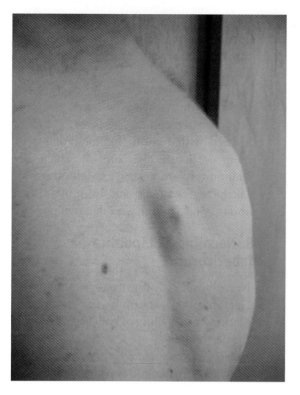

Figure 8-23   Lipoma on mid-back region.

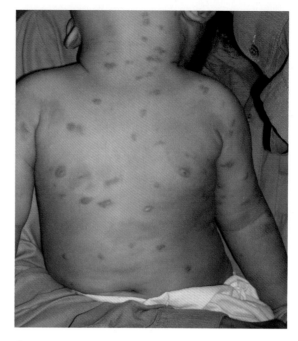

Figure 8-24   Mastocytosis (urticaria pigmentosa) in an infant.

in diameter; may be solitary (most common) or multiple.

- Most are located on the trunk (back and neck), thighs or arms.

- Typically subcutaneous but may occur around internal organs.

- At least seven categories: solitary, diffuse, symmetrical (Madelung disease, associated with diabetes, obesity and alcoholism), familial multiple lipomatosis, adiposis dolorosa (extremely painful lesions), angiolipomas and hibernomas (brown lipomas).

- Rarely symptomatic; no treatment required except for cosmetic reasons.

25. Mastocytosis (Urticaria Pigmentosa)

- Disorder characterized by mast cell proliferation and accumulation within various organs, most commonly the skin.

- Consists of at least seven forms, of which cutaneous mastocytosis is only one; cutaneous mastocytosis consists of four forms, of which urticaria pigmentosa is the most common; causes numerous oval red-brown wheals, patchy macules or maculopapular lesions.

- When the lesions are rubbed or stroked, they become edematous, erythematous and appear as hives; this is called the Darier sign and is caused by the degranulation of mast cells when they are manipulated or damaged.

- May be self limited; patients are usually advised to avoid substances that induce mast cell mediator release, such as salicylates, crawfish, lobster, alcohol, spicy foods, hot beverages, and cheese.

- Advise patients to avoid certain physical stimuli, including emotional stress, temperature extremes, physical exertion, bacterial toxins, envenomation by insects to which the patient is allergic, and rubbing, scratching, or traumatizing the lesions of cutaneous mastocytosis.

26. Miliaria

- Also known as sweat rash, prickly heat, and miliaria rubra.

- Due to plugging of sweat glands by dead skin cells; results in local inflammation due to trapped sweat (itching, tingling or prickly sensation).

- Seen as a rash of small red papules, often in skin folds, such as under the breast, in the neck area and scrotum; may also occur on the face.

- May be difficult to distinguish from herpes zoster infection at first since both present

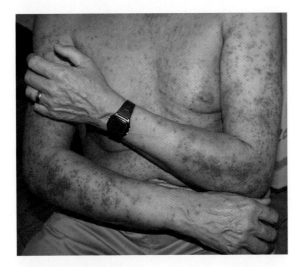

Figure 8-25 Miliaria.

with paresthesia and occur as red papules (at least initially).

- Most cases resolve spontaneously; advice should be provided regarding avoidance, skin hygiene and use of cool clothing; symptoms may be relieved using camphor, menthol or calamine.

27. Morphea

- Also known as localized scleroderma (no involvement of internal organs)—like other rheumatic diseases, affect females more than males (3:1).
- Thickened, hardened plaques of skin and subcutaneous tissue (one form may pre-

sent with bullae, but most lesions are hardened plaques); lesions may vary in color but are often red-violet.

- Usually very localized but may also be widespread; when mild, may go unnoticed, unreported, or even when seen clinically, unrecognized and undiagnosed.
- Treated with typical rheumatologic regimen: corticosteroids, anti-malarials, immunomodulators (such as Methotrexate).
- Likely represents an autoimmune disease and may have familial tendency.

28. Necrobiosis Lipoidica Diabeticorum

- Necrobiosis = death (*nekros*) of life (*bios*).
- Necrobiosis = condition of gradual degeneration and swelling of collagen bundles in the dermis.
- In diabetics, associated with necrobiosis of connective tissue and elastic tissue.
- Associated with discoloration and ulceration of skin.
- Considered common in diabetics.

29. Neurotic Excoriation

- Compulsive skin picking or scratching, resulting in excoriation or erosion; entirely a psychological condition with a dermatological manifestation (scratching is conscious and may even be ritualistic).
- Typically occur on areas that can be reached by a patient: upper back, extensor surfaces of extremities (such as elbow), and the face.
- Usually an adult condition; generally more females than males.

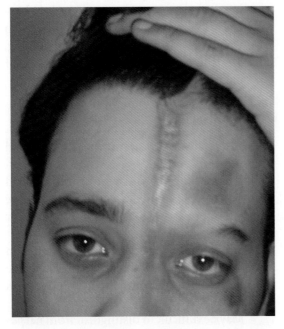

Figure 8-26 Coup de sabre in Morphea.

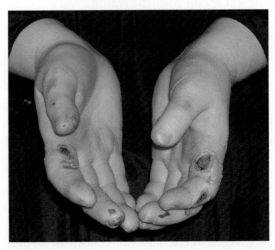

Figure 8-27 Neurotic excoriations inflicted on the hands of a housewife.

- 9-10% of pruritus is related to neurotic excoriation; must be differentiated from other causes of similar lesions and picking, such as uremic pruritus and scabies.
- Typically associated with other psychological or psychiatric conditions as a comorbidity; treatment is directed to the underlying condition.

30. Nevus (plural, Nevi; including Mongolian Spots)

- Benign proliferation of melanocytes typically resulting in brown macules; usually congenital but may be acquired, usually at puberty; dysplastic lesions should be carefully observed for changes in appearance suggestive of neoplasm.
- Nevus anemicus is not a proliferation of melanocytes but is considered a form of nevus; in this case there are white macules seen on the back and chest, usually in females; the condition is benign and due to local vasoconstriction of blood vessels.
- Nevus sebaceus is another variety which results in a hairless patch on the scalp or face and is not related to melanocytes, but

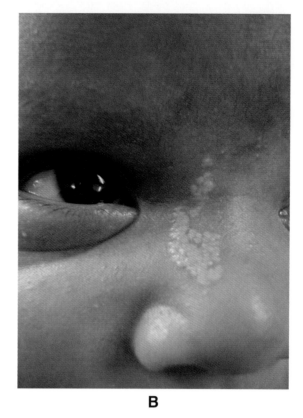

B

Figure 8-28 (B) Nevus sebaceous.

is rather a hamartomatous lesion consisting of sebaceous glands.
- One in ten people has at least one mole that appears atypical and could be dysplastic; dysplastic moles may be irregular in shape and color, larger than common moles, and they may have a scaly or irregular surface.
- Mongolian spots (congenital melanocytic nevi) are sometimes seen over the sacral region appearing as benign blue-black to grey patches often with terminal hairs.

31. Panniculitis

- A group of diseases associated with inflammation of subcutaneous fat; can either affect fat cells themselves (lobular) or the septa between the cells (septal).
- Lobular and septal forms may both be either accompanied by vasculitis or not, hence the characterization of four forms: lobular with vasculitis (examples, leprosy and Crohn's disease), lobular without vasculitis (examples, panniculitis due to infection or trauma, post-steroid panniculitis), septal with vasculitis (examples, superficial thrombophlebitis and cutaneous polyarteritis nodosa),

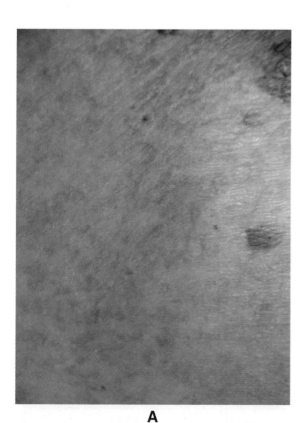

A

Figure 8-28 (A) Blue nevi.

and septal without vasculitis (examples, necrobiosis lipoidica, erythema nodosum, morphea, and granuloma annulare).

- Skin feels thickened and woody to touch; may exhibit reddish or brown pigmentation and nodules or lumps under the skin.
- May be tender to touch; following the resolution of the inflammation, the skin may exhibit a depression due to lipodystrophy.
- Treat underlying conditions; also rest, elevation and compression may help relieve symptoms.

32. Pemphigus (Pemphigus Vulgaris)

- Serious, often fatal, autoimmune condition of skin and mucous membranes.
- Onset 40-60 years of age, starts in oral mucosa.
- Painful skin (bullae) and oral (erosion) lesions; may develop over months.
- Must be treated aggressively with immunosuppressant drugs.
- Lesions may be widespread and affect scalp, face, chest, groin, back.

33. Perlèche

- Angular cheilitis, erosion and cracks in the skin due to moisture trapped at angles of mouth from sagging skin, usually in the elderly (also called angular stomatitis, and cheilosis).
- Not life-threatening, but causes constant discomfort and may lead to infection and ulceration.
- May also be due to nutritional deficiency, particularly riboflavin and iron; a good

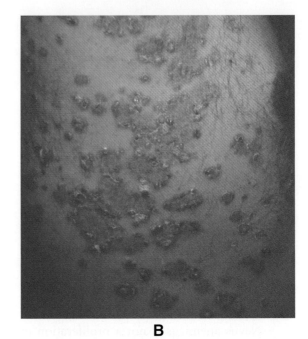

B

Figure 8-29 (B) Pemphigus vulgaris.

rule of thumb is to ensure that a B-vitamin complex is taken.
- Pain may be eased by simple application of petroleum jelly.
- In susceptible individuals, lesions may become infected with *Candida albicans*.

34. Porphyria Cutanea Tarda

- Patients complain of fragile skin with frequent vesicles and bullae following minor trauma.
- May be acquired (Type I, due to drugs, estrogens or alcohol) or hereditary (Type II).

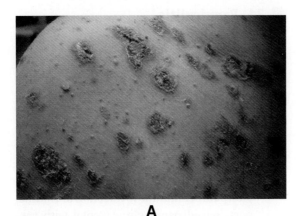

A

Figure 8-29 (A) Erosions with significant crusting in a case of pemphigus vulgaris.

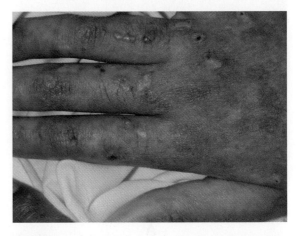

Figure 8-30 Lesions of porphyria cutanea tarda presenting on the right hand.

- Photosensitivity leads to bullae and vesicles on hands and feet; remainder of skin generally normal and may suntan normally.
- Liver enzyme abnormality leads to deficient production of hemoglobin and increased circulating porphyrins which cause the photosensitivity and skin lesions.
- Treated by avoiding alcohol and by regular phlebotomies, to reduce circulating iron and porphyrins.

35. Prurigo Nodularis

- Multiple pruritic nodules on arms or legs; often excoriated due to itching as a result of intense pruritis.
- Begin as papules (often pigmented) around hair follicles and progress to nodules followed by intense itching.
- May be associated with systemic disease such as liver disease, autoimmune disease.
- Repetitive scratching may result in lichenification, hyperpigmentation and hyperkeratosis; lesions may not heal and become repeatedly scaly, crusted and scabbed.
- Treatment is difficult and aimed at stopping the itching/scratching cycle; UVB light therapy may help.

36. Pseudofolliculitis Barbae

- Razor bumps occurring in up to 60% of African-American men; may lead to pustules and abscesses.
- Shaved hair or whiskers curve and grow back into the skin resulting in inflammation and keloid formation.
- The condition is curative by allowing the beard to grow and avoiding close shaving.
- A number of specialized shaving creams and oils targeted at African-American men are commonly available in pharmacies.
- This is to be distinguished from folliculitis barbae which is a true infection of a hair follicle due to a viral or bacterial infection.

37. Pseudoxanthoma Elasticum

- Rare genetic disease, more common in females, begins in childhood and progresses, leading to soft, lax skin with wrinkled, hanging folds affecting the skin of the neck,

axillae and groin (NOTE—lesions begin on lateral neck with plucked chicken or cobblestone appearance).
- The skin lesions are asymptomatic and of cosmetic concern only, but changes in the elastic fibers in the retina, and gastrointestinal and cardiovascular systems can be very serious (and potentially life-threatening).
- Early detection is very important to effect lifestyle changes that minimize complications of extracutaneous manifestations; adolescents who have been diagnosed with PE should avoid weight-lifting or contact sports.
- Begins with small yellow papules, usually linear or reticular, which eventually coalesce to form a plaque.
- Regular exercise and a diet low in fat and calcium (only 600-1200 mg/day) are recommended to minimize cardiovascular

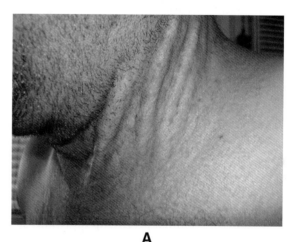

A

Figure 8-31 (A)   Pseudoxanthoma elasticum (neck).

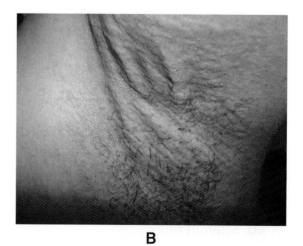

B

Figure 8-31 (B)   Pseudoxanthoma elasticum (axilla); note the sagging skin due to loss of elasticity.

complications; cigarette smoking exacerbates the progress of the disease; vitamins A, C, and E and zinc supplements may reduce the risk of retinal or gastrointestinal hemorrhage.

38. Pyoderma Gangrenosum

- Mostly seen in patients 40-60 years old.
- Necrotic ulcers occur on the legs leading to chronic wounds; initially appearing as small lesions similar to bug bites, they can progress to large ulcers several inches in diameter.
- Rarely leads to death but chronic wounds lead to pain and scarring.
- Usually associated with immune deficiency states; about 50% occur in patients with Crohn's disease, ulcerative colitis and rheumatoid arthritis.
- Treatment aimed at underlying disease and usually includes corticosteroids and drugs used to treat rheumatic disease; ulcers require specialized wound care.

39. Rocky Mountain Spotted Fever

- The most severe tick-borne rickettsial illness in the US; caused by infection with the bacteria *Rickettsia rickettsii*; can be serious or fatal especially if diagnosis is delayed (death occurs in 3-5% of patients).
- Onset of symptoms occurs 1-2 weeks after a tick bite; initial presentation includes fever, headache, myalgia followed by a macular or maculopapular rash.
- Rash is centripetal, that is beginning in extremities and moving inward towards trunk; maculopapular and/or petechial rash (35-60% of patients) may cover a large area; 10-15% of patients do not develop a rash.
- Has been seen in virtually every state, not only in the Rocky mountain area.
- Antibiotic therapy must be started immediately upon diagnosis or strong suspicion; Doxycycline and chloramphenicol are commonly used drugs.

40. Scleroderma

- Chronic autoimmune disease causing atrophic sclerosis of skin and connective tissue associated with organs and blood vessels.
- Diffuse form (systemic sclerosis) causes widespread skin lesions; localized form usually only causes lesions on face and fingers.
- Localized form may be associated with other conditions: CREST syndrome = calcinosis of skin, Raynaud's phenomenon, esophageal disease leading to heartburn, sclerodactyly, and telangiectasia.
- Another form: Morphea, consists of linear skin lesions and no organ involvement (see condition #27).
- Drug treatment is complex and specialized; application of heat may help reduce skin hardening.

41. Spider Bites

- 98-99% of spider bites are harmless, resulting in red papules; in the other 1-2% injury may occur from either toxins (neurotoxic venom from a Black Widow bite) or tissue necrosis and infection (necrotic venom from a Brown Recluse bite).
- Many skin disorders are initially wrongly diagnosed as bites from the Brown Recluse spider, such as pyoderma gangrenosum, bacterial infections, Lyme disease, diabetic ulcers and squamous cell carcinoma.
- Black Widow spider (*Latrodectus*) has characteristic hourglass marking; Brown Recluse spider (*Loxosceles recluse*) has characteristic violin shaped marking (fiddleback spider); Brown Recluse spider also has 6 eyes, 3 in each of two rows which makes it easier to identify.
- Brown Recluse spider bite is initially painless and erythema develops within 6-12 hours, progressing to a large necrotic lesion within a few days; treatment is symptomatic and includes cleansing of the wound; may require skin grafts to close the large necrotic ulcer.
- Black Widow spider bite (lactrodectism) results in neurotoxic signs and symptoms: headache, severe cramps, anxiety, diaphoresis, cardiac abnormalities, hypertension and shock; treatment includes analgesics, prevention of muscle cramps and occasionally, the use of a specific antivenom.

42. Stevens-Johnson Syndrome

- A form of toxic epidermal necrolysis; can be life-threatening; involves cell death and separation of epidermis from dermis; begins as macular rash that develops into papules, vesicles, bullae, urticarial plaques, or confluent erythema.

- Cause can be idiopathic (about 50% of cases), infection, or toxic reaction to drugs; cases have been reported following cocaine use.
- Treatment is supportive and patients are treated in the same manner of patients with severe burns; offending drug use must be stopped immediately; the use of corticosteroids is controversial.
- Mortality is 5% in cases where 10% or less of the skin is involved; blindness and visual impairment is a common outcome.
- Mortality may be predicted with a severity-of-illness scale called the SCORTEN scale, which includes age, associated malignancy, heart rate, serum BUN (blood urea nitrogen), area of skin involved, serum bicarbonate and serum glucose.

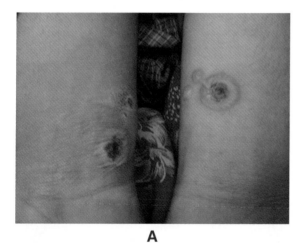

A

Figure 8-32 (A)   Stevens-Johnson syndrome due to drug reaction.

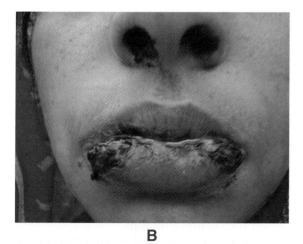

B

Figure 8-32 (B)   Mucocutaneous involvement in Stevens-Johnson syndrome from penicillin sensitivity.

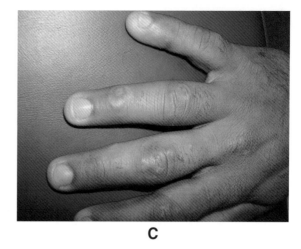

C

Figure 8-32 (C)   Early signs of Stevens-Johnson syndrome presenting on the hand.

43. Sweets Syndrome (Acute Febrile Neutrophilic Dermatosis)

- Sudden onset of fever and tender erythematous macules, papules and plaques.
- A reactive condition, often associated with hematologic disease (such as leukemia) or rheumatologic disease (such as rheumatoid arthritis) and to be considered a marker of internal disease (20% are associated with malignancy).
- Two constant features of diagnosis = typical clinically observed eruption and histologic presence of neutrophilic dermal infiltrate (in papules).
- Skin lesions occur particularly on the backs of hands and fingers, rarely on trunk.
- Must be treated promptly with systemic corticosteroids (skin lesions will generally resolve within 3-9 days of treatment).

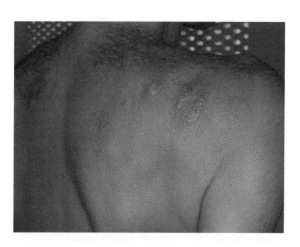

Figure 8-33   Sweets syndrome.

44. Syringoma

- Harmless sweat duct tumors usually around the eyelids or on cheeks but may also be found on axillae, vulva and penis.
- Appear as 1-3 mm small firm, round skin-colored or yellow papules.
- Must be differentiated from xanthelasma on eyelids, or basal cell carcinoma on face and cheeks.
- May be associated with Down's syndrome and diabetes mellitus.
- No treatment required but they may be removed for cosmetic reasons using laser therapy.

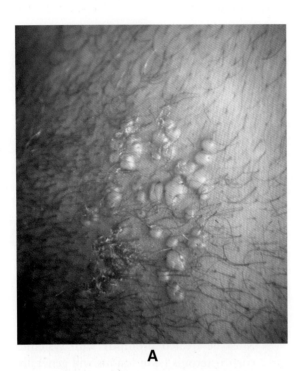

A

Figure 8-34 (A) Classical flesh shaped papules of syringomas.

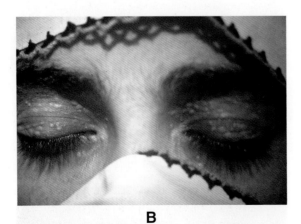

B

Figure 8-34 (B) Syringomas in the facial region.

45. Telangiectasia

- Refers to a visibly dilated blood vessel or vessels on the skin and mucous membranes; they are generally meaningless but may be associated with a variety of conditions (some serious).
- Found in numerous inherited or congenital conditions including Louis Bar syndrome (inherited ataxia-telangiectasia), nevus flammeus, xeroderma pigmentosa, and hereditary hemorrhagic telangiectasia (Osler-Weber-Rendu syndrome).
- Simple telangiectasia may be caused by alcohol use, aging and exposure to the sun.
- Acquired causes include venous hypertension, acne rosacea, CREST syndrome, chronic use of topical corticosteroids; spider angiomas are associated with hepatic cirrhosis, pregnancy and high estrogen levels in liver disease.
- Treatment is by sclerotherapy (injection of sclerosant agent) and laser.

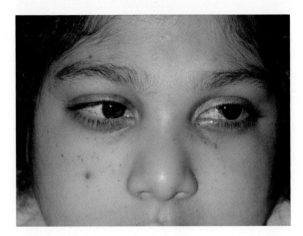

Figure 8-35 Telangiectasia in the eyes of a patient with hereditary ataxia.

46. Telogen Effluvium

- Non-scarring alopecia with acute diffuse hair shedding; can also have a chronic form but more commonly an acute disorder.
- Associated with reaction to physiologic, metabolic or hormonal stress or medication use.
- Recovery is usually complete and spontaneous within 6 months.
- Telogen refers to the resting stage of the hair growth cycle (about 3 months) as

compared to anagen, the growth stage of the cycle (about 3 years)—in other words, a given hair may grow for 3 years, rest for 3 months and then shed, making room for a new hair out of the same follicle; at any given time, 5-15% of hair is in telogen.

- No treatment is required unless an underlying condition exists; any reversible cause of hair shedding, such as poor diet, iron deficiency, hypothyroidism, or medication use should be corrected.

47. Toxic Epidermal Necrolysis (TEN, Lyell's Syndrome)

- A life threatening dermatological condition considered to be a more severe form of Stevens-Johnson syndrome; may involve up to 30% or more of the skin surface (in contrast to SJS which usually affects 10% or less).
- Condition is caused by the death of keratinocytes resulting in the separation of epidermis and dermis.
- A history of medication use is present in 95% of cases; a wide variety of medications can cause TEN; TEN may also occur after immunization or in association with some infections.
- Syndrome begins with 1-2 weeks of fever and illness resembling an upper respiratory infection; this is followed by the appearance of a macular rash which becomes widespread, painful and within hours the epidermis can be peeled away from the underlying dermis.
- There are 3 levels of treatment: first, withdraw suspected causative drugs and manage patient supportively in a burn unit or

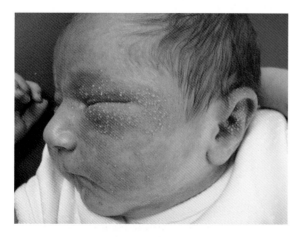

Figure 8-36 Toxic epidermal necrolysis.

intensive care unit; second, intravenous immunoglobulin; third, the use of specialized medications to stimulate cell growth.

48. Trichotillomania

- An impulse control disorder characterized by a compulsive urge to pull out hair (scalp hair, eyebrows, nose hair, pubic hair or other body hair).
- Usually begins during the teen years and can be triggered by stress or depression; affects females more than males.
- Dermatologically considered as a traumatic alopecia.
- Treatment is often ineffective and may involve psychiatry, medication, and self-monitoring; patients often present with a complex psychological profile.
- Generally, treatment is more effective in younger patients.

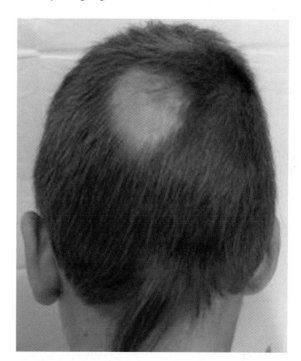

Figure 8-37 Forced pulling of hair in trichotillomania.

49. Tuberous Sclerosis

- Rare multisystem autosomal dominant genetic disease resulting in multisite hamartomas.
- Symptoms may vary and be widespread depending on the organs and tissues involved; typically they include seizures, developmental delay, behavioral problems and skin abnormalities.

- Cutaneous manifestations include angiofibromas, fibrous plaques, collagenomas (shagreen patches), periungual fibromas (Koenen tumors), gingival fibromas, dental enamel pits, hypopigmented macules (ash-leaf and confetti), and cafè-au-lait macules.
- Common presenting symptoms and signs include hypopigmented macules (ash leaf spots), seizures, and facial angiofibromas (on the nose and cheeks in a butterfly distribution).
- This is a complex disorder and treatment typically involves antiepilepsy medication; prognosis is good unless renal function is compromised, although patients are typically mentally and behaviorally challenged.

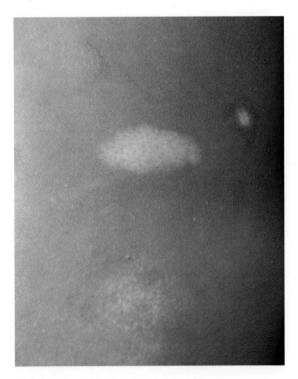

Figure 8-38 Ash leaf macules in tuberous sclerosis.

50. Venous Leg Ulcers

- Due to ineffiency of venous valves in the leg veins and responsible for up to 90% of chronic wounds in the legs.
- Most venous ulcers can be managed by compression bandages applied by those with special training, such as nurses specializing in leg ulcers.
- Considerable research has been done on leg ulcers because of the magnitude of this problem among the elderly and long-term hospital patients.
- The Bisgaard regimen for treatment: education, elevation, elastic compression, and evaluation.
- Keeping patients active and treating underlying conditions such as obesity and poor nutrition is important in preventing leg ulcer.

General References

Arnold L Harry. *Diseases of the Skin Clinical Dermatology*, 8th ed. Philadelphia, PA: W.B Saunders Company, 1990.

Bickley LS. *Bates Guide to Physical Examination and History Taking*, 9th ed. Chicago, IL Lippincott Williams and Wilkins, 2007.

Burns DA, Breathnach SM, Cox N, Griffiths CE. *Rook's Textbook of Dermatology*, 7th ed. Oxford, UK. Blackwell Publishing, 2004.

Fitzpatrick JE, Morelli JG. *Dermatology Secrets*. 3rd ed. Philadelphia, PA. Mosby. 2006.

Habif TP. *Skin Disease: Diagnosis and Treatment*. 2nd ed. Philadelphia, PA, Elsevier Mosby; 2005.

Kumar Vinay et. al. (ED) *Robins Pathologic Basis of Disease* 7th ed Philadelphia, PA Elsevier 2005.

Mackie RM. *Clinical Dermatology* 4th ed. New York, NY, Oxford Press 2004.

Oyelowo Tolu. *Mosby's Guide to Women's Health: A Handbook for Health Professionals*, 1st ed. St. Louis, MO, Mosby Elsevier, 2007.

Wolff Klaus, et al. *Fitzpatrick's Color Atlas &Synopsis of Clinical Dermatology*. New York, NY, McGraw-Hill, 2005.

Sample Case Studies with Discussion Questions

Case Study 1

A 40-year-old female visits your office on Thursday morning for a routine visit related to her chronic back pain. She feels she may also be "coming down with the flu" as she feels generally achy, tired and had difficulty sleeping last night. Further questioning reveals that she and her family were camping during the previous week and that she got numerous insect bites. She asks you if that might have anything to do with the way she is feeling.

You ask about any particularly noticeable bites and she shows you a red annular lesion on her left lower abdomen, approximately 2 cm in diameter.

Questions for discussion:

1. What is the most likely diagnosis?
2. If your diagnosis is correct, what might you expect over the following weeks if this patient had not been diagnosed and treated?
3. Is this condition communicable? Is it reportable?
4. Name several serious sequelae that may result from lack of treatment, or ineffective treatment of this condition.
5. Describe the treatment for this condition.

Case Study 2

A 35-year-old male visits your office with a headache and general malaise. His symptoms include an upset stomach and generalized myalgia and he admits that he has been stressed lately (work and financial stress) so he wouldn't be surprised to find out that he had the flu. On examination, you note a small macular lesion on the right lateral aspect of his forehead that he believes is an insect bite that he received after doing yard work on the weekend. As you palpate the region of this lesion, he complains that it feels a little odd ("both itchy and sore at the same time"), and is actually quite tender to light touch.

Questions for discussion:

1. What is the most likely diagnosis?
2. What is the likely course of this patient's condition?
3. Is this condition contagious?
4. Describe some other common presentations of this condition.
5. Why is the patient's stress level significant in this case?

Case Study 3

An overweight 48-year-old female patient visits your office complaining of mid-back pain. Her condition appears to be occupationally related since she is sitting at a computer for long hours every day. Her general health is otherwise quite good, although she is concerned about her weight and her apparent inability to control it. On examination of her thoracic spine and paraspinal tissues, you palpate an oval mass approximately 3 cm. by 5 cm. over her right scapula. Palpation reveals this mass to be mobile, rubbery and slightly tender. Upon questioning, the patient states that she had been unaware of this mass. Your attention to it causes some distress and anxiety for the patient.

Questions for discussion:

1. What is the most likely diagnosis?
2. What other conditions might be considered in the differential diagnosis?
3. How will you advise this patient?
4. What physical findings might cause you to reconsider your diagnosis?
5. What is the most common site of these lesions?

Case Study 4

A 45-year-old female complains of lower back pain, neck pain and bilateral upper extremity paresthesia. These symptoms had been present for the past 4 months. She was diagnosed with neurofibromatosis type 1 (NF-1) in childhood. Multiple café-au-lait spots were noted on her face and trunk. Spinal examination revealed scoliosis and multiple areas of segmental dysfunction. She was treated with manipulation and physical therapy which resulted in a marked reduction in her pain and paresthesia.

Questions for discussion:

1. What concerns would you have as a chiropractor in treating this patient?
2. Can this patient's scoliosis be corrected?
3. What is likely causing the paresthesia in the upper extremities?
4. This patient chooses to continue seeing you for ongoing management of recurrent pains and stiffness. What symptomatic changes might cause you concern?
5. What is this patient's long term prognosis?

Case Study 5

A 25-year-old nurse presents with a fever, malaise and headache—all flu-like symptoms. Her physical exam is normal. She is treated symptomatically without significant relief. Within 2 days, she develops a pruritic macular rash on her face, neck and trunk. She works in the neurologic department of a major urban hospital. She has recently cared for a 62-year-old male patient in the hospital who underwent spinal surgery. Following his surgery, the nurse noted that he was worried, anxious, and under a great deal of stress regarding his health because his income was the primary financial resource of his family. Shortly after this, he developed multiple pruritic vesicles over his abdomen and flank area. The nurse reports contact with this patient including positioning him in bed and changing his surgical dressings. She did not wear protective gloves during much of this work. She too reports being under considerable stress related to career decisions and family pressures. Her childhood history is unremarkable and she admits to having had chickenpox (varicella) at age 5 during an outbreak involving her and her two siblings.

Questions for discussion:

1. What is the most likely diagnosis?
2. This case was reported in the literature as an unusual and notable case. Why?
3. What factors might have played a role in the etiology of the nurse's disease?
4. Is this disease communicable? Is it reportable?
5. What precautions should be taken with suspected contagious lesions?

Case Study 6

A 47-year-old African-American female visits your office with her 17-year-old daughter. She was diagnosed with vitiligo when she was 23 years of age. Her lesions are mainly on her fingers and on her cheeks. Although the lesions have not subsided they have not progressed to other areas of the body.

Questions for discussion:

1. What is vitiligo?
2. How do the lesions look in vitiligo?
3. Is this condition communicable?
4. What layer of the skin is affected in vitiligo?
5. Should this patient be concerned about her daughter developing vitiligo?

Case Study 7

A 55-year-old male engineer who has been in excellent health periodically visits your chiropractic office for chronic back pain. Over the last couple of visits you notice a black mole that is changing color. Further questioning with the patient reveals that his wife had noticed the mole increasing in size. The mole is neither painful nor pruritic and upon your enquiry he reports of no other symptoms. Upon examination you found the mole is asymmetrical.

Questions for discussion:

1. What is the most likely diagnosis or differential diagnosis?
2. What would you suggest to this patient as a chiropractor?
3. Is this condition communicable?
4. List the ABCD's for melanoma.
5. With his dermatology condition, what treatment options are available for this patient?

Case Study 8

A 42-year-old male hairdresser visits your chiropractic office for low back pain and expresses concern over a thick rash on his elbows and knees. He says that his dandruff has gone bad and it has become embarrassing for him to attend social events. He also informs you that he is starting to isolate himself in his own apartment. He acknowledges that his back pain is getting better with chiropractic care but his knee pain has gotten worse.

Questions for discussion:

1. What is the most likely diagnosis or differential diagnosis?
2. What would you suggest to this patient as a chiropractor?
3. Is this condition communicable?
4. With his dermatology condition, what treatment options are available for this patient?
5. Which emollients or natural treatment can chiropractors suggest for dry skin?

Case Study 9

A 16-year-old high school student visits your office and is complaining of itching (pruritus) in the scalp over the past 3 months. She says that she has used many dandruff shampoos and hair products but her itching has progressed. She is constantly scratching her scalp and becoming concerned about her condition.

Questions for discussion:

1. What is your differential diagnosis?
2. What would you do to make a more definitive diagnosis?
3. Could this condition be communicable? If so what measures would you take since she is a high school student?
4. With her dermatology condition, what treatment options are available for this patient?
5. Which over-the-counter medications can you suggest for this patient?

Case Study 10

During a chiropractic adjustment you notice a 35-year-old male has huge ring shaped lesions at the back. You question him and he explains that his back itches significantly and that his girlfriend has had similar symptoms. He says that he used several soaps and creams on his back, but both he and his girlfriend are frustrated that the itching has not yet subsided.

Questions for discussion:

1. What is the most likely cutaneous fungal infection is he suffering from?
2. Is this condition communicable or has to be reported?
3. What other areas of the body would you enquire or observe in this patient?
4. Would you treat this patient or refer him to a dermatologist?
5. What diagnostic tests would a dermatologist used?

Discussion Points

Case Study 1

1. *What is the most likely diagnosis?*

   Lyme disease

2. *If your diagnosis is correct, what might you expect over the following weeks if this patient had not been diagnosed and treated?*

   The condition would progress through 3 stages: initial—within 3-32 days (flu-like symptoms and characteristic skin lesion), second stage—within 2-12 weeks (carditis, dyspnea, dizziness, palpitations, possibly facial paralysis and meningitis), third or chronic stage—up to 2 years (arthritis, lymphadenopathy and possibly neurological symptoms).

3. *Is this condition communicable? Is it reportable?*

   It is not communicable. Depending on the jurisdiction, laws may require the reporting of Lyme disease to local or state public health departments.

4. *Name several serious sequelae that may result from lack of treatment or ineffective treatment of this condition?*

   Chronic recurrent symptoms may represent untreated disease or ineffective treatment. Often there are recurrent symptoms without objective findings. Antibiotics are not indicated or generally effective for Lyme disease sequelae. Sequelae may include neurological conditions (such as facial palsy, meningitis, encephalitis and peripheral neuropathy), cardiac manifestations, and rheumatologic manifestations (such as synovitis, arthralgia and myalgia).

5. *Describe the treatment for this condition.*

While not a treatment, it is important to note that promptly removing a tick from the skin may be an effective preventive measure. Patients in endemic areas should be advised accordingly. Treatment of serologically confirmed and symptomatic cases includes oral broad spectrum antibiotics. If serious neurological or cardiac symptoms are present, parenteral antibiotic treatment may be required. There is no current evidence supporting the use of antibiotics in the treatment of asymptomatic seropositive patients.

Case Study 2

1. *What is the most likely diagnosis?*

Herpes zoster or shingles.

2. *What is the likely course of this patient's condition?*

Following the observation of the isolated macule would be a patch of macules which, over a period of a few days become vesicles. Eventually the vesicles burst and form scabs which eventually crust over and fall off, occasionally leaving a small scar or hyperpigmentation. During these phases the patient may complain of tingling, burning and occasionally intense pain in the affected area (which in this case is the frontal branch of the ophthalmic portion of the trigeminal nerve).

3. *Is this condition contagious?*

Herpes zoster is caused by a previously dormant virus in nerve ganglia. Hence, it is not contagious as a cause of herpes zoster in another person. However, the same virus also causes varicella, or chicken pox. According to the CDC, patients with shingles are contagious to people who have not yet had chicken pox. During the vesicular stage, the vesicular fluid contains the virus and contact with this fluid should be avoided by a person who has never had chicken pox. Safe practice includes covering vesicular patches to avoid this possibility. Once the vesicles have burst and crusted over, there is no danger of contagion.

4. *Describe some other common presentations of this condition.*

This condition can occur virtually anywhere in the body that is supplied by a sensory nerve, but most commonly occurs on the trunk (hence the name *zoster*, which means girdle). Common locations are along the path of an intercostal nerve, on the thigh or groin, and in the distribution of the ophthalmic branch of the trigeminal nerve.

5. *Why is the patient's stress level significant in this case?*

Stress is thought to play a role in the etiology of this condition. The virus remains latent in the sensory ganglia following exposure to chicken pox or varicella. For most people, the latency lasts a lifetime, but stress can interfere with the immune system and lead to the virus becoming active. Common examples are stress caused by chronic disease, particularly diabetes and malignancy, and stress caused by severe personal or social issues such as marital distress, violence and financial pressure.

Case Study 3

1. *What is the most likely diagnosis?*

Benign lipoma

2. *What other conditions might be considered in the differential diagnosis?*

A number of other benign and malignant tumors such as hibernomas, lipoblastomas, liposarcomas, and neurofibromas might be considered in evaluating painless or tender rubbery subcutaneous masses. Epidermoid cysts may occasionally cause this same presentation.

3. *How will you advise this patient?*

Once the diagnosis of a benign lipoma is made, you can advise this patient that the lesion is not dangerous or ominous and that it will likely remain generally asymptomatic. Benign lipoma is by far the most common soft tissue tumor accounting for about 50% of these tumors. Surgical removal is usually only advocated for cosmetic reasons. There is a remote possibility of a liposarcomas arising from a lipoma, usually in middle-aged or older adults. The patient should be advised to report any changes in size or discomfort level.

4. *What physical findings might cause you to reconsider your diagnosis?*

If the mass is nonmobile and painful (beyond the level of moderate pressure tenderness which is seen in most lipomas) you should suspect liposarcomas. Nerves can be compressed by a growing liposarcomas which can also cause symptoms, usually pain.

Occasionally the skin above these lesions can become indurated or ulcerated.

5. *What is the most common site of these lesions?*

Benign lipomas can appear virtually anywhere in the body where fat cells are located. The most common sites are in subcutaneous tissue, but they can occur in the palate, tongue, larynx, parotid gland, and even bone and tendon sheaths. By far the most common sites of simple benign lipomas are in the area of the posterior neck, shoulder and scapular regions and the back. They can also be seen occasionally on the arms and forearms.

Case Study 4

1. *What concerns would you have as a chiropractor in treating this patient?*

You would be concerned with the possibility of spinal instability as a result of large neurofibromas located in the intervertebral foramina as well as the possibility of bone cysts.

2. *Can this patient's scoliosis be corrected?*

There is no evidence that the scoliosis resulting from neurofibromatosis can be corrected other than through surgical intervention. The cause of scoliosis in neurofibromatosis is unknown but thought to be due to a localized neurofibromatous tumor eroding and infiltrating bone.

3. *What is likely causing the paresthesia in the upper extremities?*

This is due to neurofibromas affecting the cervical nerve roots. This patient's cervical spine MRI revealed neurofibromas on every nerve root bilaterally from C1 to C7. It also showed multiple extramedullary masses from C1-C2-C3 with moderately severe spinal cord compression down to C6 level. This would certainly be responsible for the paresthesia.

4. *This patient chooses to continue seeing you for ongoing management of recurrent pains and stiffness. What symptomatic changes might cause you concern?*

In 3-5% of cases, a neurofibroma can degenerate into a neurofibrosarcoma. This most commonly occurs in a large neurofibroma particularly in the arm or leg. This may be suspected if a neurofibroma becomes more tender, or larger, or associated with symptoms attributable to local tissue erosion. You would also be alert to the possibility of intracranial

tumors resulting in neurological symptoms and ophthalmic symptoms.

5. *What is this patient's long term prognosis?*

Neurofibromatosis is rarely fatal other than in those who develop metastatic neurofibrosarcoma. There is the possibility of intracranial tumors either developing or enlarging, causing symptoms. Vertebral bone erosion due to dural ectasis can cause spinal instability, particularly in those who underwent surgery with instrumentation at a young age. Long bone involvement (thinning of the cortex) may lead to tibial fractures with nonunion, occasionally resulting in amputations. Finally, the multiple café-au-lait spots and often disfiguring neurofibromas can lead to considerable psychological stress that is best treated professionally.

Case Study 5

1. *What is the most likely diagnosis?*

Recurrent varicella.

2. *This case was reported in the literature as an unusual and notable case. Why?*

The patient apparently had varicella as a five year old child. In most cases this produces lifelong immunity. The patient was born in 1978 and therefore it is unlikely that she had smallpox (variola) since it was virtually eradicated at that time. The diagnosis of varicella is relatively easy, especially during family outbreaks. This case demonstrates that under certain conditions, varicella may recur.

3. *What factors might have played a role in the etiology of the nurse's disease?*

There are several factors: her male patient's vesicular lesions were caused by herpes zoster and the fluid within them contains varicella-zoster virus (VZV); she handled this patient without using protective gloves; she was under considerable stress which would have weakened her own immune response.

4. *Is this disease communicable? Is it reportable?*

Varicella (chickenpox) is highly contagious. In most jurisdictions, chickenpox is a reportable disease. In 2003, the Centers for Disease Control (CDC) recommended that it be reportable nationwide. States have generally complied with this recommendation; however, a few only require the reporting of chickenpox related deaths.

5. *What precautions should be taken with suspected contagious lesions?*

In any suspected case of contagion, protective measures should be taken, such as wearing a mask and gloves. Frequent hand washing using an appropriate soap is strongly recommended. The case reported was a notable one, as has been described, and resulted in a strong recommendation that hospital and health care workers receive an adult VZV vaccine, whether or not they report a previous incidence of chickenpox.

Case Study 6

1. *What is vitiligo?*

Vitiligo is a pigmentation disorder in which melanocytes in the skin, the mucous membranes, and the retina are destroyed.

2. *How do the lesions look in vitiligo?*

Hypopigmented macules and patches mainly on the hands, knees, feet, face and hair.

3. *Is this condition communicable?*

Vitiligo is not a contagious condition and is highly mistaken as a contagious infection.

4. *What layer of the skin is affected in vitiligo?*

Stratum basale of the epidermis.

5. *Should she be concerned about her daughter developing vitiligo?*

Vitiligo could be hereditary. Clinicians can explain that vitiligo is an autoimmune response and that she should observe any emerging vitiligo lesions in her daughter. Early treatment can sometimes help.

Case Study 7

1. *What is the most likely diagnosis or differential diagnosis?*

Melanoma, seborrheic keratoses or lentigines can all be considered.

2. *What would you suggest to this patient as a chiropractor?*

The patient could be at a risk of melanoma and needs to be referred urgently to a dermatologist/dermatologic surgeon where timely biopsies can be performed to rule out various stages of melanoma. If diagnosed

with melanoma, the patient needs to undergo radical surgery.

3. *Is this condition communicable?*

Melanomas are neither contagious nor communicable.

4. *List the ABCD's for melanoma.*

Asymmetry

Border

Color

Diameter

5. *Based on your diagnosis, what treatment options are available for this patient?*

Topical treatment is not effective, neither any naturopathic treatment. Surgical intervention is quickly required and surgical excision can be considered for smaller benign lentigines.

Case Study 8

1. *What is the most likely diagnosis or differential diagnosis?*

More likely the patient is suffering from psoriasis, scalp psoriasis, seborrheic dermatitis or eczemas.

2. *What would you suggest to this patient?*

Psoriasis and eczemas are chronic and long standing conditions that require constant treatment under a dermatologist. After suggesting some naturopathic or over-the-counter products for treatment chiropractors should write a comprehensive referral.

Topical treatments can be suggested such as use of over-the-counter topical steroids (sparing use of), salicylic acid can all be starting treatments.

3. *Is this condition communicable?*

Psoriasis and eczema are not communicable diseases.

4. *Based on your diagnosis, what treatment options are available for this patient?*

There are numerous natural treatment options for psoriasis and eczema. These can be chronic and difficult conditions to treat but persistence and carefully observing your patient's response can be valuable clues as to which treatments may be beneficial. Topical emollient ointments may be used, and the possible recommended treatments include salicylic acid, coal tar related products, topical zinc oxide and evening primrose oil, and an antiinflammatory diet low in red meat, saturated fats and refined sugars, with B vitamin supplementation.

5. *Which emollients or naturopathic treatment can chiropractors suggest for dry skin?*

Petrolatum jelly (white soft paraffin), zinc oxide paste may be applied to skin to relieve itchiness of psoriasis, evening primrose oil applied to cracked and sore skin can help promote healing. Chick weed, chamomile, calendula, St. John's Wort, and goldenseal can be applied topically to the skin to promote healing of cracked, painful, or dry skin.

Case Study 9

1. *What is your differential diagnosis?*

Seborrheic dermatitis, pediculosis capitis, scalp psoriasis and tinea capitis will form main differential diagnosis.

2. *What would you do to make a more definitive diagnosis?*

Rule out fungal infection by observing under Wood lamp. If there is no scaling, rule out seborrheic eczema and psoriasis. If you observe nits, a definitive diagnosis of pediculosis (lice) can be made.

3. *Could this condition be communicable? If so, what measures would you take since this patient is a high school student?*

Fungal infections and pediculosis are communicable diseases. Schools have to be notified and the condition has to be reported. Your patient should be advised to stay at home and in addition you should check if anyone else in the family has contracted a similar skin condition.

4. *What treatment options are available for this patient?*

Getting rid of the lice and eggs is critical in the treatment of pediculosis. Everyone in the family or group, whether showing symptoms or not, should be treated at the same time to stop the spread of lice. This also includes sexual partners, close friends, and class-

mates of this patient. Nits could be removed by combing or using egg remover gels. Hair could be saturated with 50:50 ratio of water and vinegar to help dislodge the lice from hair shafts.

Good personal hygiene and washing all clothes and bedding should be always recommended.

5. *Using the textbook, which over-the-counter medications can you suggest for this patient?*

Hair clean oil spray kills lice in 15 minutes. Neem and tea tree oil applications have shown some results. Vaseline, mayonnaise or pomades can be applied to scalp overnight and washed next day with a shampoo although multiple treatments are required. Some over-the-counter medications like antihistamines can be considered for oral treatment to control itching.

Case Study 10

1. *What is the most likely cutaneous fungal infection is he suffering from?*

Tinea corporis.

2. *Is this condition communicable?*

Yes, most cutaneous tinea infections are contagious and can recur after treatment.

3. *What other areas of the body would you enquire or observe in this patient?*

Scalp, neck, skin creases, nails, hands and feet and enquiry about rash between the thighs all are important sites for infection.

4. *Would you treat this patient or refer him to a dermatologist?*

A topical antifungal can be tried but the patient should be referred to a dermatologist to prevent reinfection and spread of infection to others.

5. *What diagnostic tests would a dermatologist order?*

Skin scrapings, Wood light lamp to aid in the diagnosis.

Sample Selected Response Questions for Self-Assessment

(Answers and page references are on page 209)

Chapter 1

1. Which is the only place in the body where arteries can be directly observed?

    A. nail beds

    B. tympanic membrane

    C. retina

    D. oral mucous membranes

2. What is the most common site for malignant melanoma in men?

    A. scalp

    B. upper back

    C. lower back

    D. lower legs

3. The ACC Chiropractic Scope and Practice Paradigm (1996) suggests that the chiropractor's ultimate target is:

    A. subluxation correction

    B. general health promotion

    C. pain management

    D. palliative care

4. The chiropractic subluxation is generally characterized by:

    A. facilitation of motoneuron pools

    B. inhibition of segmental motor pathways

    C. loss of sensation

    D. all of the above

5. Early research by osteopaths showed that the skin overlying somatic dysfunction exhibited:

    A. increased temperature

    B. excessive dryness

    C. redness

    D. none of the above

6. What is the only organ or organ system proven to function abnormally when associated with somatic dysfunction?

    A. skin

    B. respiratory tract

    C. thyroid gland

    D. colonic mucosa

7. The neurophysiological goal of spinal manipulation, while not completely understood, is likely to be:

    A. elimination of segmental sympatheticotonia

    B. elimination of segmental sympatheticatonia

    C. stimulation of motoneuron pools

    D. none of the above

Chapter 2

8. A common dermatological response to an allergic reaction is:

    A. psoriasis

    B. urticaria

    C. rosaceous

    D. vitiligo

9. Dry skin resulting from loss of moisture due to cold weather, swimming in chlorinated pools, exposure to wind, washing with harsh soaps, chaffing and poor humidity control in air conditioned spaces will present with:

    A. dermatitis

    B. ichthyoids

    C. pruritus

    D. all the above

10. The sun delivers three forms of ultraviolet (UV) light rays. _____ is /are absorbed by the ozone layer.

    A. UVA

    B. UVB

    C. UVC

    D. UVB and UVC

11. The SPF number is used to calculate the exposure time before the skin starts to burn. If you typically start to burn in full sunlight in 20 minutes and apply a SPF 15 lotion, you will be protected for _____ minutes.

    A. 30

    B. 150

    C. 200

    D. 300

12. What is the best advice you can give a patient with soft, weak and brittle nails who has chipped the nail polish?

    A. cut the chipped area back

    B. remove the nail polish and reapply it

    C. leave it alone

    D. apply another layer of polish

13. Regulation of tattooing is under local jurisdiction but the ink is subject to _____ regulation as a cosmetic and color additive.

    A. EPA

    B. FDA

    C. OSHA

    D. FFA

14. When educating a patient to prevent folliculitis and ingrown hairs associated with shaving, the following tip would be beneficial:

    A. use an electric razor

    B. use a double or triple blade razor

    C. pull skin tight when shaving

    D. shave every day when a break out occurs

15. The enzyme tyrosinase plays a role in the formation of normal melanin and contains which mineral?

    A. copper

    B. manganese

    C. zinc

    D. magnesium

16. Follicular hyperkeratosis or raised bumps around hair follicles primarily on backs of arms and sides of thighs is associated with _____ deficiency.

    A. vitamin B1

    B. vitamin B2

    C. vitamin A

    D. vitamin K

17. Bruising is associated with _____ deficiency.

    A. vitamin B1

    B. vitamin B2

    C. vitamin A

    D. vitamin K

Chapter 3

18. The skin is _____ in origin.

    A. ectodermic

    B. endodermic

    C. mesodermic

    D. none of the above

19. The melanocytes are located in the _____ layer of the skin.

    A. corneal

    B. granular

    C. spinous

    D. basal

20. The structure right beneath the nail bed is the _____.

    A. lunula

    B. nail cuticle

    C. hyponichium

    D. nail root

21. The layer that is gives palms and soles the thickness is the _____.

    A. epidermis

    B. dermis

    C. subcutaneous

    D. none of the above

22. The sweat glands in the skin are innervated by sympathetic system that releases _____.

    A. epinephrine

    B. acetylcholine

    C. dopamine

    D. norepinephrine

23. The immunity provided by the skin is by the _____ cells.
    A. melanocytic
    B. Langherans
    C. epithelial
    D. fibroblastic

24. The structures that detect vertical indentation or dimpling in the skin are _____.
    A. Meissner's corpuscles
    B. Pacinian corpuscles
    C. Ruffini's corpuscles
    D. Merkel's discs

25. The sensory structures in the dermis that detect pressure changes are called:
    A. Meissner's corpuscles
    B. Pacinian corpuscles
    C. Ruffini's corpuscles
    D. Merkel's discs

26. All of the following are functions of the skin EXCEPT _____.
    A. synthesis of Vitamin D
    B. lipid storage
    C. synthesis of Vitamin A
    D. excretion of waste

Chapter 4

27. The thickening of the skin is known as ___.
    A. lichenification
    B. atrophy
    C. fissure
    D. excoriation

28. The main lesion that develops when a normal person is scratched gently with a pencil tip is a _____.
    A. patch
    B. nodule
    C. wheal
    D. excoriation

29. A flat skin lesion less than 1cm is known as a _____.
    A. macule
    B. papule
    C. vesicle
    D. patch

30. The difference between bullae and vesicles is that bullae _____.
    A. contain pus
    B. are larger in size
    C. are same as pustules
    D. resemble large macules

31. If a nodule grows larger than 3 cm then it is labeled as a _____.
    A. patch
    B. bulla
    C. tumor
    D. pustule

32. Small macules coalesce or combine to form _____.
    A. patches
    B. plaques
    C. tumors
    D. pustules

33. Telangiectasias are defined as superficial _____.
    A. patches
    B. papules
    C. vesicles
    D. blood vessels

34. All of the following skin lesions can cause superficial loss of epidermis EXCEPT:
    A. erosion
    B. excoriation
    C. purpura
    D. ulcer

35. All of the following skin lesions can arise from the dermis to the epidermis EXCEPT:
    A. nodule
    B. macule
    C. tumor
    D. abscess

36. Scale is a flake of _____ that can be separated from epidermal layer:
    A. epidermis
    B. dermis
    C. intra-dermis
    D. subcutaneous

37. All of the following are fluid filled lesions EXCEPT:

    A. cyst
    B. vesicle
    C. nodule
    D. pustules

38. When skin thickens and appears as a bark of tree, these lesions are known to have _____.

    A. excoriated
    B. ulcerated
    C. scratched
    D. lichenified

Chapter 5

39. Rocky Mountain spotted fever is caused by:

    A. *Borrelia burgdorferi*
    B. *Francisella tularensis*
    C. *Mycobacterium balnei*
    D. *Rickettsia rickettsii*

40. Lyme disease is caused by:

    A. *Borrelia burgdorferi*
    B. *Francisella tularensis*
    C. *Mycobacterium balnei*
    D. *Rickettsia rickettsii*

41. The following are commonly found in a dermatological history:

    A. use of folk remedies
    B. use of over-the-counter medications
    C. self-medication
    D. all of the above

42. The Latin word *scabere*, from which the word scab is derived, means:

    A. a plaque
    B. to scratch
    C. skin disease
    D. sword-like

43. Which of the following is associated with severe itching?

    A. melanoma
    B. syringoma
    C. vitiligo
    D. obstructive jaundice

44. Which of the following is NOT commonly associated with rheumatologic disease?

    A. ocular symptoms
    B. fatigue
    C. candidiasis
    D. vasculitis

45. Dermatological misdiagnosis may be caused by:

    A. doctor fatigue
    B. diagnostic overconfidence
    C. fear
    D. all of the above

46. The four cardinal elements of any physical examination are:

    A. history, examination, laboratory testing and diagnostic imaging
    B. inspection, palpation, percussion, auscultation
    C. head and neck, chest, abdomen and extremities
    D. none of the above

47. Hirsutism is:

    A. an endocrinological disease
    B. the result of excessive endorphins
    C. excessive distribution of hair
    D. gonadal atrophy

48. Wood's lamp examination involves:

    A. the use of an ultraviolet light source
    B. tangential lighting in a darkened room
    C. immunofluoroscence
    D. a specialized procedure reserved for allopathic dermatologists

Chapter 6

49. Lesser Trelat is a sign of internal malignancy with numerous multiple eruptive lesions of _____.

    A. psoriasis
    B. eczema
    C. seborrheic keratoses
    D. seborrheic dermatitis

50. In 50% of patients, increase in uric acid levels is associated with _____.
    A. psoriasis
    B. eczema
    C. seborrheic keratoses
    D. melanomas

51. Which of the following statements is true for pediculosis pubis?
    A. It develops quickly into malignant melanoma
    B. It is a form of scabies
    C. It is a sexually transmitted disease
    D. It is a disease of predominant itching in feet

52. In measles the Koplik's spots are mainly formed on/in the _____.
    A. head
    B. mouth
    C. trunk
    D. legs

53. Flea bites can be transmitted from _____.
    A. flies
    B. mosquitoes
    C. dogs
    D. birds

54. The skin disease that has risen with HIV infection is _____.
    A. measles
    B. psoriasis
    C. seborrheic keratoses
    D. eosinophilic folliculitis

55. All of the following can resemble skin abscess EXCEPT:
    A. psoriasis
    B. furuncle
    C. cysts
    D. carbuncle

56. The main cause of carbuncle is _____.
    A. staphylococci
    B. streptococci
    C. tinea
    D. melanoma

57. Xanthoma is a condition where _____.
    A. uric acid levels are high
    B. there are numerous papules on the face
    C. fat is deposited in the skin
    D. dark tan colored lesions are found mainly in the armpits

58. Which of the following statement is NOT TRUE for seborrheic dermatitis?
    A. chronic self-limiting condition
    B. presented as dry, flaky skin that may be white or yellow in color
    C. may also cause itching due to the flaking off of the epidermal layer
    D. frequently degenerates into an erosive malignancy

59. All of the following conditions could result mainly in red plaques EXCEPT:
    A. psoriasis
    B. herpes simplex
    C. contact eczema
    D. atopic eczema

60. Which of the following will NOT cause atopic dermatitis/eczema?
    A. dust mites
    B. food
    C. chemical irritants
    D. *Sarcoptes scabei*

61. All of the following are lesions of psoriasis EXCEPT:
    A. plaques
    B. pustules
    C. lipomas
    D. papules

62. Tinea pedis is a fungal infection of the _____.
    A. hand
    B. foot
    C. finger
    D. body

63. The most likely cause of velvety hyperpigmented thick warty patches in the arms and neck of a diabetic male would be _____.

    A. melasma
    B. vitiligo
    C. pityriasis alba
    D. acanthosis nigricans

64. The most likely cause of brown hyperpigmented patches over the face of a 34-year-old female with no systemic symptoms is _____.

    A. melasma
    B. vitiligo
    C. pityriasis alba
    D. tinea

65. Which of following is an incorrect statement about keloids?

    A. It is a disease mainly of blood vessels.
    B. It can have a genetic predisposition.
    C. It has shiny rounded smooth skin lesions that could be itchy.
    D. When exposed to sunlight it can cause skin cancer.

66. Impetigo can be caused by _____.

    A. sunlight
    B. infected towels
    C. autoimmune disorders
    D. stress

67. Melanoma occurs _____ times more frequently in Caucasians than in African Americans.

    A. 5
    B. 10
    C. 20
    D. 100

68. The C of the ABCD in the diagnosis of melanoma is _____.

    A. cancer
    B. chancre
    C. color
    D. coating

69. Pityriasis rosea is a _____ condition.

    A. highly infectious
    B. self limiting
    C. cancerous
    D. mainly bacterial

70. A recurrent dermatitis that can happen in response to sun exposure is _____.

    A. pityriasis alba
    B. psoriasis
    C. seborrheic keratosis
    D. polymorphous light eruption

71. Scabies is caused from mites that can infect _____.

    A. furniture
    B. clothing
    C. humans
    D. all of the above

72. Cutaneous lupus erythematosus is caused by _____.

    A. bacteria
    B. fungi
    C. autoimmunity
    D. mites

73. The best way to diagnose basal cell carcinoma is to _____.

    A. observe the symptoms carefully
    B. quickly send for biopsy
    C. reassure the patient and send home
    D. apply topical creams

74. Which of the following are cause(s) of hyperhidrosis:

    A. caffeine
    B. tuberculosis
    C. obesity
    D. all of the above

75. All of the following are TRUE for vitiligo EXCEPT:

    A. it may be hereditary
    B. there are dark hyperpigmented patches
    C. could be triggered by sunburn and extreme stress
    D. melanocytes destroy themselves

76. The best possible way to diagnose tinea barbae would be to _____.

    A. identify itching
    B. look at the lesions that are easy to diagnose
    C. use a Wood's lamp and microscopy to aid in diagnosis
    D. discard the lesions as tinea is self limiting

77. Acne is a common skin disorder that has _____ lesions.

    A. papular
    B. nodulocystic
    C. pustular
    D. all of the above

78. Symptoms from herpes infections are intense and the skin lesions are mainly _____.

    A. painless
    B. cystic
    C. vesicular
    D. like basal cell carcinoma

79. Squamous cell carcinoma forms a _____ , nodular, scale like lesion.

    A. painless
    B. cystic
    C. vesicular
    D. crusty

80. In contact dermatitis, lesions would resemble others forms of dermatitis and eczema. The most important information to differentiate contact eczema would be _____.

    A. history of itching
    B. history of contact
    C. history of autoimmune disorders
    D. history of systemic symptoms like fever, nausea and vomiting

81. Rosacea resembles acne, but in rosacea the etiology is _____.

    A. unknown
    B. mainly bacterial
    C. due to herpes simplex
    D. malignant melanoma

82. Candidiasis can occur in mainly in the _____.

    A. hair
    B. armpits and thigh creases
    C. teeth
    D. all of the above

83. The disease caused by a pox virus and has characteristic umblicated flesh like papule is known as _____.

    A. herpes simplex
    B. chicken pox
    C. measles
    D. molluscum contagiosum

84. Von Recklinghausen's disease is also known as _____.

    A. hemangioma
    B. thrombophlebitis
    C. neurofibromatosis
    D. psoriasis and eczema

Chapter 7

85. Cryotherapy stings and may be painful at the time of application and for a variable period afterwards. In rare cases, it may cause a permanent change such as:

    A. redness
    B. milia
    C. hypopigmentation
    D. hyperpigmentation

86. Which form of dermabrasion and exfoliation is not only very effective at removing dead skin cells, but is also effective in stimulating the circulatory system?

    A. dermabrasion
    B. microdermabrasion
    C. skin brushing
    D. chemical exfoliation

87. Electrolysis, laser and pulsed light forms of hair removal heat up the follicle forcing the hair into the resting phase or _____ phase.

    A. anagen
    B. catagen
    C. telagen
    D. miogen

88. A hot Epsom Salt sitz bath would best treat _____.
    A. acne
    B. muscle spasms
    C. a splinter
    D. folliculitis

89. When treating warts electrophoretically with salicylic acid the _____ electrode will promote the entry of the acid into the tissue.
    A. positive
    B. negative
    C. both
    D. neither

90. UV light facilitates some of the chemical reactions in the skin cells such as the formation of Vitamin D. Which of the UV bands is/are most active in this process?
    A. UVA
    B. UVB
    C. UVC
    D. UVA and UVB

91. External use of almond oil has many benefits for the skin and can be especially useful in the treatment of conditions that are characteristically _____.
    A. dry and scaly
    B. wet and seeping
    C. red and inflamed
    D. swollen and hot

92. Lanolin may be effective for all of the following conditions EXCEPT _____.
    A. xerosis
    B. chapped lips
    C. acne
    D. diaper rash

93. Mineral oil is a clear, odorless liquid that is a derivative of _____.
    A. vegetable oil
    B. wool grease
    C. nut oil
    D. petroleum

94. Toxic responses to olive oil include:
    A. allergic contact dermatitis
    B. urticaria
    C. seborrhea dermatitis
    D. psoriasis

95. Evening Primrose oil is a source of:
    A. EPA
    B. DHA
    C. GLA
    D. AA

96. Scabies mites are usually killed by the Tea Tree Oil within _____ hour(s) after application.
    A. 1
    B. 3
    C. 5
    D. 7

97. Petroleum jelly is a very safe, nontoxic substance that can be used as a:
    A. lubricant in latex gloves
    B. moisturizer around open flames
    C. sun block
    D. conjunctival lubricant

98. Vitamin A has multiple actions. Of the following which is NOT an action of Vitamin A?
    A. protects cells from oxidative damage
    B. acts as a hormone to activate genes
    C. required for formation of retinal pigment
    D. acts as a sun block

99. Vitamin D is considered a(n) _____.
    A. prohormone
    B. hormone
    C. cofactor
    D. enzyme

100. Vitamin E is not a single compound, but a group of _____ isomers.
    A. 2
    B. 4
    C. 6
    D. 8

101. The National Institutes of Health recognizes _____ as a possible complication from a colloidal silver toxicity.

    A. argyria
    B. cyanosis
    C. rubor
    D. dolor

102. Epsom Salt is a magnesium salt whose chemical name is _____.

    A. magnesium citrate
    B. magnesium sulfate
    C. magnesium gluconate
    D. magnesium carbonate

103. The mechanism by which potassium iodide functions is uncertain, however it is thought that it primarily affects _____ activity.

    A. neutrophil
    B. lymphocyte
    C. monocyte
    D. eosinophil

104. Prolonged exposure to baking soda may _____.

    A. burn the skin
    B. dry out the skin
    C. blister the skin
    D. moisturize the skin

105. Chronic topical exposure to zinc oxide may result in skin irritation and a(n) _____ skin eruption generally in the axilla, inner thigh, inner arm, scrotal, pubic, rectal, and perineal arcas.

    A. maculo-papular
    B. papulo-pustular
    C. vesiculo-bullous
    D. ulcerative

106. Oral use of Aloe Vera may lead to abdominal cramps and diarrhea when there is a high concentration of _____.

    A. aloin
    B. lignin
    C. salicylic acid
    D. sterols

107. Vinegar contains acetic acid. The pH of a 5% acetic acid solution is _____ which is less acidic than lemon juice but more acidic than tomato juice.

    A. 2.0
    B. 2.4
    C. 2.8
    D. 3.2

108. Black walnuts are high in proteins and fatty acids and also are rich in _____.

    A. magnesium
    B. manganese
    C. copper
    D. zinc

109. Allergic reaction to Burdock may occur in patients who are also allergic to related plants such as _____.

    A. garlic
    B. onion
    C. marigold
    D. roses

110. Allergic reaction to Calendula may occur in patients who are also allergic to related plants such as _____.

    A. garlic
    B. onion
    C. daisy
    D. lily

111. The flavonoids of chamomile are considered to have _____ qualities.

    A. antispasmodic
    B. antibacterial
    C. antifungal
    D. antihelminthic

112. Nordihdroguaiaretic acid (NDGA) is considered the most active component of chaparral and is considered to have _____ activity.

    A. antispasmodic
    B. antibacterial
    C. antifungal
    D. antihelminthic

113. The pyrrolizidine alkaloids that are present in comfrey are considered to be toxic substances to the _____.
    A. kidney
    B. spleen
    C. liver
    D. pancreas

114. Cornstarch may be used to treat the symptoms of which of the following conditions?
    A. measles
    B. mumps
    C. scabies
    D. lice

115. Elderberry contains anthocyanins, which are powerful _____ phytochemicals.
    A. antiinflammatory
    B. antibacterial
    C. antiviral
    D. antioxidant

116. Allicin, the best known active component of garlic, is a(n) _____ sulphur compound.
    A. oxygenated
    B. nitrogenated
    C. hydrogenated
    D. hydrolysed

117. Allergic reactions to ginger may occur in patients who are also allergic to related plants such as _____.
    A. garlic
    B. rosemary
    C. chamomile
    D. turmeric

118. Eclectic physicians in the United States used goldenseal for its antiseptic, antiinflammatory and _____ qualities.
    A. analgesic
    B. astringent
    C. antiviral
    D. antioxidant

119. The *Camellia sinensis* is an Asian shrub whose dried leaves are used to make _____ tea.
    A. green
    B. black
    C. white
    D. red

120. _____ are in the family of *Rutaceae* and grow on a small evergreen tree.
    A. black walnuts
    B. almonds
    C. olives
    D. lemons

121. Oatmeal has been used to treat different types of skin conditions due to the exfoliating and soothing benefits from its _____ property.
    A. emollient   C.   nutritive
    B. astringent   D.   aromatic

122. Onions are a rich source of the trace mineral _____.
    A. zinc
    B. copper
    C. chromium
    D. manganese

123. Undecylenic acid is an eleven carbon mono-unsaturated fatty acid derived commercially from _____.
    A. almond
    B. corn oil
    C. castor oil
    D. olive oil

124. White Willow may cause dryness, peeling, flushing and redness of the skin in patients allergic to _____.
    A. ibuprofen
    B. aspirin
    C. naproxen
    D. acetaminophen

125. Witch Hazel is an extract produced from the _____ and _____ of the shrub.
    A. leaves, roots
    B. leaves, bark
    C. flowers, roots
    D. flowers, bark

126. The combination of neomycin, polymyxin and bacitracin in a common antibiotic cream is effective against:
    A. Gram positive bacteria
    B. Gram negative bacteria
    C. Gram positive and negative bacteria
    D. neither Gram positive or negative bacteria

127. The primary component of calamine lotion is _____.
    A. zinc oxide
    B. iron oxide
    C. magnesium oxide
    D. aluminum oxide

128. Dermatogical side effects of topically applied hydrocortisone may include:
    A. hyperpigmentation
    B. hypopigmentation
    C. hypertrophy
    D. atrophy

129. The _____ action of hydrogen peroxide helps loosen up dead tissue, debris and pus.
    A. astringent
    B. effervescent
    C. antibacterial
    D. antiviral

130. Dimethylsulfoxide, or DMSO, is a natural substance derived from wood pulp that has _____ effects.
    A. antiviral
    B. antibacterial
    C. antihelminthic
    D. antifungal

131. Menthol has actions that are antipruritic, antiseptic, analgesic and cooling. One of its actions stimulates _____ receptors in the skin.
    A. cold
    B. heat
    C. pain
    D. position

132. Topically applied talcum powder is _____.
    A. absorbable and nontoxic
    B. non-absorbable but toxic
    C. absorbable and toxic
    D. non-absorbable and nontoxic

133. Normal saline (____ saline solution) is an isotonic solution.
    A. 0.7%
    B. 0.9%
    C. 1.1%
    D. 1.7%

134. The general consensus of studies using urea suggests that lotions and salves containing _____ or more are the most effective.
    A. 5%
    B. 10%
    C. 15%
    D. 20%

Chapter 8

135. "Sunspots" on fair-skinned persons are known by what name?
    A. Miliaria
    B. Morphea
    C. Actinic keratosis
    D. Sweet syndrome

136. Alopecia areata is caused by _____.
    A. an auto-immune process
    B. a genetic disorder
    C. chemotherapy
    D. chronic fungal infection

137. The name pemphigus comes from a Greek word meaning what?
    A. sloughing off
    B. breaking out in blisters
    C. scratching
    D. hideous

138. A patient has recently returned from one month in Florida and is complaining of very itchy skin on his abdomen, which has some signs of secondary infection from scratching. Which of the following is among your most likely diagnoses?

    A. cutaneous larva migrans
    B. Bowen's disease
    C. Linear IgA disease
    D. Erythema multiforme

139. What condition is associated with gluten sensitivity and causes intense itching around the elbows and knees?

    A. mastocytosis
    B. Grover's disease
    C. dermatitis herpetiformis
    D. pemphigus vulgaris

140. A number of skin conditions can cause a butterfly rash on the face. Which of the following is one of them?

    A. lentigo
    B. epidermolysis bullosa
    C. pemphigoid
    D. erysipelas

141. What does the term *annular* mean, with respect to dermatological disease?

    A. ring shaped
    B. snake-like
    C. itchy
    D. thick

142. What is the name of the skin disorder most commonly associated with acquired immune deficiency syndrome?

    A. Bowen's disease
    B. Kaposi's sarcoma
    C. Grover's disease
    D. erythema nodosum

143. Lentigines are also known as:

    A. razor bumps
    B. liver spots
    C. rodent ulcers
    D. skin tags

144. When mast cells are damaged by rubbing or stroking the skin, they become degranulated, causing edema and erythema. In some patients, this condition may be aggravated by substances that induce mast cell mediator release, such as alcohol and shellfish. What is the name of this condition?

    A. toxic epidermal necrolysis
    B. epidermolysis bullosa
    C. urticaria pigmentosa
    D. eythema multiforme

145. What is the most likely cause of the skin-picking associated with neurotic excoriation?

    A. an underlying psychiatric disorder
    B. an underlying liver disorder
    C. an associated parasitic condition
    D. a hereditary skin condition

146. Which of the following is associated with the greatest mortality?

    A. bullous pemphigoid
    B. morphea
    C. linear IgA disease
    D. pemphigus vulgaris

147. What is the name of a skin condition associated with systemic disease that can cause intense and chronic pruritis?

    A. dermatitis herpetiformis
    B. Kawasaki's disease
    C. mastocytosis
    D. prurigo nodularis

148. What disease leads to lax skin, with wrinkled, hanging folds particularly in the neck and axillae?

    A. syringoma
    B. pseudoxanthoma elasticum
    C. granuloma annulare
    D. Grover's disease

149. What is the name of the severe life-threatening form of Stevens-Johnson syndrome?

    A. pyoderma gangrenosum

    B. pemphigus

    C. toxic epidermal necrolysis

    D. necrobiosis lipoidica diabeticorum

150. The Bisgaard regimen for venous ulcers does NOT contain which of the following?

    A. Education

    B. Rest

    C. Elastic compression

    D. Elevation

▨ Answers to Selected response Questions

1. C, reference page 1

2. B, reference page 1

3. B, reference page 3

4. A, reference page 4

5. D, reference page 4

6. A, reference page 5

7. A, reference page 5

8. B, reference page 7

9. D, reference page 8

10. C, reference page 8

11. D, reference page 9

12. C, reference page 10

13. B, reference page 10

14. A, reference page 12

15. A, reference page 12

16. C, reference page 13

17. D, reference page 13

18. C, reference page 29

19. D, reference page 30

20. C, reference page 32

21. A, reference page 29

22. B, reference page 31

23. B, reference page 31

24. D, reference page 31

25. B, reference page 31

26. C, reference page 31

27. A, reference pages 33–34

28. C, reference pages 33–34

29. A, reference pages 33–34

30. B, reference pages 33–34

31. C, reference pages 33–34

32. A, reference pages 33–34

33. D, reference pages 33–34

34. C, reference pages 33–34

35. B, reference pages 33–34

36. A, reference pages 33–34

37. C, reference pages 33–34

38. D, reference pages 33–34

39. D, reference page 46

40. A, reference page 46

41. D, reference page 46

42. B, reference page 46

43. D, reference page 47

44. C, reference page 47

45. D, reference page 48

46. B, reference page 49

47. C, reference page 49

48. A, reference page 50

49. C, reference pages 69–70

50. A, reference page 53

51. C, reference page 107

52. B, reference page 129

53. C, reference page 109

54. D, reference page 93

55. A, reference pages 94–97

56. A, reference page 94

57. C, reference page 71

58. D, reference pages 56–57

59. B, reference page 122

60. D, reference pages 63–64

61. C, reference pages 53–54

62. B, reference page 103

63. D, reference page 116

64. A, reference page 115

65. A, reference pages 72–73

66. B, reference page 95

67. C, reference page 83

68. C, reference page 85

69. B, reference page 66

70. D, reference page 130

71. D, reference page 110

72. C, reference page 119

73. B, reference page 81

74. D, reference page 131

75. B, reference page 117

76. C, reference pages 102–103

77. D, reference page 86

78. C, reference page 122

79. D, reference page 80

80. B, reference page 64

81. A, reference page 88

82. B, reference page 100

83. D, reference page 127

84. C, reference pages 77–78

85. C, reference page 140

86. C, reference page 140

87. C, reference page 141

88. B, reference page 142

89. B, reference page 142

90. B, reference page 143

91. A, reference page 143

92. C, reference page 144

93. D, reference page 144

94. A, reference page 145

95. C, reference page 146

96. B, reference page 146

97. C, reference page 147

98. D, reference page 147

99. A, reference page 147

100. D, reference page 148

101. A, reference page 149

102. B, reference page 149

103. A, reference page 149

104. C, reference page 150

105. B, reference page 150

106. A, reference page 151

107. B, reference page 151

108. B, reference page 152

109. C, reference page 152

110. C, reference page 153

111. A, reference page 153

112. B, reference page 153

113. C, reference page 154

114. A, reference page 154

115. D, reference page 155

116. A, reference page 155

117. D, reference page 156

118. B, reference page 156

119. A, reference page 156

120. D, reference page 157

121. A, reference page 157

122. C, reference page 157

123. C, reference page 158

124. B, reference page 158

125. B, reference page 158

126. C, reference page 159

127. A, reference page 159

128. D, reference page 160

129. B, reference page 160

130. A, reference page 160

131. A, reference page 161

132. D, reference page 161

133. B, reference page 161

134. B, reference page 162

135. C, reference page 169

136. A, reference page 170

137. B, reference page 171

138. A, reference page 172

139. C, reference page 173

140. D, reference page 174

141. A, reference page 174

142. B, reference page 174

143. B, reference page 177

144. C, reference page 179

145. A, reference page 180

146. D, reference page 182

147. D, reference page 183

148. B, reference page 183

149. C, reference page 187

150. B, reference page 188

Photo Credits

Figure 6-33 (A-B) *Col. Nasser Dar, LMH, Lahore, Pakistan.* **104**

Figure 6-33 (H) *Paulk, David and Donna M. Agnew, Physician Assistant Review Guide. © 2010 Jones and Bartlett Publishers, LLC.* **104**

Figure 6-33 (I) *Col. Nasser Dar, LMH, Lahore, Pakistan.* **104**

Figure 6-33 (M) *Col. Nasser Dar, LMH, Lahore, Pakistan.* **105**

Figure 6-33 (N) *Paulk, David and Donna M. Agnew, Physician Assistant Review Guide. © 2010 Jones and Bartlett Publishers, LLC.* **105**

Figure 6-34 (A) *Dr. Azeem Alam Khan, Consultant Dermatologist, Islamabad, Pakistan.* **108**

Figure 6-35 (A-B) *Col. Nasser Dar, LMH, Lahore, Pakistan.* **109**

Figure 6-36 (B-C) *Col. Nasser Dar, LMH, Lahore, Pakistan.* **111**

Figure 6-37 *Courtesy of James Gathany/CDC.* **112**

Figure 6-38 *Courtesy of Leonard V. Crowley, M.D., Biology Department, Century College.* **114**

Figure 6-39(A) *© DermQuest.com. Used with permission from Galderma SA.* **115**

Figure 6-40 (A) *Col. Nasser Dar, LMH, Lahore, Pakistan.* **116**

Figure 6-41 (A) *Dr. Azeem Alam Khan, Consultant Dermatologist, Islamabad, Pakistan.* **117**

Figure 6-42 *© Rob Byron/ShutterStock, Inc.* **119**

Figure 6-43 (A) *Col. Nasser Dar, LMH, Lahore, Pakistan.* **120**

Figure 6-44 (A) *Col. Nasser Dar, LMH, Lahore, Pakistan.* **121**

Figure 6-45 (A-B) *Col. Nasser Dar, LMH, Lahore, Pakistan.* **124**

Figure 6-46 (A-B) *Paulk, David and Donna M. Agnew, Physician Assistant Review Guide. © 2010 Jones and Bartlett Publishers, LLC.* **125**

Figure 6-46 (C) *Col. Nasser Dar, LMH, Lahore, Pakistan.* **125**

Figure 6-46 (D-E) *Col. Nasser Dar, LMH, Lahore, Pakistan.* **126**

Figure 6-47 (A) *Paulk, David and Donna M. Agnew, Physician Assistant Review Guide. © 2010 Jones and Bartlett Publishers, LLC.* **127**

Figure 6-47 (B) *Col. Nasser Dar, LMH, Lahore, Pakistan.* **127**

Figure 6-48 (A-B) *Col. Nasser Dar, LMH, Lahore, Pakistan.* **130**

Figure 6-49 (A) *Col. Nasser Dar, LMH, Lahore, Pakistan.* **130**

Figure 6-50(A) *© DermQuest.com. Used with permission from Galderma SA.* **131**

Figure 8-1 *Paulk, David and Donna M. Agnew, Physician Assistant Review Guide. © 2010 Jones and Bartlett Publishers, LLC.* **170**

Figure 8-2 (A-B) *Paulk, David and Donna M. Agnew, Physician Assistant Review Guide. © 2010 Jones and Bartlett Publishers, LLC.* **170**

Figure 8-3 *© Jens Stolt/ShutterStock, Inc.* **171**

Figure 8-4 *Paulk, David and Donna M. Agnew, Physician Assistant Review Guide. © 2010 Jones and Bartlett Publishers, LLC.* **171**

Figure 8-5 *Col. Nasser Dar, LMH, Lahore, Pakistan.* **171**

Figure 8-6 *Paulk, David and Donna M. Agnew, Physician Assistant Review Guide. © 2010 Jones and Bartlett Publishers, LLC.* **172**

Figure 8-7 *Paulk, David and Donna M. Agnew, Physician Assistant Review Guide. © 2010 Jones and Bartlett Publishers, LLC.* **172**

Figure 8-8 *© DermQuest.com. Used with permission from Galderma SA.* **172**

Figure 8-9 *© DermQuest.com. Used with permission from Galderma SA.* **173**

Figure 8-10 *Col. Nasser Dar, LMH, Lahore, Pakistan.* **173**

Figure 8-11 *© DermQuest.com. Used with permission from Galderma SA.* **173**

Figure 8-12 *© DermQuest.com. Used with permission from Galderma SA.* **174**

Figure 8-13 *Col. Nasser Dar, LMH, Lahore, Pakistan.* **174**

Figure 8-14 *Col. Nasser Dar, LMH, Lahore, Pakistan.* **174**

Figure 8-15 (A) *Paulk, David and Donna M. Agnew, Physician Assistant Review Guide. © 2010 Jones and Bartlett Publishers, LLC.* **175**

Figure 8-15 (B-C) *Col. Nasser Dar, LMH, Lahore, Pakistan.* **175**

Figure 8-16 *Col. Nasser Dar, LMH, Lahore, Pakistan.* **175**

Figure 8-17 *© DermQuest.com. Used with permission from Galderma SA.* **176**

Figure 8-18 *Courtesy of National Cancer Institute.* **176**

Figure 8-19 *Col. Nasser Dar, LMH, Lahore, Pakistan.* **177**

Figure 8-20 *© DermQuest.com. Used with permission from Galderma SA.* **177**

Figure 8-21 (A-B) *Col. Nasser Dar, LMH, Lahore, Pakistan.* **178**

Figure 8-22 *Col. Nasser Dar, LMH, Lahore, Pakistan.* **178**

Figure 8-24 *Col. Nasser Dar, LMH, Lahore, Pakistan.* **179**

Figure 8-25 *Col. Nasser Dar, LMH, Lahore, Pakistan.* **180**

Figure 8-26 *Dr. Azeem Alam Khan, Consultant Dermatologist, Islamabad, Pakistan.* **180**

Figure 8-27 *Col. Nasser Dar, LMH, Lahore, Pakistan.* **180**

Figure 8-28 (A-B) *Col. Nasser Dar, LMH, Lahore, Pakistan.* **181**

Figure 8-29 (A-B) *Col. Nasser Dar, LMH, Lahore, Pakistan.* **182**

Figure 8-30 *Col. Nasser Dar, LMH, Lahore, Pakistan.* **182**

Figure 8-31 (A-B) *Col. Nasser Dar, LMH, Lahore, Pakistan.* **183**

Figure 8-32 (A-C) *Col. Nasser Dar, LMH, Lahore, Pakistan.* **185**

Figure 8-33 *Col. Nasser Dar, LMH, Lahore, Pakistan.* **185**

Figure 8-34 (A-B) *Col. Nasser Dar, LMH, Lahore, Pakistan.* **186**

Figure 8-35 *Col. Nasser Dar, LMH, Lahore, Pakistan.* **186**

Figure 8-36 *Col. Nasser Dar, LMH, Lahore, Pakistan.* **187**

Figure 8-37 *Dr. Azeem Alam Khan, Consultant Dermatologist, Islamabad, Pakistan.* **187**

Figure 8-38 *Col. Nasser Dar, LMH, Lahore, Pakistan.* **188**

Index